T0257036

CLINICAL HANDBOOK OF
Pediatric Endocrinology

CLINICAL HANDBOOK OF

Pediatric
Endocrinology
Second Edition

Elizabeth K. Babler · ARNP, PhC, CDE
Kelly J. Betts · RN-BC, MNS(c), Ed.D(c)
Jan A. Courtney · RN, MSN
Betty M. Flores · RN, MS, PNP-BC, CCRP
Catherine Flynn · RN, MSN, CPNP, CDE
Michele Lamerson · RN, MS, CPNP
Gail Neuenkirchen · RN, MS, CPNP
Nancy Ann Varni · RN, MS, MBA, CPNP
Deborah B. Welch · RN, MSN
Deborah D. Worley · RN, MSN, PNP-BC, CDE

Quality Medical Publishing, Inc.
2013 • St. Louis, Missouri

Printed in the United States of America

This book presents current scientific information and opinion pertinent to medical professionals. It does not provide advice concerning specific diagnosis and treatment of individual cases and is not intended for use by the layperson. Medical knowledge is constantly changing. As new information becomes available, changes in treatment, procedures, equipment, and the use of drugs become necessary. The editors/authors/contributors and the publisher have, as far as it is possible, taken care to ensure that the information given in this text is accurate and up to date. However, readers are strongly advised to confirm that the information, especially with regard to drug usage, complies with the latest legislation and standards of practice. The authors and publisher will not be responsible for any errors or liable for actions taken as a result of information or opinions expressed in this book.

The publishers have made every effort to trace the copyright holders for borrowed material. If they have inadvertently overlooked any, they will be pleased to make the necessary arrangements at the first opportunity.

PUBLISHER: Karen Berger
EDITORIAL DIRECTOR: Michelle Berger
PRODUCTION: Carolyn Reich
COVER DESIGN: David Berger

Quality Medical Publishing, Inc.
2248 Welsch Industrial Court
St. Louis, Missouri 63146
Telephone: 1-800-348-7808
Website: http://www.qmp.com

LIBRARY OF CONGRESS CATALOGING-IN-PUBLICATION DATA

Clinical handbook of pediatric endocrinology / Elizabeth K. Babler ... [et al.]. -- 2nd ed.
    p. ; cm.
  Includes bibliographical references and index.
  ISBN 978-1-57626-282-5 (pbk.)
  I. Babler, Elizabeth K.
  [DNLM: 1. Endocrine System Diseases--Handbooks. 2. Child. 3. Growth Disorders--
Handbooks. WS 39]
  LC Classification not assigned
  618.924--dc23
                              2012047438

QM/QM/UG
5 4 3 2 1

Act as if what you do makes a difference. It does.
WILLIAM JAMES

We dedicate this handbook
to those who came before us and showed us the way,
to all who are serving in the field of pediatric endocrinology now,
and to those who will choose this amazing specialty in the future

CONTRIBUTORS

Elizabeth K. Babler, ARNP, PhC, CDE
Pediatric Nurse Practitioner, Department of Pediatric Endocrinology,
Mary Bridge Children's Health Center, Tacoma, Washington

Kelly J. Betts, RN-BC, MNSc, Ed.D(c)
Assistant Dean for Baccalaureate Education, Assistant Professor, College of Nursing,
University of Arkansas for Medical Sciences, Little Rock, Arkansas

Jan A. Courtney, RN, MSN
President, Synergy Clinical Research LLC, Millstadt, Illinois

Betty M. Flores, RN, MS, PNP-BC, CCRP
Pediatric Nurse Practitioner, Children's Hospital & Research Center Oakland,
Oakland, California

Catherine Flynn, RN, MSN, CPNP, CDE
Pediatric Endocrine Nurse Practitioner, Pediatric Endocrinology and Diabetes Clinic,
University Medical Center, Las Vegas, Nevada

Michele Lamerson, RN, MS, CPNP
Corcept Therapeutics, Menlo Park, California

Gail Neuenkirchen, MS, RN, CPNP
Pediatric Nurse Practitioner, Department of Anesthesiology,
Children's Hospital Colorado; Instructor, Department of Anesthesiology,
University of Colorado–Denver, Aurora, Colorado

Nancy Ann Varni, RN, MS, MBA, CPNP
Pediatric Nurse Practitioner, Department of Endocrinology and Diabetes,
Children's Hospital of Orange County, Orange, California

Deborah B. Welch, RN, MSN
Instructor, School of Nursing, Mississippi College, Clinton, Mississippi

Deborah D. Worley, RN, MSN, PNP-BC, CDE
Diabetes Educator, Apex, North Carolina

PREFACE TO THE SECOND EDITION

When our group worked on the first edition of this clinical handbook, we had no idea that it would be such an overwhelming success. Not in our wildest dreams did we think that there would be a second edition. Yet here we are, years later.

This work would not have been possible without the continued dedication of the authors who returned to help us. Thank you for your hard work and for what you have brought to our specialty.

We also wish to thank those pediatric endocrinologists who kindly lent their medical expertise in reviewing our work. Thank you for your support with this project and for what you have taught us over the years.

We must not overlook extending thanks also to those who have used this tool in their clinical practice. You made the first edition a success. Our efforts have been for you, and we hope that you will continue to find our "little" handbook helpful.

Jan A. Courtney
Deborah D. Worley

PREFACE TO THE FIRST EDITION

As with all things related to endocrinology, nothing is ever simple. The idea for a succinct aid to endocrinology nurses blossomed into a comprehensive handbook that can serve as a quick reference tool for health care professionals in pediatric hospitals and offices. This handbook has been four years in the making, and the collaborators embody the dedication, tenacity, and knowledge of the endocrinology nursing world. We are indebted to them for their time and effort in this production. We also wish to thank those endocrinologists who have graciously reviewed the handbook as medical experts.

Jan A. Courtney
Helen B. Carney
Denise B. Haydar

CONTENTS

❶ GENERAL ENDOCRINE ASSESSMENT

The initial visit for any child seen for an endocrine abnormality should begin with a thorough history and physical examination.

HISTORY

The history areas to be covered include the following:

1. **Prenatal History**
   a. Prenatal care
   b. Problems during the pregnancy, labor, or delivery
   c. Tobacco, alcohol, drug, medication use
2. **Birth History**
   a. Where birth occurred: city, state, hospital, home
   b. Type of delivery, instruments used, Apgar scores if known
   c. Neonatal course: length of hospitalization, NICU stay, oxygen or ventilator use, GI problems, infections, jaundice
3. **Hospitalizations**
   a. Any overnight hospitalizations
   b. Course of stay: illness, length, complications
4. **Surgeries**
   a. Reason and type
   b. Recovery and complications
5. **Primary Care Provider**
   a. Last physical examination
   b. Recent lab tests or X-rays
   c. Availability of records for review
6. **Accidents/Injuries**
7. **Medications**
8. **Immunizations**
9. **Allergies**
10. **Family History**
    a. Parental heights and age at menarche/growth spurt
    b. Heights of other family members as appropriate
    c. History of chronic disease in family members: parents, siblings, grandparents, aunts, uncles, cousins
       1. Allergies/asthma
       2. Arthritis
       3. Blood or bleeding problems
       4. Cancer
       5. Diabetes
       6. Growth problems

   7. Heart problems
   8. High blood pressure
   9. High cholesterol
   10. Seizures
   11. Thyroid disorders
   12. Drug/alcohol abuse
   13. Mental illness
   14. Menstrual irregularities
   15. Infertility
   16. Obesity
   17. Early or delayed puberty

11. Social History
 a. People in household
 b. Insurance
 c. Employment status

12. Developmental History
 a. Age of developmental milestones: rolling, walking, speech, toilet training
 b. School performance: grade level and grades
 c. Behavior in school—any change
 d. Teasing or bullying by others
 e. Attention to class work
 f. Ability to follow rules

13. Nutrition
 a. Breast milk, formula, amount of cow's milk, length of feeding
 b. Daily eating pattern
 c. Special meal plan
 d. Snacks
 e. Amount of juice and soda
 f. Fast food
 g. Problems with chewing, swallowing, eating, drinking
 h. Vomiting related to nutrition

14. Activities
 a. Daily activity
 b. Physical education
 c. Participation in organized activities: sports, dance, etc.
 d. Restrictions on activity
 e. Television/computer habits

15. Review of Systems
 a. Neurologic/headaches
 b. Ear/sinus infections
 c. Heart problems
 d. Decreased energy

e. Abnormal weight gain or loss
f. Seizures
g. Dental problems
h. Asthma/pneumonia
i. Change in growth rate
j. Body odor/acne
k. Vision problems/glasses or contacts
l. Late eruption of teeth
m. Constipation/diarrhea/abdominal pain
n. Increased thirst/urination
o. Sleep problems
p. Other

16. Any other information that the family would like to share

PHYSICAL EXAMINATION

The physical examination may consist of the following:

1. Vital Signs
   a. Weight in children: This should be obtained in light clothing and without shoes. Infants should be weighed without clothes or a diaper. Scales should be routinely calibrated for accuracy. (For normal values see p. 9 and Growth Charts, pp. 442-449.)
   b. Length: Supine measurement is used until age 24 months (or 36 months if birth-to-36 month chart is used). Fully extend the body by holding the head in midline, grasp the knees together, and push down gently until the legs are fully extended. The head should be touching firmly at the top of the measuring device. The heels should be placed on the footboard when the measurement is taken. Having a parent hold the head helps maintain the body in alignment. (For normal values see p. 9 and Growth Charts, pp. 442-449.)
   c. Height: Measurement used when children are standing upright.
   d. Arm span: The arm span should be done with the patient standing against a flat wall with the arms spread out as far as possible, creating a 90-degree angle with the torso. Measure the distance between the distal ends of the middle phalanges to determine the arm span. (For normal values see p. 10.)
   e. Head circumference: Obtained until third birthday and thereafter as appropriate. (For normal values see p. 9.)
   f. Upper-to-lower body segment ratio: Measure the distance between the upper body and the symphysis pubis and the floor with the patient standing against a flat wall in the correct position for measuring a height.

    g. Sitting height: Used to measure upper segment. Using a Harpenden sitting table, have the patient sit on the table with the back of the knees touching the table. The vertical unit is moved close to the patient's back. The entire back and back of the head must touch the vertical surface. The measurement is indicated on the counter. The standing height to sitting height ratio (relative sitting height) is calculated and multiplied by 100. (For normal values see pp. 10-11.)

    h. Chest circumference.

    i. Heart rate. (For normal values see p. 11.)

    j. Respiratory rate. (For normal values see p. 11.)

    k. Blood pressure. (For normal values see pp.12-21.)

2. **Growth Charts**

    a. When plotting weight, height, and length measurements, it is important to calculate the child's exact age. An infant should be plotted to the week of age and a child to the month of age (see Growth Charts, pp. 442-444 and 446-448).

    b. The height/length, weight, and head circumference should be plotted on the appropriate growth chart for age, sex, and/or genetic syndrome (see Growth Charts, pp. 442-444 and 446-448).

    c. If a length was obtained, it should be plotted on the chart for birth to 36 months. If a height was obtained, it should be plotted on the chart for 2 to 18 years.

    d. Head circumference should be plotted on the appropriate growth chart (see Growth Charts, pp. 443 and 447).

3. **Calculations**

    a. Body surface area can be calculated using either the nomogram or Mosteller's formula (see p. 430).

    b. Body mass index can be calculated (see p. 425).

    c. Growth velocity (see p. 431).

    d. Target height (see p. 431).

4. **Pubertal Development: Tanner Staging**

Stages of Breast Development (Fig. 1.1)

1 Preadolescent; elevation of papilla only

2 Breast bud; elevation of breast and papilla as small mound; enlargement of areolar diameter

3 Further enlargement and elevation of breast and areola; no separation of their contours

4 Projection of the areola and papilla to form secondary mound above level of breast

5 Mature stage; projection of papilla only as a result of recession of areola to contour of breast

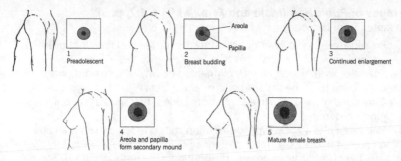

Figure 1.1 Tanner stages of breast development in females. (This figure was published in The Harriet Lane Handbook, Custer JW, Rau RE, eds, Adolescent Medicine, pp 132-134, Copyright Elsevier, 2009.)

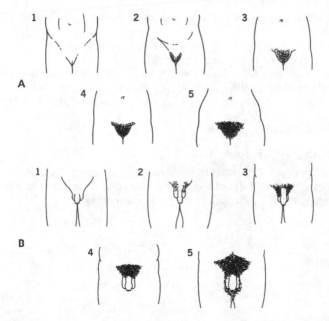

Figure 1.2 **A,** Tanner stages of pubic hair development in females. **B,** Tanner stages of pubic hair and genital development in males. (This figure was published in The Harriet Lane Handbook, Custer JW, Rau RE, eds, Adolescent Medicine, pp 132-134, Copyright Elsevier, 2009.)

GENERAL ENDOCRINE ASSESSMENT

Stages of Pubic Hair (Male and Female) (Fig. 1.2, p. 5)

(adapted from Namour[1])

1 Preadolescent: vellus over pubes no further developed than that over the abdominal wall
2 Sparse growth of long, slightly pigmented downy hair, straight or only slightly curled, chiefly at the base of penis or along labia
3 Considerably darker, coarser, and more curled; hair spreads sparsely over junction of pubes
4 Hair resembles adult in type; distribution still considerably less than adult; no spread to medial surfaces of thighs
5 Adult in quantity and type with distribution of horizontal pattern
6 Spread up the linea alba; "male escutcheon"

Stages of Genital Development (Male) (see Fig. 1.2)

(adapted from Namour[1])

1 Preadolescent; testes, scrotum, and penis about the same size as in early childhood
2 Enlargement of scrotum and testes; skin of scrotum reddens and changes in texture; little or no enlargement of penis
3 Enlargement of penis, first mainly in length; further growth of testes and scrotum
4 Increased size of penis with growth in breadth and development of glans; further enlargement of testes and scrotum and increased darkening of scrotal skin
5 Genitalia adult in size and shape

Penile Length (Fig. 1.3, Table 1.1)

a. Measure from the pubic ramus to the tip of the glans penis. Traction should be applied along the length of the penis until increased resistance is met.
b. A penile length of >2.5 SD below the mean is abnormal.

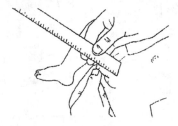

Figure 1.3 Measuring penile length. (Reprinted from Hall JG, Froster-Iskenius UG, Allanson JE. Handbook of Normal Physical Measurements. Oxford: Oxford University Press, 1990, p 320. By permission of Oxford University Press.)

Table 1.1 Mean Stretched Penile Length (cm)

Age	Mean ± SD	−2.5 SD
Birth		
30-wk gestation	2.5 ± 0.4	1.5
34-wk gestation	3.0 ± 0.4	2.0
Full term	3.5 ± 0.4	2.5
0-5 mo	3.9 ± 0.8	1.8
6-12 mo	4.3 ± 0.8	2.1
1-2 yr	4.7 ± 0.8	2.6
2-3 yr	5.1 ± 0.9	3.0
3-4 yr	5.5 ± 0.9	2.9
4-5 yr	5.7 ± 0.9	3.4
5-7 yr	6.0 ± 0.9	3.8
7-9 yr	6.3 ± 1.0	3.8
9-10 yr	6.3 ± 1.0	3.8
10-11 yr	6.4 ± 1.1	5.0
Adult	13.3 ± 1.6	4.0

This table was published in The Harriet Lane Handbook, Custer JW, Rau RE, eds, Endocrinology, p 296, Copyright Elsevier, 2009.

Testicular Development (Table 1.2)

Use of an orchidometer is the most accurate way to measure testicular volume.

Table 1.2 Testicular Size

Corresponding Age (yr)	Length (cm) (mean ± SD)	Volume (mL) (approximate)	Tanner Stage
8-10	2.0 ± 0.5	2	1
10-12	2.7 ± 0.7	5	2
12-14	3.4 ± 0.8	10	3
14-16	4.1 ± 1.0	20	4
16-18	5.0 ± 0.5	29	5
18-20	5.0 ± 0.3	29	

This table was published in The Harriet Lane Handbook, Custer JW, Rau RE, eds, Endocrinology, p 296, Copyright Elsevier, 2009.

Table 1.3	Clitoral Size	
	Width (mm)	Length (mm)
Newborn	5	10-15
Early childhood	2-5	
8-13 yr	2-5	
>13 yr	<10	15-20

This table was published in Atlas of Pediatric Physical Diagnosis, 3rd ed. Murray PA, Davis HA, Hamp M. In Zitelli BJ, Davis HA, eds, p 528, Copyright Elsevier, 1997.

5. Physical Findings (Tables 1.3 through 1.11)

   a. General: Appearance, development, alertness, short- and long-term memory
   b. Head: Anterior and posterior fontanel, shape, forehead, hair pattern and distribution
   c. Eyes: Conjunctivae, sclera, pupils (equal, round, reaction to light, accommodation), confrontational visual fields, fundi, vision
   d. Ears: Pinna, placement, external auditory canals, tympanic membranes, gross hearing
   e. Nose: Nares patent, discharge
   f. Throat: Palate intact, pharynx, uvula, dentition (Table 1.5)—normal for age
   g. Neck: Supple, lymphadenopathy, thyroid (palpable, size, nodules)
   h. Lungs: Respiratory rate, lung sounds (normal or abnormal)
   i. Cardiovascular: Heart rate, normal S1 and S2, murmurs, sinus arrhythmia, abnormal heart sounds, peripheral pulses
   j. Abdomen: Bowel sounds, enlarged liver or spleen, masses or tenderness
   k. Pubertal development: Tanner stage (See Figs. 1.1 and 1.2; Tables 1.1 through 1.3.)
   l. Musculoskeletal: Range of motion, muscle strength, deficits, scoliosis
   m. Neurologic: Cranial nerves, deep tendon reflexes, gross and fine motor skills
   n. Extremities: Range of motion, reflexes
   o. Skin: Temperature, color, texture, lesions, rash

Table 1.4 Normal Values for Growth and Development

Weight

Weight loss first few days: 5%-10% of birth weight
Regain birth weight in 7-14 days
Average weight gains:
  6-8 oz/wk for the first 5-6 mo
  3-4 oz/wk until 1 yr
  4-6 lb/yr between yr 2 and puberty

Height/Length

0-3 mo	10-11 cm
3-6 mo	9-10 cm
6-9 mo	4-5 cm
9-12 mo	3-4 cm
1-2 yr	10-11 cm
2-3 yr	7-8 cm
3 yr-puberty	5-6 cm

Head Circumference

Increases 2 cm/mo for first 3 mo
1 cm/mo from 4 to 12 mo
10 cm total growth for the rest of life

Table 1.5 Dental Development: Chronology of Primary and Secondary Teeth

	Age at Eruption		Age at Shedding	
	Maxillary	Mandibular	Maxillary	Mandibular
Primary Teeth				
Central incisors	6-8 mo	5-7 mo	7-8 yr	6-7 yr
Lateral incisors	8-11 mo	7-10 mo	8-9 yr	7-8 yr
Cuspids (canines)	16-20 mo	16-20 mo	11-12 yr	9-11 yr
First molars	10-16 mo	10-16 mo	10-11 yr	10-12 yr
Second molars	20-30 mo	20-30 mo	10-12 yr	11-13 yr
Secondary Teeth				
Central incisors	7-8 yr	6-7 yr		
Lateral incisors	8-9 yr	7-8 yr		
Cuspids (canines)	11-12 yr	9-11 yr		
First premolars (bicuspids)	10-11 yr	10-12 yr		
Second premolars (bicuspids)	10-12 yr	11-13 yr		
First molars	6-7 yr	6-7 yr		
Second molars	12-13 yr	12-13 yr		
Third molars	17-22 yr	17-22 yr		

This table was published in Nelson Textbook of Pediatrics, 18th ed, Feigelman S. In Kliegman RM, Behrman RE, Jenson HB, Stanton BF, eds, p 47, Copyright Elsevier, 2007.

Table 1.6 Arm Span: Normal Ranges for Arm Span

Sex	Age	Arm Span
Girls	11-14 yr	Shorter than height
Boys	10-11 yr	Shorter than height
Females	Adult	1.2 cm > height
Males	Adult	5.3 cm > height

Adapted from Carrillo AA, Recker BF. Reference charts used frequently by endocrinologists in assessing the growth and development of youth. In Lifshitz F, ed. Pediatric Endocrinology, 5th ed. New York: Marcel Dekker, 2003. (With permission from Marcel Dekker, Inc.)

Table 1.7 Sitting Heights

Age	Standing Height (inches)		Sitting Height (absolute)		Sitting Height (relative)	
	M	F	M	F	M	F
Birth	20.2	19.9	13.6	13.4	67.3	67.3
3 mo	24.1	23.7	15.8	15.6	65.6	65.7
6 mo	26.4	26.0	16.9	16.7	64.1	64.2
9 mo	28.1	27.6	17.7	17.4	63.1	63.2
12 mo	29.5	29.0	18.4	18.1	62.3	62.4
18 mo	31.9	31.4	19.4	19.1	60.9	61.0
2 yr	33.9	33.4	20.3	20.0	59.8	59.9
3 yr	37.3	36.7	21.7	21.4	58.2	58.3
4 yr	40.2	39.6	22.9	22.5	57.0	56.9
5 yr	42.7	42.2	23.9	23.6	56.0	55.9
6 yr	45.0	44.6	24.9	24.6	55.2	55.2
7 yr	47.2	46.8	25.8	25.5	54.6	54.5
8 yr	49.2	48.9	26.6	26.4	54.1	54.0
9 yr	51.2	50.9	27.5	27.3	53.7	53.6
10 yr	53.2	53.0	28.3	28.1	53.2	53.0
11 yr	55.2	55.3	29.2	29.1	52.9	52.6
12 yr	57.1	57.6	30.0	30.3	52.6	52.6
13 yr	58.9	59.7	30.9	31.5	52.4	52.8

Adapted from Carrillo AA, Recker BF. Reference charts used frequently by endocrinologists in assessing the growth and development of youth. In Lifshitz F, ed. Pediatric Endocrinology, 5th ed. New York: Marcel Dekker, 2003. (With permission from Marcel Dekker, Inc.)

Table 1.7 Sitting Heights—cont'd

Age	Standing Height (inches)		Sitting Height (absolute)		Sitting Height (relative)	
	M	F	M	F	M	F
14 yr	60.7	61.4	31.7	32.5	52.3	52.9
15 yr	62.4	62.5	32.8	33.0	52.5	52.9
16 yr	64.0	63.2	33.7	33.4	52.7	52.9
17 yr	65.4	63.7	34.5	33.6	52.8	52.8
18 yr	66.6	64.0	35.1	33.8	52.7	52.8
19 yr	67.5	64.0	35.5	33.8	52.6	52.8
20 yr	68.0	64.0	35.7	33.8	52.5	52.8

Table 1.8 Heart Rate: Age-Specific Heart Rates

Age	2%	Mean	98%
0-7 days	95	125	160
1-3 wk	105	145	180
1-5 mo	110	145	180
6-11 mo	110	135	170
1-3 yr	90	120	150
4-5 yr	65	110	135
6-8 yr	60	100	130
9-11 yr	60	85	110
12-16 yr	60	85	100
>16 yr	60	80	100

This table was adapted from The Harriet Lane Handbook, Custer JW, Rau RE, eds, Cardiology, p 188, Copyright Elsevier, 2009.

Table 1.9 Respiratory Rate

Age	Rate (breaths/min)
0-1 yr	24-38
1-3 yr	22-30
4-6 yr	20-24
7-9 yr	18-24
10-14 yr	16-22
14-18 yr	14-20

This table was published in The Harriet Lane Handbook, Custer JW, Rau RE, eds, Pulmonology, p 624, Copyright Elsevier, 2009.

GENERAL ENDOCRINE ASSESSMENT

1

Table 1.10 Blood Pressure Levels for Girls by Age and Height Percentile

| Age (yr) | BP Percentile | Systolic BP (mm Hg) | | | | | | |
| | | Percentile of Height | | | | | | |
		5th	10th	25th	50th	75th	90th	95th
1	50th	83	84	85	86	88	89	90
	90th	97	97	98	100	101	102	103
	95th	100	101	102	104	105	106	107
	99th	108	108	109	111	112	113	114
2	50th	85	85	87	88	89	91	91
	90th	98	99	100	101	103	104	105
	95th	102	103	104	105	107	108	109
	99th	109	110	111	112	114	115	116
3	50th	86	87	88	89	91	92	93
	90th	100	100	102	103	104	106	106
	95th	104	104	105	107	108	109	110
	99th	111	111	113	114	115	116	117
4	50th	88	88	90	91	92	94	94
	90th	101	102	103	104	106	107	108
	95th	105	106	107	108	110	111	112
	99th	112	113	114	115	117	118	119
5	50th	89	90	91	93	94	95	96
	90th	103	103	105	106	107	109	109
	95th	107	107	108	110	111	112	113
	99th	114	114	116	117	118	120	120
6	50th	91	92	93	94	96	97	98
	90th	104	105	106	108	109	110	111
	95th	108	109	110	111	113	114	115
	99th	115	116	117	119	120	121	122
7	50th	93	93	95	96	97	99	99
	90th	106	107	108	109	111	112	113
	95th	110	111	112	113	115	116	116
	99th	117	118	119	120	122	123	124

From National Heart, Lung, and Blood Institute as a part of the National Institutes of Health and the U.S. Department of Health and Human Services.
Available at *http://www.nhlbi.nih.gov/guidelines/hypertension/child_tbl.pdf*. Accessed July 22, 2009.
The 90th percentile is 1.28 SD, 95th percentile is 1.645 SD, and the 99th percentile is 2.326 SD over the mean.

Diastolic BP (mm Hg)

Percentile of Height						
5th	10th	25th	50th	75th	90th	95th
38	39	39	40	41	41	42
52	53	53	54	55	55	56
56	57	57	58	59	59	60
64	64	65	65	66	67	67
43	44	44	45	46	46	47
57	58	58	59	60	61	61
61	62	62	63	64	65	65
69	69	70	70	71	72	72
47	48	48	49	50	50	51
61	62	62	63	64	64	65
65	66	66	67	68	68	69
73	73	74	74	75	76	76
50	50	51	52	52	53	54
64	64	65	66	67	67	68
68	68	69	70	71	71	72
76	76	76	77	78	79	79
52	53	53	54	55	55	56
66	67	67	68	69	69	70
70	71	71	72	73	73	74
78	78	79	79	80	81	81
54	54	55	56	56	57	58
68	68	69	70	70	71	72
72	72	73	74	74	75	76
80	80	80	81	82	83	83
55	56	56	57	58	58	59
69	70	70	71	72	72	73
73	74	74	75	76	76	77
81	81	82	82	83	84	84

(continued)

GENERAL ENDOCRINE ASSESSMENT ❶

Table 1.10   Blood Pressure Levels for Girls by Age and Height Percentile—cont'd

Age (yr)	BP Percentile	Systolic BP (mm Hg)						
		Percentile of Height						
		5th	10th	25th	50th	75th	90th	95th
8	50th	95	95	96	98	99	100	101
	90th	108	109	110	111	113	114	114
	95th	112	112	114	115	116	118	118
	99th	119	120	121	122	123	125	125
9	50th	96	97	98	100	101	102	103
	90th	110	110	112	113	114	116	116
	95th	114	114	115	117	118	119	120
	99th	121	121	123	124	125	127	127
10	50th	98	99	100	102	103	104	105
	90th	112	112	114	115	116	118	118
	95th	116	116	117	119	120	121	122
	99th	123	123	125	126	127	129	129
11	50th	100	101	102	103	105	106	107
	90th	114	114	116	117	118	119	120
	95th	118	118	119	121	122	123	124
	99th	125	125	126	128	129	130	131
12	50th	102	103	104	105	107	108	109
	90th	116	116	117	119	120	121	122
	95th	119	120	121	123	124	125	126
	99th	127	127	128	130	131	132	133
13	50th	104	105	106	107	109	110	110
	90th	117	118	119	121	122	123	124
	95th	121	122	123	124	126	127	128
	99th	128	129	130	132	133	134	135
14	50th	106	106	107	109	110	111	112
	90th	119	120	121	122	124	125	125
	95th	123	123	125	126	127	129	129
	99th	130	131	132	133	135	136	136
15	50th	107	108	109	110	111	113	113
	90th	120	121	122	123	125	126	127
	95th	124	125	126	127	129	130	131
	99th	131	132	133	134	136	137	138

The 90th percentile is 1.28 SD, 95th percentile is 1.645 SD, and the 99th percentile is 2.326 SD over the mean.

Diastolic BP (mm Hg)

Percentile of Height

5th	10th	25th	50th	75th	90th	95th
57	57	57	58	59	60	60
71	71	71	72	73	74	74
75	75	75	76	77	78	78
82	82	83	83	84	85	86
58	58	58	59	60	61	61
72	72	72	73	74	75	75
76	76	76	77	78	79	79
83	83	84	84	85	86	87
59	59	59	60	61	62	62
73	73	73	74	75	76	76
77	77	77	78	79	80	80
84	84	85	86	86	87	88
60	60	60	61	62	63	63
74	74	74	75	76	77	77
78	78	78	79	80	81	81
85	85	86	87	87	88	89
61	61	61	62	63	64	64
75	75	75	76	77	78	78
79	79	79	80	81	82	82
86	86	87	88	88	89	90
62	62	62	63	64	65	65
76	76	76	77	78	79	79
80	80	80	81	82	83	83
87	87	88	89	89	90	91
63	63	63	64	65	66	66
77	77	77	78	79	80	80
81	81	81	82	83	84	84
88	88	89	90	90	91	92
64	64	64	65	66	67	67
78	78	78	79	80	81	81
82	82	82	83	84	85	85
89	89	90	91	91	92	93

(continued)

GENERAL ENDOCRINE ASSESSMENT ❶

Table 1.10 Blood Pressure Levels for Girls by Age and Height Percentile—cont'd

		Systolic BP (mm Hg)						
		Percentile of Height						
Age (yr)	BP Percentile	5th	10th	25th	50th	75th	90th	95th
16	50th	108	108	110	111	112	114	114
	90th	121	122	123	124	126	127	128
	95th	125	126	127	128	130	131	132
	99th	132	133	134	135	137	138	139
17	50th	108	109	110	111	113	114	115
	90th	122	122	123	125	126	127	128
	95th	125	126	127	129	130	131	132
	99th	133	133	134	136	137	138	139

The 90th percentile is 1.28 SD, 95th percentile is 1.645 SD, and the 99th percentile is 2.326 SD over the mean.

Table 1.11 Blood Pressure Levels for Boys by Age and Height Percentile

		Systolic BP (mm Hg)						
		Percentile of Height						
Age (yr)	BP Percentile	5th	10th	25th	50th	75th	90th	95th
1	50th	80	81	83	85	87	88	89
	90th	94	95	97	99	100	102	103
	95th	98	99	101	103	104	106	106
	99th	105	106	108	110	112	113	114
2	50th	84	85	87	88	90	92	92
	90th	97	99	100	102	104	105	106
	95th	101	102	104	106	108	109	110
	99th	109	110	111	113	115	117	117
3	50th	86	87	89	91	93	94	95
	90th	100	101	103	105	107	108	109
	95th	104	105	107	109	110	112	113
	99th	111	112	114	116	118	119	120

From National Heart, Lung, and Blood Institute as a part of the National Institutes of Health and the U.S. Department of Health and Human Services.
Available at *http://www.nhlbi.nih.gov/guidelines/hypertension/child_tbl.pdf*. Accessed July 22, 2009.
The 90th percentile is 1.28 SD, 95th percentile is 1.645 SD, and the 99th percentile is 2.326 SD over the mean.

Diastolic BP (mm Hg)

Percentile of Height

5th	10th	25th	50th	75th	90th	95th
64	64	65	66	66	67	68
78	78	79	80	81	81	82
82	82	83	84	85	85	86
90	90	90	91	92	93	93
64	65	65	66	67	67	68
78	79	79	80	81	81	82
82	83	83	84	85	85	86
90	90	91	91	92	93	93

Diastolic BP (mm Hg)

Percentile of Height

5th	10th	25th	50th	75th	90th	95th
34	35	36	37	38	39	39
49	50	51	52	53	53	54
54	54	55	56	57	58	58
61	62	63	64	65	66	66
39	40	41	42	43	44	44
54	55	56	57	58	58	59
59	59	60	61	62	63	63
66	67	68	69	70	71	71
44	44	45	46	47	48	48
59	59	60	61	62	63	63
63	63	64	65	66	67	67
71	71	72	73	74	75	75

(continued)

GENERAL ENDOCRINE ASSESSMENT ❶

Table 1.11 Blood Pressure Levels for Boys by Age and Height Percentile—cont'd

		Systolic BP (mm Hg)						
		Percentile of Height						
Age (yr)	BP Percentile	5th	10th	25th	50th	75th	90th	95th
4	50th	88	89	91	93	95	96	97
	90th	102	103	105	107	109	110	111
	95th	106	107	109	111	112	114	115
	99th	113	114	116	118	120	121	122
5	50th	90	91	93	95	96	98	98
	90th	104	105	106	108	110	111	112
	95th	108	109	110	112	114	115	116
	99th	115	116	118	120	121	123	123
6	50th	91	92	94	96	98	99	100
	90th	105	106	108	110	111	113	113
	95th	109	110	112	114	115	117	117
	99th	116	117	119	121	123	124	125
7	50th	92	94	95	97	99	100	101
	90th	106	107	109	111	113	114	115
	95th	110	111	113	115	117	118	119
	99th	117	118	120	122	124	125	126
8	50th	94	95	97	99	100	102	102
	90th	107	109	110	112	114	115	116
	95th	111	112	114	116	118	119	120
	99th	119	120	122	123	125	127	127
9	50th	95	96	98	100	102	103	104
	90th	109	110	112	114	115	117	118
	95th	113	114	116	118	119	121	121
	99th	120	121	123	125	127	128	129
10	50th	97	98	100	102	103	105	106
	90th	111	112	114	115	117	119	119
	95th	115	116	117	119	121	122	123
	99th	122	123	125	127	128	130	130

The 90th percentile is 1.28 SD, 95th percentile is 1.645 SD, and the 99th percentile is 2.326 SD over the mean.

Diastolic BP (mm Hg)

Percentile of Height						
5th	**10th**	**25th**	**50th**	**75th**	**90th**	**95th**
47	48	49	50	51	51	52
62	63	64	65	66	66	67
66	67	68	69	70	71	71
74	75	76	77	78	78	79
50	51	52	53	54	55	55
65	66	67	68	69	69	70
69	70	71	72	73	74	74
77	78	79	80	81	81	82
53	53	54	55	56	57	57
68	68	69	70	71	72	72
72	72	73	74	75	76	76
80	80	81	82	83	84	84
55	55	56	57	58	59	59
70	70	71	72	73	74	74
74	74	75	76	77	78	78
82	82	83	84	85	86	86
56	57	58	59	60	60	61
71	72	72	73	74	75	76
75	76	77	78	79	79	80
83	84	85	86	87	87	88
57	58	59	60	61	61	62
72	73	74	75	76	76	77
76	77	78	79	80	81	81
84	85	86	87	88	88	89
58	59	60	61	61	62	63
73	73	74	75	76	77	78
77	78	79	80	81	81	82
85	86	86	88	88	89	90

(continued)

GENERAL ENDOCRINE ASSESSMENT ❶

Table 1.11 Blood Pressure Levels for Boys by Age and Height Percentile—cont'd

Age (yr)	BP Percentile	Systolic BP (mm Hg)						
		Percentile of Height						
		5th	10th	25th	50th	75th	90th	95th
11	50th	99	100	102	104	105	107	107
	90th	113	114	115	117	119	120	121
	95th	117	118	119	121	123	124	125
	99th	124	125	127	129	130	132	132
12	50th	101	102	104	106	108	109	110
	90th	115	116	118	120	121	123	123
	95th	119	120	122	123	125	127	127
	99th	126	127	129	131	133	134	135
13	50th	104	105	106	108	110	111	112
	90th	117	118	120	122	124	125	126
	95th	121	122	124	126	128	129	130
	99th	128	130	131	133	135	136	137
14	50th	106	107	109	111	113	114	115
	90th	120	121	123	125	126	128	128
	95th	124	125	127	128	130	132	132
	99th	131	132	134	136	138	139	140
15	50th	109	110	112	113	115	117	117
	90th	122	124	125	127	129	130	131
	95th	126	127	129	131	133	134	135
	99th	134	135	136	138	140	142	142
16	50th	111	112	114	116	118	119	120
	90th	125	126	128	130	131	133	134
	95th	129	130	132	134	135	137	137
	99th	136	137	139	141	143	144	145
17	50th	114	115	116	118	120	121	122
	90th	127	128	130	132	134	135	136
	95th	131	132	134	136	138	139	140
	99th	139	140	141	143	145	146	147

The 90th percentile is 1.28 SD, 95th percentile is 1.645 SD, and the 99th percentile is 2.326 SD over the mean.

Diastolic BP (mm Hg)

Percentile of Height						
5th	10th	25th	50th	75th	90th	95th
59	59	60	61	62	63	63
74	74	75	76	77	78	78
78	78	79	80	81	82	82
86	86	87	88	89	90	90
59	60	61	62	63	63	64
74	75	75	76	77	78	79
78	79	80	81	82	82	83
86	87	88	89	90	90	91
60	60	61	62	63	64	64
75	75	76	77	78	79	79
79	79	80	81	82	83	83
87	87	88	89	90	91	91
60	61	62	63	64	65	65
75	76	77	78	79	79	80
80	80	81	82	83	84	84
87	88	89	90	91	92	92
61	62	63	64	65	66	66
76	77	78	79	80	80	81
81	81	82	83	84	85	85
88	89	90	91	92	93	93
63	63	64	65	66	67	67
78	78	79	80	81	82	82
82	83	83	84	85	86	87
90	90	91	92	93	94	94
65	66	66	67	68	69	70
80	80	81	82	83	84	84
84	85	86	87	87	88	89
92	93	93	94	95	96	97

❷ ADRENAL DISORDERS

OVERVIEW

The adrenal gland is located above the kidneys bilaterally. It is made up of two endocrine tissues: the cortex and the medulla. The outer portion, the adrenal cortex, is responsible for the production of glucocorticoids (cortisol), mineralo-corticoids (aldosterone, deoxycorticosterone), and the sex hormones (DHEA, androstenedione). The inner portion is the adrenal medulla. Here the catecholamines epinephrine, norepinephrine, and dopamine are manufactured (Fig. 2.1).

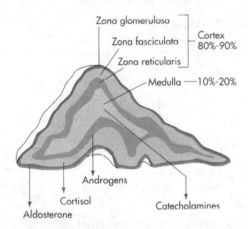

Figure 2.1 The adrenal gland. (From Porterfield S, ed. Endocrine Physiology. St Louis: Mosby–Year Book, 1997. With permission from Elsevier.)

HISTORY

General history with attention to:

- Change in overall appearance
- Increase in appetite, salt craving
- Change in weight and/or growth velocity
- Headache, visual disturbances
- GI concerns: nausea and vomiting, constipation or diarrhea, anorexia, polydipsia, vague abdominal pain or distention, peptic ulcer
- Weakness, fatigue, muscular pain
- Darkening skin color

- Nervousness, insomnia, euphoria, depression, sweating, tremor, anxious appearance
- Onset of puberty, menarche and menstrual patterns, development
- Polyuria and enuresis
- Poor wound healing, infection, diabetes
- Current medications
- Autoimmune disorders, malignancies
- Pituitary disease or hormone deficiency resulting from metastatic disease, trauma, or surgery
- Sustained hypertension, orthostatic hypotension
- Family history of endocrine disorders

PHYSICAL EXAMINATION

General examination with attention to:

- Overall appearance, face, and body shape/proportion
- Mental status, reflexes
- Blood pressure
- Weight and height, growth velocity
- Skin turgor, acne, striae, hirsutism, skin discolorations or pigmentation, edema, vitiligo
- Shape of abdomen, distention
- Appearance of genitalia appropriate for sex and age
- Tanner stage appropriate for age
- Muscle tone, strength

CONGENITAL ADRENAL HYPERPLASIA

Congenital adrenal hyperplasia (CAH) is an inherited enzymatic defect in the pathway between the conversion of cholesterol to cortisol, resulting in over-production of the sex hormones. It is inherited in an autosomal recessive fashion. There are many different types of CAH depending on where the enzymatic block is located in the adrenal steroid pathway. Fig. 2.2 shows the adrenal steroid pathway.

The different types of CAH and rates of occurrence are listed below:

1. 21-hydroxylase (most common; 90%-95%)
    a. Salt loser: a more severe form associated with hyponatremia and hyperkalemia (75%)
    b. Non–salt-losing or simple virilized: a less severe form (25%)
    c. Nonclassical or late onset: no genital ambiguity at birth in females

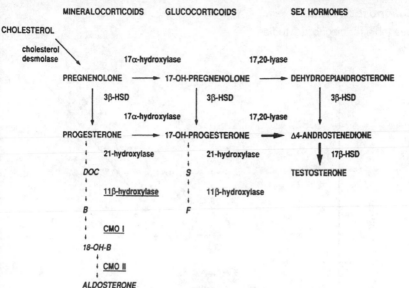

Figure 2.2 The adrenal steroid pathway. (From New M, Ghizzoni L, Speiser PW. Update on congenital adrenal hyperplasia. In Lifshitz F, ed. Pediatric Endocrinology, 3rd ed. New York: Marcel Dekker, 1996. With permission from Marcel Dekker.)

B, Corticosterone; *CMO,* corticosterone methyloxidase; *DOC,* deoxycorticosterone; *F,* cortisol; *HSD,* hydroxysteroid dehydrogenase; *S,* 11-deoxycortisol.

2. 11-beta hydroxylase (5%-8%)
3. 3-beta hydroxysteroid dehydrogenase (<2%)
4. 17 alpha hydroxylase/17, 20 lyase (<2%)
5. 20, 22 hydroxylase (cholesterol desmolase) (rare)

The non–salt-losing or simple virilized type of CAH, as well as the nonclassical or late-onset type, do not have a mineralocorticoid deficiency; therefore electrolytes are stable. Depending on the degree of severity of the defect, children may present in the neonatal period with ambiguous genitalia and/or salt wasting or may only be discovered later with hyperandrogenic symptoms, such as precocious adrenarche, advanced bone age, and accelerated growth. Female adolescents with irregular menses, polycystic ovary syndrome (PCOS), acne, and hirsutism should be evaluated for nonclassical 21-OH deficiency.

ADRENAL DISORDERS

Diagnostic Testing

See table for diagnostic studies.

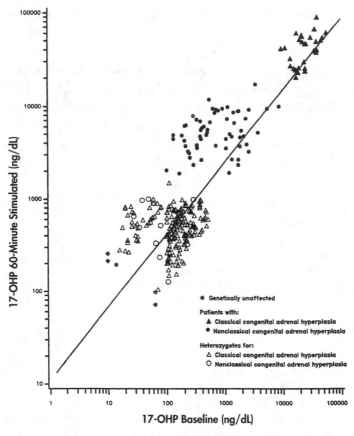

Figure 2.3 17-OHP nomogram for the diagnosis of steroid 21–hydroxylase deficiency: 60-minute cortrosyn stimulation test. The data for this nomogram were collected between 1982 and 1991 at the Department of Pediatrics, The New York Hospital–Cornell Medical Center, New York. (From New M, Ghizzoni L, Speiser PW. Update on congenital adrenal hyperplasia. In Lifshitz F, ed. Pediatric Endocrinology, 3rd ed. New York: Marcel Dekker, 1996. With permission from Marcel Dekker.)

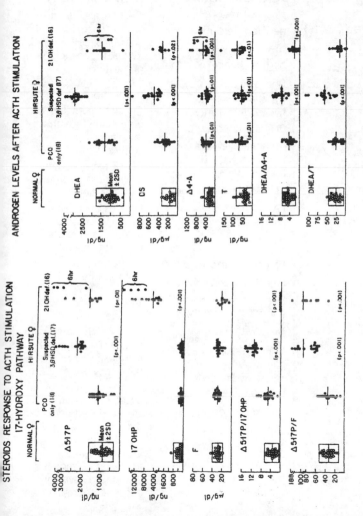

Figure 2.4 Use the 60-minute stimulated hormone level to complete the figure.

KEY Δ5-17P = 17-OHP Pregnenolone   T = Testosterone
17-OHP = 17-OHP Progesterone   F = Cortisol   Δ4-A = Androstenedione

ADRENAL DISORDERS ❷

From Pang SY, Lerner AJ, Stoner E, et al. Late-onset adrenal steroid 3 beta-hydroxysteroid dehydrogenase deficiency. I. A cause of hirsutism in pubertal and postpubertal women. J Clin Endocrinol Metab 60:428-439, 1985. With permission from The Endocrine Society.

DIAGNOSIS	CLINICAL FINDINGS	DIAGNOSTIC FINDINGS

Congenital Adrenal Hyperplasia (CAH)

Incidence
21-OH Deficiency (only)

Classic
1:12,000

Nonclassical
1:100 (all Caucasians)
1:30 (Ashkenazi Jews)

Pertinent History

Elevated 17-OHP on newborn screening

Ambiguous genitalia at birth in the female infant

Unexplained hyponatremia and/or hyperkalemia and/or hypoglycemia

Vomiting, dehydration in the neonatal period (more likely presentation in the male infant)

Precocious adrenarche

Irregular menses, acne, hirsutism

Physical Findings

Precocious adrenarche with advanced bone age and accelerated growth

Acne with hirsutism

Unexplained hyponatremia/hyperkalemia and dehydration in the newborn period

Ambiguous genitalia

Diagnostic Tests

CAH Profile 6 (cortisol, androstenedione, Specific S, DHEA, DOC, 17-OH pregnenolone, progesterone, 17-OH progesterone, testosterone)

Check sodium and potassium if electrolyte imbalance is a consideration.

Check plasma renin activity if salt-wasting is a consideration.

In cases of ambiguous genitalia: chromosome analysis, genitogram, pelvic ultrasound

Cortrosyn stimulation test for adrenal androgens if nonclassical 21-OH deficiency is a consideration

The 17-OHP nomogram can be utilized in the diagnosis of 21-OH deficiency (see Fig. 2.3).

For the diagnosis of late onset 3 beta-dyhydroxysteroid dehydrogenase deficiency, use Fig. 2.4. The diagnosis is indicated when all of the following hormones are 2 standard deviations above the normal mean:
Δ5-17P
Δ5-17P ÷ 17-OHP
Δ5-17P ÷ F
DHEA

Medications

Hydrocortisone is used in growing children and given either tid or bid depending on the age of the child.

In emergency situations, injectable Solu-Cortef is advisable.

Prednisone or dexamethasone is used when growth is complete. (See steroid equivalency chart on p. 424.)

Fludrocortisone acetate is used in the salt-losing form of CAH. This is needed if the plasma renin activity is high, even if the sodium level is normal.

Other

Salt is used during the first year of life since infant formulas are relatively salt-poor. Sodium chloride tablets of ½ to 1 g/day is generally all that is required for the first year of life.

Referral to a pediatric urologist if ambiguous genitalia are present

Referral to a geneticist

Nursing Considerations

The salt should be dissolved in the water used to make the formula so that the salt is distributed evenly throughout the day.

Parents should be educated that during illness, accident, surgery, immunizations, or other times of stress, steroid stress doses should be utilized. *Doses may be doubled or tripled based on institutional policy.*

A letter for stress dosing of both the hydrocortisone and the Solu-Cortef should be given to the family. Instructions should include medication doses and specifics about when to double or triple the dose. The family can share the letter with a school nurse or emergency department in case of emergency.

(continued)

Monitor BP, height, and weight at every visit.

Monitor for cushingoid symptoms at every visit.

Monitor for signs of inappropriate virilization prior to attaining puberty as well as at puberty.

If there is inappropriate linear growth, monitor bone age.

Re-evaluate for adequate suppression every 3 to 4 months with appropriate labs:

21-OH, non–salt-losing: 17-OHP and androgen levels

21-OH, salt-losing: 17-OHP, plasma renin activity, androgen levels

11-beta-OH: Plasma renin activity and either an 11-deoxycortisol (Compound S) or 11-deoxycorticosterone (DOC)

3-beta-HSD: 17-OH Pregnenolone, dehydroepiandrosterone (DHEA). If salt wasting is present, also check the plasma renin activity.

17-hydroxylase: Plasma renin activity and either DOC or Compound B

20-hydroxylase: ACTH. If salt wasting is present, also check the plasma renin activity.

ADRENAL DISORDERS

②

MANAGEMENT/EDUCATION	EVALUATION

Parents should have injectable hydrocortisone at home for emergency administration in the event of an illness (during which the child cannot tolerate oral medications). Following the injection, families should call their endocrinologist for further instructions.

At all times the child should wear a medical ID tag that reads "Adrenal Insufficiency—Takes Cortisol."

Transition to Adulthood

Once skeletal maturity is attained, prednisone or dexamethasone can be used rather than hydro-cortisone to achieve better suppression.

Since CAH is transmitted in an autosomal recessive pattern of inheritance, prospective parents may wish to determine if they carry the gene mutation for 21-OH deficiency. Testing can be performed by a genetics specialist.

During pregnancy it is still possible to minimize the degree of virilization that a female child may be born with and decrease the need for or degree of postnatal repair required. This is done by treating the mother with dexamethasone starting before the eighth week of gestation. Intervention should occur within the first 6-7 weeks of fetal life. Dexametha-sone suppresses excessive androgen production of the fetus. Once the sex of the fetus is known, dexamethasone is continued only if the fetus is female and affected (see Fig. 2.5).

1. **Pre-pregnancy:**

   Blood samples from <u>mother</u>, <u>father</u> and <u>affected sib</u> for:

   a) SEROLOGIC TESTING for HLA antigens.

   b) HYBRIDIZATION ANALYSIS using
      1. HLA Class I and II cDNA probes. Characteristic RFLPs (restriction fragment length polymorphisms) detected by molecular probes identify HLA antigens with greater specificity.
      2. Oligonucleotide probes synthesized to correspond to and directly identify the occurrence of known mutations in the active 21-hydroxylase gene sequence.

      Molecular analysis is becoming increasingly available but is not yet a part of standard laboratory evaluation. Oligonucleotide probes are still highly experimental.

   c) ACTH STIMULATION TESTING measuring 17α-hydroxyprogesterone in serum (or saliva) at 0 min (baseline) and 60 min after administration of Cortrosyn (0.25 mg i.v.) will reveal distinct hormonal responses according to 21-hydroxylase genotype.

      Once the 21-hydroxylase deficiency-linked HLA types for the pedigree have been determined, the detection of both marker haplotypes together in a genotype is presumptive diagnosis of affected status.

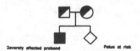

Severely affected proband   Fetus at risk

2. **In pregnancy:**

FETAL AGE	DIAGNOSTIC TEST	THERAPY
a) 8 to 10 days	Pregnancy test (β-hCG assay)	start: dexamethasone 20 μg/(kg·d)
b) 9 or 10 weeks	CHORIONIC VILLUS BIOPSY	
	i) HLA serotypes (Class I) of cultured villus cells	if affected: continue
	ii) Hybridization analysis	
	iii) Metabolic assay (hormonal testing)	
	iv) Cell culture karyotype to ascertain fetal sex	if M: stop
c) 15 to 18 weeks	AMNIOCENTESIS (if CVB risk is unacceptable; also if genotyping by CVB has been equivocal)	
	i) HLA serotyping of cultured amniotic fluid (fetal) cells	(as above)
	ii) sex determination	(as above)
	iii) hormonal testing (17-hydroxyprogesterone RIA) if not under treatment	

Figure 2.5 Algorithm depicting prenatal management of pregnancy in families at risk for a fetus affected with 21-OH deficiency. (From New MI, del Balso P, Crawford C, et al. The adrenal cortex. In Kaplan S, ed. Clinical Pediatric Endocrinology. Philadelphia: WB Saunders, 1990. With permission from Elsevier Science.)

PHEOCHROMOCYTOMA

Pheochromocytoma is a rare childhood tumor that can originate in any chromaffin tissue in the body but most commonly is located in the right adrenal gland. The peak incidence is between 9 and 12 years of age. One must differentiate this tumor from a neuroblastoma.

Diagnostic Testing

See table for diagnostic studies.

DIAGNOSIS	CLINICAL FINDINGS	DIAGNOSTIC FINDINGS
Pheochromocytoma **Incidence** Rare	**Pertinent History** Complaints of intermittent symptoms of catecholamine effects: weakness, sweating, flushing pallor, palpitations Complaints of intermittent abdominal pain and distention, chronic constipation, nervousness, visual disturbances, polydipsia, polyuria, enuresis, forceful heartbeat, anxiety or feelings of impending death, tremor, fatigue, exhaustion, chest pain, weight loss **Physical Findings** Sustained hypertension, orthostatic hypotension, headache, sweating, nausea, vomiting, visual disturbances, weight loss, anxious appearing, pale, weak, emotionally labile, tremor, tachycardia, acrocyanosis with cold extremities, hyperglycemia, glucosuria, increased free fatty acids, convulsions	**Laboratory Tests** 24-hour urine for vanillylmandelic acid (VMA), norepinephrine, epinephrine, metanephrine, and normetanephrine. Elevations should be confirmed by at least one repeated test (See Tables 2.1 and 2.2 for norms.) MRI or CT scan to localize the tumor Metaiodobenzylguanidine scintigraphy for recurrent or metastatic disease

MANAGEMENT/EDUCATION	EVALUATION
Excision, if possible	Following surgical removal, 24-hour urine for VMA catecholamines and their metabolites should be checked yearly for 5 years if asymptomatic or sooner if symptomatic.
Pharmacologic preparations such as phentolamine, prazosin, phenoxybenzamine are used to inhibit catecholamine synthesis and establish adrenergic blockade.	
After alpha receptor blockade has been established, propranolol may be used to control marked tachycardia.	If surgery is not an option, chronic long-term medical management is necessary using alpha blockade and metyrosine.
	The 24-hour urine studies should be repeated at intervals to assess medical management.
	Also evaluate for one of the familial syndromes such as multiple endocrine neoplasia type 2 (MEN2) or von Hippel-Lindau.

2

ADRENAL DISORDERS

Table 2.1 Urinary Excretion of Catecholamines and VMA by Healthy Children

µg per 24 hours

Age	NE		E		VMA	
	Mean	SD	Mean	SD	Mean	SD
Birth to 1 yr	10.6	3.4	1.3	1.2	569	309
1 through 5 yr	18.8	7.0	3.2	2.7	1348	443
6 through 15 yr	37.4	16.6	4.8	2.4	2373	698
Over 15 yr	50.7	15.7	7.1	3.3	3192	669

µg per sq M per 24 hours

Age	NE		E		VMA	
	Mean	SD	Mean	SD	Mean	SD
Birth to 1 yr	41.1	15.3	4.7	3.3	2021	1121
1 through 5 yr	27.9	8.9	4.9	4.4	2001	571
6 through 15 yr	31.2	15.7	4.3	1.9	2133	378
Over 15 yr	30.5	8.1	4.3	1.9	1931	389

From New MI, del Balso P, Crawford C, et al. The adrenal cortex. In Kaplan S, ed. Clinical Pediatric Endocrinology. Philadelphia: WB Saunders, 1990. With permission from Elsevier Science.
E, Epinephrine; *NE,* norepinephrine; *VMA,* vanillylmandelic acid (3-methoxy-4-hydroxymandelic acid).

Table 2.2 Urinary Excretion of Catecholamine Metabolites by Normal Children

µg per mg Creatinine

Age	VMA		HVA		M + NM	
	Mean	SD	Mean	SD	Mean	SD
1-12 mo	6.9	3.2	12.9	9.58	1.64	1.32
1-2 yr	4.7	2.22	12.6	6.26	1.68	1.13
2-5 yr	3.95	1.72	7.58	3.56	1.25	0.77
5-10 yr	3.3	1.40	4.7	2.66	1.13	0.78
10-15 yr	1.91	0.77	2.5	2.42	0.60	0.48
15-18 yr	1.4	0.61	1.0	0.65	0.24	0.23

From New MI, del Balso P, Crawford C, et al. The adrenal cortex. In Kaplan S, ed. Clinical Pediatric Endocrinology. Philadelphia: WB Saunders, 1990. With permission from Elsevier Science.
HVA, Homovanillic acid; *M,* metanephrine; *NM,* normetanephrine; *VMA,* vanillylmandelic acid (3-methoxy-4-hydroxymandelic acid).

ADDISON'S DISEASE (Primary Adrenocortical Insufficiency)

Addison's disease is a condition caused by the partial or complete failure of adrenocortical function. The onset is usually gradual, over a period of weeks or months. All general functions of the adrenal cortex are lost—glucocorticoid, mineralocorticoid, and androgenic. Rare in pediatrics. Tuberculosis infection is no longer a common cause as in previous generations. Idiopathic adrenal atrophy, which usually results from an autoimmune disorder, is presently the most common cause of Addison's disease. Other causes include metastatic malignancy or lymphoma, adrenal hemorrhage, infections (TB, CMV, fungi, histoplasmosis, coccidioidomycosis), adrenoleukodystrophy, infiltrative disorders, amyloidosis, hemochromatosis, congenital adrenal hyperplasia, familial glucocorticoid deficiency, and drugs (ketoconazole, metyrapone, aminoglutethimide, trilostane, mitotane, etomidate).

Since the majority of cases are related to autoimmune disease, the patient may often have other associated autoimmune disorders, such as diabetes mellitus type 1, oophoritis, parathyroid or thyroid deficiency, and/or pernicious anemia. Other disorders seen in patients with Addison's disease include malabsorption, hypogonadism, chronic active hepatitis, vitiligo, alopecia, or chronic monilial infections of the skin. If the cause is an autoimmune disorder, then positive adrenal antibodies will be found. Ninety percent (90%) of adrenal tissue must be nonfunctioning before clinical signs are manifested. If cause is related to an infection, there may be signs of the infection in other sites of the body. Due to the adrenal cortex's crucial role in the body's response to stress, the patient may exhibit or report anxiety, restlessness, irritability, and confusion.

2

ADRENAL DISORDERS

DIAGNOSIS	CLINICAL FINDINGS	DIAGNOSTIC FINDINGS
Addison's Disease (Primary adrenocortical deficiency)	**Pertinent History**	**Laboratory Tests**

Addison's Disease (Primary adrenocortical deficiency)

Pathologic condition

Affecting both adrenal glands

Glucocorticoid, mineralocorticoid, and androgenic functions are lost

Pertinent History

Other autoimmune disorder

Headache

Diaphoresis

Generalized weakness

Anorexia, nausea, and vomiting

Irritability, apathy, negativism

Increased sleeping, listlessness

Salt craving

Hypotension, fainting, dizziness

Amenorrhea

Physical Findings

Weight loss, ↑ pulse rate, hypotension, dehydration, tremors, ↓ muscle strength, ↓ pubic/axillary hair, vitiligo

Hyperpigmentation of the buccal mucosa, skin folds, pressure areas, and areolas

Laboratory Tests

Rapid ACTH stimulation test

↓ Cortisol

↓ 17-OHCS

↓ 17-KS

↑ ACTH

↓ Glu

↓ Na^+

↑ K^+

↑ $Ca+$

↑ BUN

↑ Creatinine

↓ HCO_3

↓ pH

ECG: Nonspecific ST-T wave abnormalities due to abnormal electrolytes

CT scan: Adrenal calcifications, adrenal enlargement

MANAGEMENT/EDUCATION	EVALUATION

Medications

Glucocorticoid and mineralocorticoid replacement therapy (See steroid equivalency chart on p. 424)

Mild androgen replacement for adolescent females to promote growth of pubic hair

Education

Teach patient/family about the disease and the following:

- Eating 3 meals/day
- Properly self-administering steroid therapy
- Increasing fluid intake
- Wearing medical identification
- Carrying emergency glucocorticoid injection kit
- Avoiding persons with infectious diseases
- Reporting adverse drug effects, such as excess weight gain, edema, marked muscle weakness, bone pain, hypertension, depression, headache, polyuria, infection
- Regular medical checkups
- When to seek medical attention

Nursing Considerations

At each visit, it is important to evaluate the patient's and family's understanding of and compliance with therapy.

The body's need for glucocorticoids increases in times of stress, such as fever, infection, dental work, emotional upset, and surgery. During these events stress doses of glucocorticoids should be utilized. *Doses may be doubled or tripled depending on institutional policy.*

EVALUATION

Follow-up assessment every 3-4 months

Adequate glucocorticoid treatment results in the disappearance of symptoms

Hyperpigmentation improves but may not disappear.

Assessment of mineralocorticoid replacement may be determined by monitoring BP, plasma renin, and electrolytes.

Transition to Adulthood

Addison's disease is incurable and requires lifelong hormone replacement of glucocorticoids and mineralocorticoids.

Review with the patient self-administration of maintenance daily dosing, sick/stress day dosing, and emergency steroid therapy.

Male hormone replacement is not usually needed, as boys with Addison's disease have very little, if any, delay in their sexual maturation.

ADRENAL DISORDERS

SECONDARY ADRENAL INSUFFICIENCY

Secondary adrenal insufficiency results when there is insufficient ACTH from the pituitary gland due to either pituitary disease or suppression of ACTH secretion by exogenous steroid administration. This occurs more commonly than Addison's disease due to the common use of synthetic steroids. Tumors of the pituitary or hypothalamus are the most common natural causes.

Diagnostic Testing

See table for diagnostic studies.

DIAGNOSIS	CLINICAL FINDINGS	DIAGNOSTIC FINDINGS
Secondary Adrenocortical Deficiency Reduced ACTH secretion Mineralocorticoid and androgenic functions of the adrenal glands are not lost. More common than Addison's disease	**Pertinent History** Weight change, nausea, vomiting, anorexia, arthralgia, weakness, fatigue, muscular pain, menarche/pubertal changes **Physical Findings** Similar to clinical features of Addison's disease *except:* Hyperpigmentation is not present Dehydration does not occur Hypotension is less prominent	**Laboratory Tests** Rapid ACTH stimulation test Metyrapone test ↓ Cortisol ↓ ACTH ↓ 11-deoxycortisol ↓ Glucose ↓ Na$^+$ N K$^+$ N BUN N Creatinine N HCO$_3$

MANAGEMENT/EDUCATION

Medications

Glucocorticoid replacement (same as for primary adrenal insufficiency)

Education

Teach patient/family about the disease and the following:

- Eating 3 meals/day
- Properly self-administering steroid therapy
- Increasing fluid intake
- Wearing medical identification
- Carrying emergency glucocorticoid injection kit
- Avoiding persons with infectious diseases
- Reporting adverse drug effects, such as excess weight gain, edema, marked muscle weakness, bone pain, hypertension, depression, headache, polyuria, infection
- Regular medical checkups
- When to seek medical attention

Nursing Considerations

Patients whose base levels of cortisol were normal in testing but produced an inappropriate metyrapone test may only need therapy at times of stress.

Patients on daily glucocorticoid maintenance therapy will also need dose increases during periods of illness or stress.

Fludrocortisone is not usually required as there is no mineralocorticoid deficiency.

Steroid therapy should be withdrawn gradually (tapering the daily dose over a period of 1 month) to avoid adrenal crisis.

EVALUATION

Follow-up assessment every 3-4 months

Adequate glucocorticoid treatment results in the disappearance of symptoms.

Overtreatment is indicated by cushingoid features such as:
- Moon face
- Reddened cheeks
- Pendulous abdomen
- Striae
- Short stature
- Excessive hair growth
- Muscle weakness

Transition to Adulthood

Need for glucocorticoid replacement may be lifelong.

Review with the patient self-administration of maintenance daily dosing, sick/stress day dosing, and emergency steroid therapy.

ADRENAL DISORDERS

CUSHING'S SYNDROME (Hyperadrenocorticism)

Cushing's syndrome is a metabolic disorder that results from excessive cortisol production by the adrenal cortex. It may also be caused by large doses of glucocorticoids for several weeks or longer, although this may be reversed when steroids are gradually discontinued. This syndrome is characterized by the inability of the body to regulate cortisol or ACTH secretion. Cushing's is unusual in infancy and childhood. Tumor of the adrenal gland is a common cause up to about age 7 years. A pituitary tumor, such as an adenoma, may be found in some patients. If overproduction is caused by a pituitary tumor, it is called *Cushing's disease*.

Diagnostic Testing

See table for diagnostic studies.

DIAGNOSIS	CLINICAL FINDINGS	DIAGNOSTIC FINDINGS
Cushing's Syndrome Characteristic group of clinical manifestations caused by excessive circulating free cortisol May be of pituitary, adrenal, ectopic, or iatrogenic cause Uncommon in children	**Pertinent History** Change in overall appearance, ↑appetite, fatigue, poor wound healing, infection, insomnia, euphoria, depression, menstrual irregularities, poor growth, ↑frequency of infection, peptic ulcer, diabetes, fractures, backache, voice deepening **Physical Findings** (see Fig. 2.6) Short stature Truncal obesity Fat pads on neck and back "Buffalo humps" Moon face Thin extremities *(continued)*	**Laboratory Tests** Dexamethasone suppression test ↓ACTH ↑Urine cortisol ↑Serum cortisol ↑17-OHCS ↑17-KS ↓K^+ ↑Na^+ **Ultrasound/CT Scan** Identify adrenal, pituitary, or nonendocrine tumor as cause. **Radiologic Studies** Identify fractures. **Bone Mineral Density** Identify osteoporosis.

MANAGEMENT/EDUCATION	EVALUATION

Medications

Replacement of pituitary hormones for patients having radiation or excision of tumor:

- GH
- ADH
- Thyroid extract
- Steroids
- Gonadotropins

Steroidogenic inhibitors

- Mitotane
- Metyrapone
- Aminoglutethimide
- Ketoconazole

Neuromodulatory effect on ACTH

- Bromocriptine
- Cyproheptadine
- Valproic acid
- Octreotide

Surgery

Removal of pituitary tumor (usually transsphenoidal route)

Unilateral or bilateral adrenalectomy—will need lifelong steroid replacement

(continued)

Follow-up assessment every 3-4 months

Monitor height/weight.

Monitor for signs of infection.

Monitor for fluid and electrolyte imbalance.

Assess patient for effective coping skills in dealing with appearance changes.

Continue assessment of education needs for side effects of medication/ surgery.

Transition to Adulthood

Patients who have a bilateral adrenalectomy will require lifelong hormone replacement of glucocorticoids and mineralocorticoids.

(continued)

DIAGNOSIS	CLINICAL FINDINGS	DIAGNOSTIC FINDINGS
(Cushing's Syndrome)	Pendulous abdomen Muscle weakness Thin skin Excessive bruising Petechiae Red cheeks ↑BP Kyphosis Hirsutism Acne Clitoral enlargement	

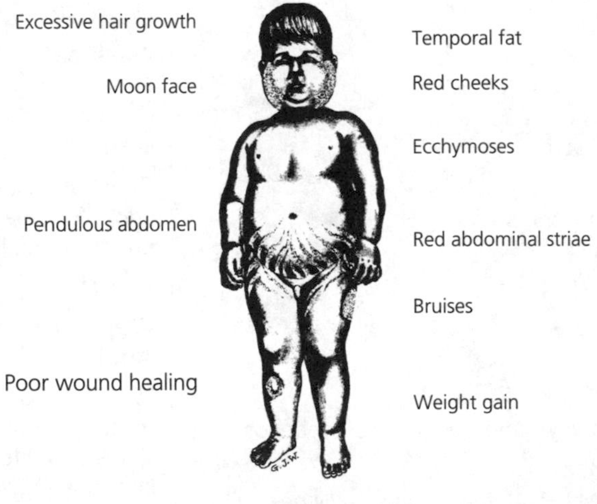

Excessive hair growth

Moon face

Pendulous abdomen

Poor wound healing

Temporal fat

Red cheeks

Ecchymoses

Red abdominal striae

Bruises

Weight gain

Figure 2.6   Characteristics of Cushing's syndrome. (From Cerasuolo K. The child with endocrine dysfunction. In Hockenberry MJ, Wilson D, eds. Wong's Nursing Care of Infants and Children, 8th ed. St Louis: Mosby Elsevier, 2007. With permission from Elsevier.)

MANAGEMENT/EDUCATION	EVALUATION
Radiation Therapy May be used for pituitary tumors **Education** Teach patient/family about the disease and treatment rationale. Discuss operative benefits and disadvantages. Postoperative teaching on drug therapy. Advise patient/family when to seek medical attention. **Nursing Considerations** Priorities for patients with Cushing's syndrome include preventing accidental injury caused by muscle weakness, preventing infection, increasing activity tolerance, and identifying and promoting coping mechanisms for dealing with changes in physical appearance.	Review with patient self-administration of maintenance daily dosing, sick/stress day dosing, and emergency steroid therapy.

RESOURCES/SUPPORT GROUPS

CUSH
PO Box 1424
Florence, AL 35631-1424
www.cush.org

Cushing's Support & Research Foundation
65 E. India Row, Suite 22B
Boston, MA 02110
www.csrf.net

John's Foundation for Cushing's Awareness
www.jfcainc.com

Magic Foundation for Children's Growth
1327 N. Harlem Avenue
Oak Park, IL 60302
(800) 432-5378
www.magicfoundation.org

Medic Alert Foundation
PO Box 1009
2323 Colorado Avenue
Turlock, CA 95380
(800) 432-5378
www.medicalert.org

National Adrenal Diseases Foundation (NADF)
505 Northern Boulevard
Great Neck, NY 11021
(516) 487-4992
www.medhelp.org/nadf

ADRENAL DISORDERS 2

BONE MINERALIZATION AND METABOLIC DISORDERS

OVERVIEW

In order for proper bone growth to occur, many factors are involved. Vitamin D metabolism is essential in the central control mechanism. There are two sources of vitamin D: cholecalciferol and ergocalciferol. Vitamin D is produced endogenously in the skin following exposure to ultraviolet radiation (cholecalciferol or vitamin D_3) or obtained exogenously from the diet (ergocalciferol or vitamin D_2). After exposure to ultraviolet B radiation, 7-dehydrocholesterol in the skin is converted to precholecalciferol and cholecalciferol. Next, either cholecalciferol or ergocalciferol is hydroxylated in the liver to 25-hydroxyvitamin D. This active metabolite increases absorption of calcium from the intestine and mobilizes calcium and phosphorus from bone.[1]

HISTORY

HPI/ROS Growth, activity, appetite/diet, motor development, muscle weakness/cramps/paresthesia, bone pain, changes in mental status, irritability, lethargy, apnea, seizures, headaches, general malaise, abdominal pain, vomiting, nausea, bowel movements, skin/hair/nail problems, thirst, nocturia/enuresis

Medical history Prematurity/low birth weight, birth hypoxia, short stature, failure to thrive, pernicious anemia, heart murmur, seizures, anticonvulsant use, prescribed and OTC medications, vitamin D supplementation provided to child, recent gastrointestinal or respiratory tract illness, fractures, bowed legs, tumors, radiation exposure

Family history History of rickets; maternal vitamin D status, maternal dietary history—especially a history of breast-feeding without vitamin D supplementation or low milk intake, maternal calcium/phosphate/PTH levels; history of familial genetic disorders

Social history Intellectual development, school performance

PHYSICAL EXAMINATION

Height, weight, head circumference (<2 years of age)

HEENT General appearance, fontanelles (anterior and posterior—open/closed, size), cranial sutures (infant), dentition, eyes (fundi, lenses), hair (consistency), other routine

Chest Shape, symmetry, thoracic base

Cardiovascular Murmur, rhythm, edema

Gastrointestinal Masses, constipation

Genitourinary Tanner staging, structural abnormalities

Neurologic Mental status, reflexes, Chvostek's sign

> NOTE Chvostek's sign: The facial nerve is tapped with a fingertip (as a hammer), 1-2 cm anterior to the earlobe below the zygomatic process. The local spasm of the facial nerve muscles is graded as (1) twitching of the upper lip (at the corner) only, (2) twitching of the lower extended portion of the lateral wall of the nose as well, (3) contraction of the muscle around the opening or the orbit of the eye as well, and (4) contraction of all the muscles on that side. A sign > grade 2 suggests hypocalcemia. The greater the grade, the more serious the condition.

Musculoskeletal Gait, bony abnormalities, muscle weakness/tetany

Skin Color, texture

RICKETS

This is a disorder of growing bone that is associated with a softening of the skeleton, particularly the epiphyses and costochondral junctions. Categories include vitamin D deficiency rickets, vitamin D-resistant (hypophosphatemic) rickets, and vitamin D-dependent rickets. Rickets is the most common form of metabolic bone disease in children.[1-4]

BONE MINERALIZATION AND METABOLIC DISORDERS

DIAGNOSIS	CLINICAL FINDINGS

Vitamin D Deficiency Rickets

Low in the United States with advent of vitamin D supplementation in diet

May occur with infants who are breast-fed or in families with special dietary habits

Higher incidence in dark-skinned individuals[5]

Pertinent History

Vegetarian diet
Breast-feeding
Prematurity/low birth weight
? Vitamin D supplementation
Sun exposure
Recent growth spurt
Seizure
Anticonvulsant use
Recent gastrointestinal or respiratory tract illness
Delayed motor development
Fatigue
Bone pain
Muscle weakness

Physical Findings

Developmental delay
Waddling gait
Failure to thrive
Skin pigmentation (dark pigmentation at greater risk)
Fractures
Bony abnormalities
  Palpable and visible enlargements of extremities of
    long bones and of costochondral junctions
  Long bones—mostly at wrists and ankles
  Costochondral junctions—enlargement bilaterally
    on thorax, "rachitic rosary"
  Tibial and femoral bowing
  Ulnar and radial bowing (severe)
  Pectus carinatum, thoracic asymmetry, widening of
    thoracic base (severe)
  Occipital thumb pressure softening (infants >3 mo)
  Enlarged sutures and fontanels
  Delayed closure of fontanel
  Occipital or parietal flattening
  Fractures
Dental abnormalities
  Delayed tooth eruption
  Enamel hypoplasia
  Early numerous caries
Altered mental status, lethargy, seizures, tetany

| DIAGNOSTIC FINDINGS | MANAGEMENT/EDUCATION | EVALUATION |

Laboratory Tests

See Table 3.1, p. 51.

Radiologic Studies

Radiography (knees, wrists, chest)—early rachitic changes on wrists and knees—cupping, fraying, and widening of the epiphyses (diffuse osteopenia); evidence of malalignment of long bones, "rachitic rosary" of costochondral junctions, "champagne cork" aspect on chest X-ray

Medications

Ergocalciferol

Occasional calcium supplementation

Education

Hypervitaminosis—hypotonia, irritability, anorexia, constipation, polyuria, polydipsia, pallor, dehydration

Fracture prevention

Dietary and lifestyle changes needed to provide recommended daily allowance (RDA) of vitamin D

Vitamin D supplementation for solely or partially breast-fed infants should begin soon after birth.[6,7,7a]

Casual daily exposure to direct sunlight without sunscreen[8]

Nursing Considerations

Record subjective history at each visit. Assessment and evaluation of drug therapy should also be elicited from the patient and family at each visit.

Follow-up assessment every 4 months

Monitor calcifediol, PTH, Ca, alkaline phosphatase at these intervals.

Therapy to continue until all physical, radiologic, and biochemical evidence of rickets has been reversed

Transition to Adulthood

Usually not a factor with appropriate vitamin D supplementation[2,3]

BONE MINERALIZATION AND METABOLIC DISORDERS

| DIAGNOSIS | CLINICAL FINDINGS | DIAGNOSTIC FINDINGS |

Vitamin D–Resistant (Hypophosphatemic) Rickets

This condition is often due to an inherited X-linked deficiency in the kidneys. It occurs more often in males than females. Large amounts of phosphorus are lost in the urine. In the absence of pertinent family history, the child usually presents between 2 and 3 years of age.[9]

Pertinent History

+ Familial history
Growth retardation
± Bone pain

Physical Findings

Waddling gait
Absence of muscular
  weakness
Bony abnormalities
  Tibial and femoral
    bowing
  Frontal bossing
  Occipital or parietal
    flattening
  Vertebral abnormalities
  Calcification of ten-
    dons and ligaments
    (later years)
  Fractures
Dental abnormalities
  Delayed tooth eruption
  Dental abscesses
  Mottled teeth
    secondary to dentin
    defects
  Early numerous caries

Laboratory Tests

See Table 3.1, p. 51.

Radiologic Studies

Radiography (knees, wrists, chest)

No "rachitic rosary"

Medications

Phosphate replacement

Calcitriol replacement

Education

Signs/symptoms of hypervitaminosis: hypotonia, irritability, anorexia, constipation, polyuria, polydipsia, pallor, dehydration

Fracture prevention

Nursing Considerations

Signs/symptoms vary. Record subjective history at each visit. Assessment and evaluation of drug therapy should be elicited from the patient and family at each visit.

Emerging Therapies

Recombinant growth hormone enhances renal phosphate reabsorption and can increase plasma phosphate concentration but remains controversial and experimental.[10,11]

Follow-up assessment every 4 months

Monitor PTH, Ca, phosphate, and alkaline phosphatase at these intervals.

Transition to Adulthood

Routine dental visits are important. Dental abscesses are common. Whether treatment with phosphate and calcitriol therapy should be continued after epiphyseal closure has not been definitively determined. Calcification of soft tissue, such as in the kidneys, may occur in adulthood. Routine ultrasounds have been advised. Calcification of tendons and ligaments may occur.[12-15]

3

BONE MINERALIZATION AND METABOLIC DISORDERS

DIAGNOSIS	CLINICAL FINDINGS	DIAGNOSTIC FINDINGS

Vitamin D–Dependent Rickets

Rare inborn error of vitamin D metabolism characterized by all classic signs of vitamin D deficiency despite adequate vitamin D intake. Does not respond therapeutically to vitamin D replacement.

Pertinent History

Normal appearance at birth

Occurrence of metabolic bone disease before 2 years of age—often before 6 months of age

History of other family members with similar condition

Osteomalacia

Mediterranean descent

Physical Findings

Same as vitamin D deficiency with additional findings possible:

Alopecia

Multiple milia

Abnormal dentition

Epidermal cysts

Laboratory Tests

See Table 3.1, p. 51.

Radiologic Studies

Same as vitamin D deficiency

MANAGEMENT/EDUCATION	EVALUATION

Medications

Calcitriol

Ergocalciferol

Calcium supplementation

Education

Signs of hypervitaminosis: hypotonia, irritability, anorexia, constipation, polyuria, polydipsia, pallor, dehydration

Fracture prevention

Dietary and lifestyle changes needed to provide recommended daily allowance (RDA) of vitamin D

Nursing Considerations

Record subjective history at each visit. Assessment and evaluation of drug therapy should also be elicited from the patient and family at each visit.

Follow-up assessment every 4 months

Monitor calcifediol, PTH, Ca, and alkaline phosphatase at these intervals.

Transition to Adulthood

May be lifelong condition, so follow-up with adult endocrinologist may be required.

Routine dental visits are indicated if dentition abnormalities present.[16]

Table 3.1   Diagnostic Laboratory Differentiation of Rickets

Type	Cause	25(OH) Vitamin D (Calcifediol)	1,25(OH)$_2$ Vitamin D (Calcitrol)	PTH	Calcium	Phosphorus
Vitamin D deficiency	↓ Endogenous vitamin D	↓	N or ↑	↑	↓	↓
Vitamin D–resistant	Defective tubular reabsorption of phosphorus	N	↑	N or ↑	N	↓
Vitamin D–dependent	↓ Activity of 24(OH), 1-alpha hydroxylase	N	↓	N or ↑	N or ↓	↓

PARATHYROID HORMONE/CALCIUM DISORDERS

Parathyroid hormone (PTH) mediates the parathyroid glands to regulate the homeostasis of calcium and phosphate concentrations in extracellular fluid through regulation of their absorption from the intestine, mobilization from the skeleton, and reabsorption from the kidneys.[17]

DIAGNOSIS	CLINICAL FINDINGS	DIAGNOSTIC FINDINGS

Hypoparathyroidism
 	
Hypoparathyroidism consists of a variety of disorders that have a deficiency of parathyroid hormone (PTH) effect. Delay in recognition of this defect may result in permanent brain dysfunction or death.
	Pertinent History
	
	Irritability
	↓ Mental function
	Dry, scaly skin
	Dry, coarse hair
	Brittle nails
	Maternal history
	Seizures
	Abdominal pain
	Tingling and numbness of hands
	Muscle cramps
	Pain
	
	Physical Findings
	
	Dull affect
	Moon-shaped face
	Shortened neck
	+ Chvostek's sign
	Shortened 4th and 5th metacarpal
	?Areas of subcutaneous bone formation
	Dental abnormalities
	  Delayed eruption of teeth
	  Blunted roots
	Cataracts
	Papiledema
	↑ Intracranial pressure
	Tetany
		Laboratory Tests
		
		↓ Ca^{2+}
		↑ Phosphate
		N or ↓ Alkaline phosphatase
		↑ HCO_3
		↓ PTH
		↓ Mg^{2+}
		
		Radiologic Studies
		
		Radiography (knees, wrists, chest)—metastatic calcification

3

Medications

Calcium supplementation

Magnesium supplementation

Calcitriol replacement

Ergocalciferol replacement

Dihydrotachysterol replacement

Education

Signs of hypocalcemia: irritability, convulsions, apnea. Contact medical personnel if occurs.

Signs of hypercalcemia: headache, ↑nocturnal urine flow, thirst, anorexia, nausea, vomiting, constipation, lethargy, weakness, and changes in mental status. Contact medical personnel if occurs.

Teach families how to perform Chvostek's test.

Sick-day precautions: adequate fluid intake, adequate food intake

Large intake of fluid is important to avoid low urine flow.

Normal food intake with avoidance of fasting is important.

Nursing Considerations

Signs/symptoms vary. Record subjective history at each visit. Assessment and evaluation of drug therapy should be elicited from the patient and family at each visit.

Follow-up assessment every 3-4 months

Monitor PTH, Ca, phosphate, magnesium, alkaline phosphatase, urinary phosphate, and general chemistries at these intervals (samples should be fasting—except for infants).

Transition to Adulthood

This is a lifelong condition, so referral to an adult endocrinologist is required. There is potential for long-term kidney damage, especially if hypercalcemia occurs. Continuation of medications and endocrine follow-up should be emphasized. If kidney damage occurs, referral to a nephrologist may be indicated.

BONE MINERALIZATION AND METABOLIC DISORDERS

DIAGNOSIS	CLINICAL FINDINGS	DIAGNOSTIC FINDINGS

Hyperparathyroidism

Increased activity of parathyroid gland

Extremely rare in children

May be detected following routine chemistry studies in asymptomatic patients.

Pertinent History

Severe malaise:
  Constipation
  Dehydration
  Vomiting
Radiation exposure
Pernicious anemia
Prematurity/small for
  gestational age
Headache
↑Nocturnal urine flow
Thirst
Anorexia
Nausea
Gastric ulcer
Lethargy
Muscle weakness
Changes in mental
  status

Physical Findings

Dehydration
Muscle weakness
↓Reflexes

Laboratory Tests

$\uparrow Ca^{2+}$
$\downarrow$ Phosphate
N or $\downarrow$ alkaline phosphatase
$\downarrow HCO_3$
$\uparrow PTH$
$\uparrow Mg^{2+}$
$\uparrow$ Urine Ca^{2+}

Radiologic Studies

Radiologic examination of parathyroid gland (MRI, CT, ultrasound, radionuclide)—abnormal parathyroid tissue

EKG

Heart block
Shortening of the ST
  segment

Medications

Acute therapy: IV normal saline and furosemide

Chronic therapy: oral furosemide

↑ Na diet

Surgery

Parathyroidectomy

Education

Signs/symptoms of hypercalcemia: headache, ↑ nocturnal urine flow, thirst, anorexia, nausea, vomiting, constipation, lethargy, weakness, changes in mental status. Contact medical personnel if occurs.

Prospect of progressive skeletal mineral loss and kidney damage

Nursing Considerations

Signs/symptoms vary. Record subjective history at each visit. Assessment and evaluation of drug therapy should be elicited from the patient and family at each visit.

Follow-up assessment every 3-4 months

Monitor PTH, Ca, phosphate, magnesium, alkaline phosphatase, urinary Ca, and general chemistries at these intervals (samples should be fasting—except for infants).[18]

Transition to Adulthood

This is a lifelong condition, so referral to an adult endocrinologist is required. There is potential for long-term kidney damage, especially if hypercalcemia occurs. Continuation of medications and endocrine follow-up should be emphasized. If kidney damage occurs, referral to a nephrologist may be indicated.

BONE MINERALIZATION AND METABOLIC DISORDERS

③

DIAGNOSIS	CLINICAL FINDINGS	DIAGNOSTIC FINDINGS

Neonatal Hypocalcemia

May result from:

- Structural anomalies of parathyroids
- Gene mutation
- Maternal hypercalcemia
- ↓ Modified or unmodified cow's milk diet
- Inability to excrete phosphate into the urine

Shortly after birth there is a physiologic fall in serum calcium concentration during the first 3 days of life. Many normal infants will have serum calcium levels that are less than 8 mg/dL.

Pertinent History

Irritability
Convulsions/seizures
Apnea
Asphyxia
Prematurity
Maternal hyperparathyroidism
DiGeorge syndrome[19,20]

Physical Findings

Myocardial dysfunction
↑ Reflexes
Chvostek's test
Tetany
Abdominal pain
Tingling and numbness of hands
Muscle cramps
Pain

Laboratory Tests

↓ Ca^{2+}
↑ Phosphate
N or ↑ Alkaline phosphatase
↓ HCO_3
↑ PTH
N or ↓ Mg^{2+}
↓ Urine Ca^{2+}

Medications

Acute phase

No treatment may be needed.

Severe phase

This is a medical emergency; consultation with a physician for treatment is required.

Chronic phase

Calcitriol, calcium supplementation if indicated

Education

Signs/symptoms of hypocalcemia: irritability, seizures, apnea. Contact medical personnel if occurs.

Large intake of fluid is important to avoid low urine flow.

Normal food intake with avoidance of fasting is important.

Nursing Considerations

Signs/symptoms vary. Record subjective history at each visit. Assessment and evaluation of drug therapy should be elicited from the patient and family at each visit.

Acute phase

Frequent serum calcium monitoring

Chronic phase

Follow-up assessment every 3-4 months

Monitor PTH, Ca, phosphate, magnesium, alkaline phosphatase, urinary Ca^{2+}, and general chemistries at these intervals (samples should be fasting—except for infants).[21]

Transition to Adulthood

Lifelong hypocalcemia may occur. If it does, referral to an adult endocrinologist is required. There is potential for long-term kidney damage, especially if hypercalcemia occurs. Continuation of medications and endocrine follow-up should be emphasized. If kidney damage occurs, referral to a nephrologist may be indicated.

BONE MINERALIZATION AND METABOLIC DISORDERS

OSTEOPOROSIS

Osteoporosis in children is a heterogeneous group of metabolic bone disorders characterized by a loss of bone mass, which is manifested by brittle skeletal changes and rarefaction of bone while maintaining normal mineral metabolism. It occurs when resorption proceeds more rapidly than bone formation. There are two periods of very rapid bone gain—from birth to 2 years of age and adolescence. During puberty, increased bone mineral content occurs. The difference in bone mass at different ages is related to resorption rates. A reduction of bone mass below the norm for age, sex, and race characterizes osteoporosis in children.[22,23]

DIAGNOSIS	CLINICAL FINDINGS	DIAGNOSTIC FINDINGS
Idiopathic Juvenile Osteoporosis Rare disorder of prepubertal children Manifests usually between 8 and 14 years of age Boys : girls ratio is 3 : 1 Non-hereditary Signs/symptoms duration: 1-4 years Reversible This condition often resolves spontaneously as the adolescent growth spurt wanes.	**Pertinent History** Bone pain—localized in lower extremities ↑ With walking Constant, dull ache (bone pain) in spine with generalized back ache Family/dietary history negative Fractures usually from minimal trauma **Physical Findings** Normal Prepubertal—Tanner 1 Possible thoracolumbar kyphosis Pigeon-chest deformity Crown/pubis to pubis/heel ratio <1.0 Loss of height Long bone deformity Limp	**Laboratory Tests** N or ↑ Ca^{2+} N Phosphate N or ↑ Alkaline phosphatase **Radiologic Studies** DXA bone density: generalized osteopenia Radiography (arms, wrists, legs, spine): Fractures of weight-bearing bones Asymmetrical widening of disc spaces

MANAGEMENT/EDUCATION	EVALUATION

No specific medical or surgical therapy. Usually spontaneous recovery occurs with onset of puberty.

Follow-up assessment every 3-4 months

Supportive Care

Non-weight-bearing, crutch walking, physical therapy

Transition to Adulthood

Self-limited disease of childhood

Medications

Calcitriol in selected patients—check with physician

Education

Self-limiting condition

Dietary changes to comply with recommended daily allowance (RDA) of vitamin D and calcium supplementation

Nursing Considerations

Reassure parents and child that condition is self-limiting with usual spontaneous recovery at onset of puberty.

Encourage follow-up and supportive care.

DIAGNOSIS	CLINICAL FINDINGS	DIAGNOSTIC FINDINGS

Osteoporosis of Immobilization

Result of long-standing immobilization

Reabsorption of bone and ↓ bone formation secondary to lack of weight bearing

Hypercalcemia common

Occasionally may have ↓ renal function

Pertinent History

Bone pain
Fractures
Length of immobilization

Immobilization Hypercalcemia

Headaches
Anorexia
Nausea and vomiting
Malaise
Abdominal pain
Constipation
Weight loss
Polydipsia
Polyuria
Seizures
Hearing loss
Hypertension

Physical Findings

Growth retardation
Bone deformity

Laboratory Tests

↑ Ca^{2+}
N Phosphate
N or ↑ Alkaline phosphatase
↓ HCO_3
N PTH
N or ↓ Mg^{2+}
↑ Urine Ca^{2+}
↓ Creatinine clearance

Radiologic Studies

DXA bone density: generalized osteopenia

Fractures of weight-bearing bones

Asymmetrical widening of disc spaces

MANAGEMENT/EDUCATION	EVALUATION

Most effective therapy is remobilization. Recovery is rapid once remobilization is established.

Medications

Prednisone 25-40 mg/m^2/24 hr for 1-2 weeks

Salmon calcitonin 2-4 IU/kg SQ

400 IU vitamin D daily

Education

Teach patient and family the importance of remobilization.

Nursing Considerations

Monitor serum Ca^{2+}, phosphate, alkaline phosphatase, and urine Ca^{2+} during immobilization.

Monitor calcium/creatinine (Ca/Cr) ratio (mg/mg).

Emerging Therapies

Pamidronate intravenous 0.5-1 mg/kg/day for 3 consecutive days every 4-6 months

Alendronate orally; dosage and frequency vary in clinical trials.[25]

Daily labs for serum Ca^{2+}, phosphate, alkaline phosphatase, and urine Ca^{2+} during immobilization

Transition to Adulthood

If immobilization is long-term, follow-up with an internist is important for hormone replacement therapy and bisphosphonate therapy.[24]

BONE MINERALIZATION AND METABOLIC DISORDERS

DIAGNOSIS	CLINICAL FINDINGS	DIAGNOSTIC FINDINGS

Glucocorticoid-Induced Osteoporosis

Long-term therapy with glucocorticoids results in rapid bone loss with subsequent fractures.

Pertinent History

Use of either high- or low-dose glucocorticoids >2 months

Physical Findings

Usual late signs:
  Thoracolumbar kyphosis
  Pigeon-chest deformity
  Crown/pubis to pubis/heel ratio <1.0
  Loss of height
  Long-bone deformity
  Limp

Laboratory Tests

↑PTH
↑Fasting urinary Ca^{2+}
↑Calcifediol (25-OH vitamin D)
↑or ↓Calcitriol (1,25 OH_2, vitamin D)

Prevention of steroid-induced bone loss important.

Medications

None currently FDA-approved for children

Treatment

Cessation of glucocorticoids if possible

Weight-bearing and isometric exercises

Maintenance of good nutritional status

Education

Weight-bearing and isometric exercises

Maintenance of good nutritional status

Nursing Considerations

Recognition of possibility of glucocorticoid-induced osteoporosis

Encourage patient and family to follow diet and exercise recommendations.

Emerging Therapies

Bisphosphonates in clinical trials[26]

Assess bone mineral density every 6 months for first year.[27]

Transition to Adulthood

Follow-up with an internist is important for hormone replacement therapy and bisphosphonate therapy.

BONE MINERALIZATION AND METABOLIC DISORDERS ❸

DISORDERS OF GLUCOSE METABOLISM

OVERVIEW

Glucose is the essential energy source of the central nervous system. Yet the central nervous system is unable to either synthesize glucose or store glycogen effectively. Even short episodes of hypoglycemia have the potential to produce focal neurologic deficits and brain dysfunction. More prolonged episodes can cause structural damage and brain death. Neonates and infants are at particularly high risk because of their relatively large ratio of brain:body mass. Several endocrine glands work in synchrony to maintain the plasma glucose concentration within a relatively narrow normal range. These include the pancreas, adrenal, and pituitary glands. Thus the body is well equipped with a number of hormonal mechanisms that maintain homeostasis and prevent hypoglycemia. However, with only one hormone available to lower blood glucose (insulin), there are fewer mechanisms for preventing hyperglycemia.

Table 4.1   Key Regulatory Hormones and Their Effect on Plasma Glucose (PG) and Tissue Metabolism

Hormone	Endocrine Gland	Site of Production	Effect	Activity
Cortisol	Adrenal	Cortex	↑PG	Stimulates lipolysis Mobilizes amino acids from muscle Inhibits glucose uptake by muscle
Epinephrine	Adrenal	Medulla	↑PG	Stimulates glycogenolysis and gluconeogenesis Stimulates lipolysis Inhibits glucose uptake by muscle Inhibits insulin release Promotes glucagon and growth hormone secretion
Glucagon	Pancreas	α-cells	↑PG	Stimulates glycogenolysis and gluconeogenesis Stimulates lipolysis
Growth hormone	Pituitary	Somatotrophs	↑PG	Inhibits glucose uptake by muscle Stimulates lipolysis
Insulin	Pancreas	β-cells	↓PG	Stimulates glycolysis and glycogenesis Stimulates protein synthesis Inhibits glycogenolysis Stimulates lipogenesis

HYPOGLYCEMIA

Neonatal hypoglycemia The definition of neonatal hypoglycemia is controversial. Plasma glucose concentrations ranging from 40 to 50 mg/dL have been suggested. Plasma glucose levels less than 60 mg/dL are unusual in healthy newborns after 24 hours of extrauterine life.[1]

Hypoglycemia in infancy/childhood Plasma blood glucose of 50 mg/dL

HISTORY

HPI/ROS Parents or caregivers of a neonate or infant may report abnormal or high-pitched cry, hypothermia, diaphoresis, poor feeding, tremors, irritability/jitteriness, an exaggerated Moro reflex, lethargy, hypotonia, seizure, abnormal eye movements, cyanosis, pallor, tachypnea, apnea, or irregular respiratory patterns. However, it is not uncommon for hypoglycemic infants to have extremely low blood glucose levels without exhibiting any of the clinical signs or symptoms listed above. Clinical manifestations that parents of older children may report include sweating, anxiety, tachypnea, weakness, headache, irritability, confusion, fatigue, abnormal behavior, amnesia, and seizures, although children may also present with asymptomatic hypoglycemia.

Medical/family/social history In neonates and infants, assess for the presence of maternal risk factors: diabetes mellitus, β-agonist tocolytic therapy, pregnancy-induced hypertension or essential hypertension, substance abuse, antepartum IV administration of glucose, a previous history of having given birth to an infant with macrosomia, hypoglycemia, and/or an unexplained neonatal death. Assess for neonatal risk factors such as small for gestational age (SGA), large for gestational age (LGA), smaller of discordant twins, perinatal distress, anoxia, hypothermia, Apgar score less than 5 at 5 or 10 minutes of life; or appropriate for gestational age or LGA infant with microphallus, an anterior midline defect (cleft lip/palate, hyper/hypotelorism, hypospadias) or omphalocele, macroglossia, or gigantism. In older infants or children, inquire about current medications and potential for ingestion of alcohol or medications known to lower blood glucose levels (sulfonylureas, salicylates).

PHYSICAL EXAMINATION

Conduct a complete physical with attention to growth parameters. In the newborn, this includes gestational age assessment and determination of appropriateness of size for gestational age. In the infant and child this includes height, weight, and head circumference (if <3 years of age).

Diagnostic testing Obtain a plasma blood glucose level at the time of symptoms or after a fast with simultaneous measurement of insulin, cortisol, and growth hormone. Also test urine for ketones.

> **NOTE** Glucose reagent strips or reflectance meters are often used as a screening tool. However, variability in procedures and limitations in meter accuracy at lower glucose levels can greatly affect the accuracy of results. When a screening value is being validated against a serum specimen, it is essential to remember that whole blood glucose concentrations are 15% lower than plasma concentrations and that venous blood concentrations are 10% to 15% lower than arterial concentrations.

Additional tests may include serum β-hydroxybutyrate, acetoacetate, and free fatty acid levels. Serum electrolytes, lactate and pyruvate, serum and urine amino acids, and organic acids may also be indicated. If an insulinoma is suspected, an abdominal ultrasound may be of value to identify its location. A CT scan or MRI of the brain may be performed to detect congenital anomalies.

> **NOTE** Neonates with prematurity, intrauterine growth retardation, or SGA, or who are the smaller of discordant twins can be readily identified by gestational size and age assessment. Management involves glucose supplementation until the neonate is able to maintain adequate hepatic glycogen reserves in the face of increased glucose utilization.

Initial management Initial efforts are directed toward collecting critical laboratory samples and prompt intervention to increase and then maintain a normal plasma glucose level.

A mini-bolus of 0.2 g/kg of dextrose should be administered by an intravenous infusion over 1 minute (2 mL/kg of 10% dextrose), followed by a continuous intravenous infusion of 8 mg/kg/minute using dextrose 10% solution. Glucose levels should be obtained 15 minutes after the bolus and while the maintenance glucose solution is infusing. If hypoglycemia recurs, a bolus of 0.5 g/kg (5 mL/kg of dextrose 10%) may be given and the maintenance infusion increased by 25%-50%.[2]

DISORDERS OF GLUCOSE METABOLISM

DIAGNOSIS	CLINICAL FINDINGS	DIAGNOSTIC FINDINGS	MGT./EDUCATION
	Presentation will vary with age of child and severity of the condition.	At time of hypoglycemia	
Adrenal Insufficiency/ ACTH Deficiency	**Pertinent History** Severe hypoglycemic symptoms **Physical Findings** See p. 38.	↓ Serum cortisol N Serum growth hormone N Serum insulin	See pp. 180-182 for more information.
Amino Acid/ Organic Acid Disorders (Including maple syrup urine disease, propionic acidemia, methylmalonic aciduria, tyrosinosis, 3-hydroxy-3 methylglutaric aciduria, glutaric aciduria, type II)	**Pertinent History** Hypoglycemia occurring after protein ingestion, Reye's syndrome–like symptoms, recurrent myoglobinuria, metabolic acidosis **Physical Findings** Myopathy, cardiomyopathy may be present.	−Urine ketones +Urine organic acids −Urine non–glucose-reducing substances ↑Glycine (serum amino acids) ↑Plasma free fatty acids	Implement protein-restricted diet. Avoid prolonged fasting. Dietary consultation.
B-cell Hyperplasia/ Adenoma	**Pertinent History** Hypoglycemia **Physical Findings** Macrosomia	↑↑ Serum insulin ↑ Serum C-peptide +Intraoperative abdominal ultrasound (may be needed to identify adenomas)	Provide glucose supplementation and physiological support until child can be sent for resection of adenoma or pancreatectomy as appropriate.

DIAGNOSIS	CLINICAL FINDINGS	DIAGNOSTIC FINDINGS	MGT./EDUCATION
Beckwith-Wiedemann Syndrome	**Pertinent History** Hypoglycemia, beta cell hyperplasia **Physical Findings** Macrosomia, ear lobe fissures, macroglossia, visceromegaly, omphalocele	↑ Serum insulin	Provide glucose supplementation and consider initiating diazoxide therapy.
Familial or Acquired Lipodystrophy	**Pertinent History** Autosomal dominant or recessive inheritance History of treatment for HIV; treatment with protease inhibitors or reverse-transcriptase inhibitors Females: Oligomenorrhea, amenorrhea, infertility **Physical Findings** Absence of normal subcutaneous fat May be generalized or limited to specific areas of body Accumulation of fat in the head and neck region beginning at puberty Prominent appearance of veins and muscles Acanthosis nigricans	Larnin A/C gene mutations ↓ HDL ↑ BP ↑ VLDL	Females more likely to develop diabetes Diet Exercise Progressive resistance training Metformin Lipid management

4

DISORDERS OF GLUCOSE METABOLISM

DIAGNOSIS	CLINICAL FINDINGS	DIAGNOSTIC FINDINGS	MGT./EDUCATION
Fructose Intolerance	**Pertinent History** Vomiting, profound hypoglycemia, and convulsions after fructose ingestion **Physical Findings** Poor growth, jaundice, hepatosplenomegaly, and hemorrhage	−Urine ketones +Urine non–glucose-reducing substances +Abnormal liver function	Implement fructose-restricted diet, including elimination of fructose-containing cough syrups and drugs.
Galactosemia	**Pertinent History** Vomiting, diarrhea, profound hypoglycemia after lactose ingestion, susceptibility to infection, bleeding tendency. Identified on newborn screening in some states **Physical Findings** Failure to thrive, jaundice, cataracts, and hepatomegaly	−Urine ketones +Urine non–glucose-reducing substances +Urine organic acids +Proteinuria	Implement galactose-free diet. Refer for cognitive screening.

DIAGNOSIS	CLINICAL FINDINGS	DIAGNOSTIC FINDINGS	MGT./EDUCATION
Glycogen Storage Diseases (Many subtypes, including glucose 6-phosphatase deficiency, types Ia, Ib, amylo-1, 6-glucosidase deficiency, type III, defects of liver phosphorylation enzyme system)	**Pertinent History** Episodes of lactic acidosis, particularly during periods of concurrent illness/fasting **Physical Findings** Growth retardation, protuberant abdomen with hepatomegaly, and tendency to bruise easily	N Serum growth hormone N Serum cortisol +Urine ketones ↑Serum lactate +Hyperlipidemia	Implement restricted diet: content will vary according to specific enzymatic defect. Consider nocturnal supplementation with glucose-containing gastric feedings.
Infant of a Diabetic Mother	**Pertinent History** Maternal diabetes **Physical Findings** Macrosomia and possible congenital malformations	↑Serum insulin N Serum growth hormone N Serum cortisol	Begin glucose supplementation and consider short-term steroid therapy until insulin secretion returns to normal.

DIAGNOSIS	CLINICAL FINDINGS	DIAGNOSTIC FINDINGS	MGT./EDUCATION
Ketotic Hypoglycemia	**Pertinent History** Patient is usually between 18 months and 5 years. This is the most common diagnosis after other causes of hypoglycemia have been ruled out. History of intercurrent illness, decreased oral intake, or prolonged fast **Physical Findings** Usually unremarkable	+Plasma acetoacetate/ β-hydroxy-butyrate +Urine ketones N Serum cortisol N Serum growth hormone N Serum insulin	Instruct the family in urine ketone testing. Initiate smaller, more frequent feedings/meals, including carbohydrate and protein. Provide anticipatory guidance for times of intercurrent illness or missed meals.
Nesidioblastosis	**Pertinent History** May have a positive family history of nesidioblastosis (if a familial form) Hypoglycemia **Physical Findings** Generally unremarkable	↑ Serum insulin +Response to glucagon challenge	Start diazoxide and, if needed, add glucagon for sudden drops in blood glucose. If hypoglycemia persists, consider adding octreotide. If octreotide is unsuccessful, consider subtotal (95%) pancreatectomy. Refer for genetic counseling if familial.

DIAGNOSIS	CLINICAL FINDINGS	DIAGNOSTIC FINDINGS	MGT./EDUCATION
Panhypo-pituitarism	**Pertinent History** Severe hypoglyce-mic symptoms **Physical Findings** Midline facial abnormalities (cleft lip/palate, poorly developed nasal septum, hypotelorism/ hypertelorism) In males: Micro-phallus, poorly de-veloped scrotum, and small testes	↓ Serum growth hormone ↓ Serum cortisol N Serum insulin +Urine ketones	See pp. 158-161 for more information.

DISORDERS OF GLUCOSE METABOLISM ❹

NURSING IMPLICATIONS

Education Instruction should be provided to a minimum of two caregivers and supplemented with clearly worded written information. Survival skill topics to be covered include recognition and treatment of acute hypoglycemic episodes, home monitoring/recording of blood glucose, and when/how to call for emergency assistance. Daily management skills to be covered include medication administration, diet planning, and medical follow-up. Since many metabolic defects can lead to mental retardation (galactosemia, for example) if not properly treated, it is essential to encourage the family to seek early intervention programs in the community to provide ongoing assessment of the child's cognitive performance.

Medications Medications can be costly and lifesaving. The medication required will depend upon the cause of hypoglycemia. Ensure that parents have the phone numbers needed to contact suppliers when they have only a week's supply left. Encourage parents to obtain a medical ID tag that lists the child's medical condition and medication used and have the child wear it at all times.

Dietary modifications Inpatient instruction may require community reinforcement. Ensure that chart notes and a copy of the educational materials given to the family are sent to the referring provider and home care nurses shortly after diagnosis and/or discharge. Special formulas needed for metabolic disorders can be costly. As such, direct parents to available state and federal resources for financial assistance.

HYPERGLYCEMIA

HISTORY

HPI/ROS Determine presence of symptoms (polyuria, polydipsia, polyphagia, weight loss, blurred vision, vomiting, and abdominal pain); nutritional state (include eating patterns, weight changes, growth, and development); pattern of daily exercise; results of any recent laboratory testing related to the diagnosis of diabetes, including blood glucose, HgbA1c, and urine testing.

Past medical history Immunization status (pneumococcal, influenza, tetanus, diphtheria); current medications; details of diabetes regimen (if previously diagnosed), including the level of self-management the patient has performed in the past; any previous diabetes education, including when and where instructed, and the presence of any known complications.

Family history Assess for presence of atherosclerosis, heart disease, diabetes, and other endocrine or autoimmune disease.

Social history Lifestyle, cultural, psychosocial, educational and economic factors that could affect the patient's management

PHYSICAL EXAMINATION

Perform a complete examination with attention to:

- *Constitutional* Heart rate, blood pressure, respiratory rate, and, if infectious process suspected, temperature
- *Growth* Height, weight, height velocity, % dehydration, estimated weight loss, if any
- *Mouth* Assess for candidiasis, dental caries or infection, and tonsillar enlargement.
- *Eyes* Funduscopic examination to evaluate for retinopathy
- *Skin* Assess hydration, presence of infections, particularly at testing or injection sites in previously diagnosed patients as well as lipoatrophy and/or lipohypertrophy of injection sites.
- *Neck* Thyroid palpation to identify enlargement that may indicate autoimmune dysfunction
- *Chest* Examine for masses; Tanner staging in females and gynecomastia in males
- *Cardiovascular* Cardiac examination, pulses
- *Respiratory* Chest and lung examination (including Tanner staging for females)
- *Gastrointestinal* Abdominal examination to identify masses or tenderness
- *Genitourinary* Sexual maturation by Tanner stage
- *Feet* Check for ingrown toenails, fungal infections, and other abnormalities.
- *Neurologic* Sensation, reflexes

INITIAL DIAGNOSIS

Diabetes is diagnosed by meeting any one of the criteria listed in Box 4.1.

Box 4.1   Criteria for the Diagnosis of Diabetes

1. A1c $\geq$6.5%. The test should be performed in a laboratory using a method that is NGSP certified and standardized to the DCCT assay.*

   OR

2. FPG $\geq$126 mg/dL (7.0 mmol/L). No caloric intake for at least 8 h.*

   OR

3. 2-hr plasma glucose $\geq$200 mg/dL (11.1 mmol/L) during an OGTT. The test should be performed as described by the World Health Organization, using a glucose load containing the equivalent of 75 g anhydrous glucose dissolved in water.*

   OR

4. In a patient with classic symptoms of hyperglycemia or hyperglycemic crisis, a random plasma glucose $\geq$200 mg/dL (11.1 mmol/L).

---

*In the absence of unequivocal hyperglycemia, criteria 1-3 should be confirmed by repeat testing.[3]
DCCT, Diabetes Control and Complications Trial; *FPG,* fasting plasma glucose; *NGSP,* National Glycohemoglobin Standardization Program; *OGTT,* oral glucose tolerance test.

DIAGNOSIS	CLINICAL FINDINGS	DIAGNOSTIC FINDINGS	MGT./EDUCATION
Type 1 Diabetes Mellitus Destruction of beta cells that usually leads to an absolute deficiency of insulin	**Pertinent History** Excessive thirst and/or hunger, polyuria, unexplained weight loss, abdominal cramps, blurred vision, severe fatigue More common in Caucasian youth **Physical Findings** Often thin with signs of dehydration	↑ Blood glucose (meeting the diagnostic criteria for diabetes mellitus) ↓ Serum insulin + Serum and urine ketones at diagnosis Presence of one or more of the following autoantibodies: • ICA • IAA • GAD_{65} • IA-2 • IA-2β With the exception of insulin autoantibodies, each of these autoantibodies is detected in approximately 70% to 80% of patients at initial diagnosis of type 1 diabetes.[4]	Initiate insulin therapy. Fluid replacement as needed Begin survival skill education: • Self-monitoring blood glucose (SMBG) • Insulin administration • Dietary modifications • Hypoglycemia recognition and treatment • School management (see p. 87) • Sick-day management (see p. 91)

DIAGNOSIS	CLINICAL FINDINGS	DIAGNOSTIC FINDINGS	MGT./EDUCATION
Type 2 Diabetes Mellitus A disorder with a combination of insulin resistance and a defect in insulin secretion	**Pertinent History** Same symptoms as with type 1 diabetes, but it is important to note that patients with type 2 diabetes are frequently asymptomatic. Children with type 2 diabetes usually have a family history of type 2 diabetes, and those with non-European ancestry (African, Hispanic, Asian, American Indian, or Pacific islander) are disproportionately represented. Maturity onset diabetes of the young (MODY) is characterized by a primary defect in insulin secretion. MODY is an autosomal dominant inheritance with onset less than 25 years of age. Occurs predominantly in Caucasians See Table 4.2 on p. 79 for types of MODY.	↑Blood glucose (meeting diagnostic criteria for diabetes mellitus) ↑ or ↓ Serum insulin ±Serum and urine ketones at diagnosis No autoantibodies present at diagnosis	Initiate therapy with either an oral agent or insulin, depending on the presentation. Fluid replacement as needed Begin survival skill education: *If starting insulin therapy,* see p. 85. *If starting an oral agent:* • SMBG • Oral agent dose/schedule • Dietary modifications • Hypoglycemia recognition and treatment (if the oral agent has the potential to cause hypoglycemia) • School management • Sick-day management • Monitor liver enzymes if oral agent has liver toxicity as potential side effect.

4

DISORDERS OF GLUCOSE METABOLISM

(continued)

DIAGNOSIS	CLINICAL FINDINGS	DIAGNOSTIC FINDINGS	MGT./EDUCATION
(Type 2 Diabetes Mellitus)	Most patients exhibit decreased insulin secretion and lean body mass; however, other MODY presentations include high insulin levels and obesity. **Physical Findings** BMI >85% percentile for age and sex[5] Weight >120% of ideal for height[5] Acanthosis nigricans and candidal infections common Although less common than in patients with type 1 diabetes mellitus, many of these children present to the clinician in diabetes ketoacidosis with signs of dehydration and weight loss.		

Table 4.2 Genetic Abnormalities Resulting in the Various MODY Forms

Type of MODY	Affected Gene	Defining Characteristics
1*	Hepatocyte nuclear factor-4-alpha (HNF4α)	• Progressive hyperglycemia • 50% reduction in serum TG • 25% reduction in serum concentrations of apolipoproteins AII, CIII, and lipoprotein-α

From Gallo l, Silverstein JH, Winter W. Other specific types of diabetes mellitus and causes of hyperglycemia. In Kappy MS, Allen DB, Geffner ME, eds. Pediatric Practice Endocrinology. New York: McGraw-Hill, 2010.
*In MODY1 and MODY3, 30% to 40% of patients eventually require insulin therapy, but can be managed for decades with sulfonylureas alone.

Table 4.2 Genetic Abnormalities Resulting in the Various MODY Forms—cont'd

Type of MODY	Affected Gene	Defining Characteristics
2†	Glucokinase (GCK)‡	• Impaired fasting glucose or impaired glucose tolerance • Less than 50% of women with MODY2 mutations will have gestational diabetes • Nonprogressive • May only require medication therapy during puberty or times of illness/stress
3*	Hepatocyte nuclear factor-1-alpha (HNF1α)	• Asymptomatic glycosuria • Progressive hyperglycemia‡
4	Insulin promoter factor-1 (IPF-1)	• Homozygous mutations result in pancreatic agenesis; heterozygous mutations cause MODY4

5	Hepatocyte nuclear factor-1-beta (HNF1β)	• Renal cysts
		• Hypoplastic glomerulocystic kidney disease
		  – Proteinuria
		  – Nondiabetic renal failure
		• Reproductive tract anomalies
		  – Vaginal aplasia
		  – Rudimentary or bicornate uterus
		  – Elevated transaminases

6	Neurogenic differentia-tion 1 (NEUROD1)	• Rare

*In MODY1 and MODY3, 30% to 40% of patients eventually require insulin therapy, but can be managed for decades with sulfonylureas alone.

†MODY2 and MODY3 are the two most prevalent forms, accounting for more than 80% of MODY patients.

‡With the exception of MODY2, all forms of MODY are secondary to mutations in transcription factors required for β-cell differentiation and insulin gene expression.

NOTE: All but MODY2 patients may develop diabetes-related vascular complications.

DISORDERS OF GLUCOSE METABOLISM

INITIAL MANAGEMENT AND FOLLOW-UP

CONCERNS	CARE/TEST	FREQUENCY
General Recommendations	• Diabetes-focused visit • Review management plan, problems, and goals.	• Every 3 months or more • Each visit
Glycemic Control	• Review medications and frequency of low blood sugar episodes. • Self-monitoring blood glucose, set and review goals • See Table 4.3, p. 84. • Weight/BMI/growth parameters	• Each visit • 3-4 times/day or as recommended • Each visit
Eye Care	• Dilated-eye exam by ophthalmologist or optometrist	• All patients 10 years and older who have had diabetes for 3-5 years should have an initial exam and then annual follow-up evaluations.
Thyroid Function	• Palpation of thyroid • Evaluation of height, weight, and height velocity • Serum thyroid function tests and thyroid-specific autoantibodies • Obtain family history of hypothyroidism.	• Each visit • Obtain at diagnosis in patients with type 1 diabetes and as indicated by thyroid gland enlargement or decreased growth velocity or alterations in insulin requirements.[4-6]

CONCERNS	CARE/TEST	FREQUENCY
Cardiovascular	• Smoking	• Assess at every visit and counsel appropriately.
	• Lipid profile	• *Children:*
		>2 years at diagnosis if family history of hypercholesterolemia or CV event or if family history unknown.
		All children who are pubertal at diagnosis
		If family history is not of concern, then first lipid screening should be performed at puberty (≥10 years).[7]
	• Blood pressure: Below 90% of ideal for age (see tables, pp. 12-21)	• Each visit
	• Exercise/diet/weight goals	• Each visit
Gastrointestinal	• Serum IgA-antiendo-mysium (EMA) and IgA-antigliadin antibodies (AGA)—often done but no national guidelines	• Obtain at diagnosis in patients with type 1 diabetes. • Consider annual rescreening using the combination of AGA and EMA testing for children <2-3 years of age and the EMA test alone for those >3 years of age.[7]

CONCERNS	CARE/TEST	FREQUENCY
Kidney Function	• Urinalysis (glucose, ketones, protein, and microscopic examination) • Urine for microalbumin >30 μg/mg creatinine or 30 mg/24 hr initiate ACE inhibitor • Serum creatinine	• At diagnosis and yearly • At puberty and after 5 years, then yearly • In children, if urine microalbumin >200 mg/24 hr
Foot Care	• Inspect feet with shoes and socks off • Comprehensive lower-extremity sensory exam	• Each visit: stress importance of daily self-exam • Yearly
Pregnancy	• Assess contraception and discuss family planning. • Preconception consult • Management of pregnancy	• At diagnosis and yearly during childbearing years • 3-4 months prior to conception • Oral diabetic agents and ACE inhibitors are *not* recommended during pregnancy.
Self-management Training	• By a professional trained both in pediatric development and childhood diabetes	• At diagnosis, then every 3-6 months or as indicated by patient's status

CONCERNS	CARE/TEST	FREQUENCY
Nutrition	• By a registered dietitian • Assess nutritional status. • Set goals. • Determine interventions: There is no one "diabetic or ADA" diet. Meal plans are recommended based on assessment and treatment goals and outcomes (examples include carbohydrate counting and exchange lists). Calories—1,000 for first year of age plus 100 calories/year until 10-12 years; after age 12 girls may need a reduction in calories unless very active, and boys may need more calories, not to exceed 2,500.[8] Total calories/day from: • Protein (10%-20%) • Saturated fats (10%) • Monounsaturated fats and carbohydrates (60%-70%)	• At diagnosis, then: • Age <18 years— every 3-6 months • Age >18 years— every 6-12 months • More often if indicated

④

DISORDERS OF GLUCOSE METABOLISM

CONCERNS	CARE/TEST	FREQUENCY
Immunizations	• Influenza vaccine • Pneumococcal (polyvalent) vaccine • Prevnar vaccine • Other vaccines to be given per CDC and AAP recommendations	• Annually (early fall) for children >6 months • Once for children ≥2 years • 2, 4, 6, and 12-15 months of age

Table 4.3 Plasma Blood Glucose and A1c Goals for Type 1 Diabetes by Age Group

Values by Age (yrs)	Before Meals (mg/dL)	Bedtime/ Overnight (mg/dL)	A1c	Rationale
Toddlers and preschoolers (0-6)	90-180	110-200	<8.5% (but >7.5%)	High risk and vulnerability to hypoglycemia
School age (6-12)	100-180	100-180	<8%	Risks of hypoglycemia and relatively low risk of complications prior to puberty
Adolescents and young adults (13-19)	90-130	90-150	<7.5%	Risk of severe hypoglycemia Developmental and psychological issues A lower goal (<7.0%) is reasonable if it can be achieved without excessive hypoglycemia.

From American Diabetes Association Position Statements. Standards of Medical Care in Diabetes—2011. Diabetes Care 34(Suppl 1):S39, 2011.

Blood Glucose (mg/dL)	HgbA1c
60	4%
90	5%
120	6%
150	7%
180	8%
210	9%
240	10%
270	11%
300	12%

Key concepts in setting glycemic goals:
- Goals should be individualized, and lower goals may be reasonable based on benefit-risk assessment.
- Blood glucose goals should be higher than those listed above in children with frequent hypoglycemia or hypoglycemia unawareness.
- Postprandial blood glucose values should be measured when there is a discrepancy between preprandial blood, glucose values, and A1c levels and to help assess glycemia in those on basal/bolus regimens.[7]

INSULIN START

Usual daily maintenance dose in children: 0.5-1.0 U/kg per 24 hours; in adolescents during growth spurt: 0.8-1.2 U/kg per 24 hours.

There are various regimens to choose from. Common initial dosing regimens include:
- Conventional split mixed: Calculate the patient's total daily dose (TDD) based on weight. Give two thirds of the TTD in the morning and one third of the TTD in the evening (dinner). Each injection should be two-thirds intermediate (NPH) and one-third short-acting (regular) or rapid-acting (lispro/aspart) insulin. Make adjustments based on BG testing results.[9]
- Basal bolus regimen. See Box 4.2 for an example of initial dosing.[10]

NURSING IMPLICATIONS

Prescription checklist for newly diagnosed patients

- Insulin or oral agent
- 30-, 50-, or 100-unit insulin syringes if using insulin (syringes with half-unit markings are available)
- Alcohol wipes for injection site preparation if using insulin

---

Box 4.2   Calculations for Starting an Intermittent Subcutaneous Insulin Regimen for a 32 kg Patient

Total daily SQ insulin dose = 0.5-1.0 units/kg/day
$0.75 \times 32 = 24$ units/day

Basal insulin dose = ½ of total daily SQ dose
$24 \div 2 = 12$ units at bedtime as glargine (Lantus) in this example

Carbohydrate coverage = 450 ÷ total daily SQ insulin dose
$450 \div 24 = 18.75$
Insulin:carbohydrate ratio is 1:18.75, or 1:20 in this example

Correction factor: 1800 rule for lispro (use 1500 for regular insulin)
1800 ÷ total daily SQ insulin dose = $1800 \div 24 = 75$

One unit of insulin lispro will decrease blood glucose 75 mg/dL, or 0.5 units will decrease blood glucose approximately 40 mg/dL. The following sliding scale applies in this example.

Blood Glucose (mg/dL)	Adjust Insulin
<70	Subtract 1 unit
71-120	No adjustment
121-160	Add 0.5 units
161-200	Add 1 unit
201-240	Add 1.5 units
Each additional increase of 40 mg/dL	Add an additional 0.5 units

Calculations are based on empirically determined formulas. Doses are adjusted once responses to starting doses are assessed. (From Ballal SA, McIntosh P. Endocrinology. In Custer JW, Rau RE, eds. The Harriet Lane Handbook. Philadelphia: Mosby Elsevier, 2009.)

- Blood glucose testing meters (1) for home use and (1) for backup (school)
- Blood glucose monitoring test strips
- Lancets and lancet device
- Urine ketone testing strips (foil-wrapped last longer, bottles only 6 months once opened)
- Glucose tabs, gel for hypoglycemia treatment
- Glucagon emergency kit for type 1 diabetes (check expiration date)
- Appropriate receptacle for needles and syringes
- Insulin pen (as indicated)

School guidelines

- Parents need to inform teachers, school nurse, bus drivers, and coaches about their child's diabetes.
- Parents/child/adolescent and school nurse or staff needs a written plan (Individualized Health Care Plan or IHP) for monitoring and hypoglycemia treatment. In addition, each student should have a signed 504 plan. (Section 504 is a federal legislation requiring the school to provide reasonable accommodations related to a child's type 1 diabetes before, during, and after school. Schools are obligated under federal law to provide this plan to all children who have a medical disability. Students have a right to a 504 plan, and parents should be insistent with the schools. Sample Section 504 plans and sample IHPs can be found through the Juvenile Diabetes Research Foundation website at *www.jdrf.org.*)
- Instruct staff in blood glucose monitoring and the appropriate timing and acceptable location for this activity.
- Provide written information on recognition of hypoglycemia, hyperglycemia, and appropriate treatment for each.
- School supplies should include a blood glucose monitor, test strips, urine ketone testing strips, insulin, syringes or insulin pen (if there is an ongoing need for insulin administration during school hours), alcohol wipes, sharps container, glucagon emergency kit (if allowed), and carbohydrate sources for snacks and emergency treatment of hypoglycemia.
- Develop an emergency medical plan (EMP) for severe hypoglycemia and other medical emergencies, including environmental disasters. Student's physician will need to sign orders for glucagon administration. Remind parents that each school staff member who interacts with the child during the school day should have a copy of the emergency plan (to be updated yearly).

Exercise guidelines

- Perform blood glucose monitoring before and after exercise
- Avoid exercise if fasting glucose levels are >250 mg/dL and ketosis is present or if glucose levels are >300 mg/dL, whether or not ketosis is present.
- Keep carbohydrate-based foods available during and after exercise.
- Ingest additional carbohydrates if preexercise glucose levels are <100 mg/dL to avoid hypoglycemia.[7]
- Postexercise hypoglycemia effects may occur after 24 hours.

4

DISORDERS OF GLUCOSE METABOLISM

Hypoglycemia

Severe hypoglycemia is a medical emergency. As such, each child should have a written plan for treatment. Teachers, coaches, and any other adults who interact with the child regularly should also be apprised of the plan. See Table 4.4 for a sample hypoglycemia protocol. Glucagon by intramuscular injection should also be considered for severe hypoglycemic episodes. An individualized educational plan (IEP) or IHP can be developed with school personnel to facilitate glucagon administration in the school setting.

Diabetic ketoacidosis

Diabetic ketoacidosis (DKA) is defined by hyperglycemia, ketonemia, ketonuria, and metabolic acidosis (pH <7.30, bicarbonate <15 mEq/L).[10] Patient's history may include polyuria, polydipsia, polyphagia, weight loss, vomiting, abdominal pain, dehydration, Kussmaul's breathing, fruity breath, change in mental status, and increased blood glucose and urine ketones.

Check blood glucose, blood gas, electrolytes, urinalysis (for glucose and ketones), and possibly HgbA1c. Consult physician immediately. Fluids, insulin, and frequent evaluation of clinical status and laboratory data of the patient are essential. Cerebral edema is the most significant complication of DKA management.[10]

Sick-day management

Patient needs to check blood glucose and ketones more frequently. Fluid intake should be increased. Additional insulin may need to be given. (See sample sick-day management in Table 4.5 on p. 91.)

Travel

Discuss the impact time changes may have on insulin administration, meal planning, and exercise. For example, when travel is eastbound, there may be a 6- to 8-hour difference, resulting in a shorter day. Background insulins, such as intermediate-acting insulins or long-acting insulins, need to be reduced. Some centers use the guideline of decreasing the dose by whatever percentage of 24 hours is lost. When travel is westbound, days will be longer. Injections of regular or lispro insulin can be added for every 4 to 6 hours (before meals) to cover the additional time.[8]

Remind patients to carry their medications, blood glucose monitoring equipment, and urine ketone testing materials when traveling, as well as some form of medical identification that shows they have diabetes. Provide prescriptions for insulin, keeping in mind that U-100 insulin is not available worldwide. Teach patients how to protect strips and insulin from extremes in temperature.

Table 4.4   Hypoglycemia: Treatment of Low Blood Sugar

| | Always check blood sugar level! | | |
Low Blood Sugar Category	Mild	Moderate	Severe
Alertness	ALERT	**NOT ALERT** **Unable to drink safely (choking risk)** Needs help from another person	**UNRESPONSIVE** **Loss of consciousness** **Seizure** **Needs constant adult help (position of safety)** *Give nothing by mouth (extreme choking risk)*
Symptoms	Mood changes Shaky, sweaty Hungry Fatigue, weak Pale	Lack of focus Headache Confused Disoriented Out of control (bite, kick) *Cannot self-treat*	Loss of consciousness Seizure
Actions to take	✓ Check BS ✓ Give 2-8 oz sugary fluid (amount age dependent) ✓ Recheck BS in 10-15 min ✓ BS <70 mg/dL, repeat sugary fluid and recheck in 10-20 min	✓ *Place in position of safety* ✓ Check BS ✓ If on insulin pump, *may* disconnect or suspend until fully recovered from low blood sugar **(awake and alert)**	✓ *Place in position of safety* ✓ Check BS ✓ If on insulin pump, disconnect or suspend until fully recovered from low blood sugar **(awake and alert)**

From Chase HP, Banion C. Low blood sugar (hypoglycemia or insulin reaction). In Chase HP, ed. Understanding Diabetes: A Handbook for People Who Are Living With Diabetes, 11th ed. Denver, CO: Paros Press, 2006.
BS, Blood sugar.

Table 4.4   Hypoglycemia: Treatment of Low Blood Sugar—cont'd

Low Blood Sugar Category	Always check blood sugar level!		
	Mild	**Moderate**	**Severe**
Actions to take—cont'd	✓ BS >70 mg/dL, (give a solid snack)	✓ Give Insta-Glucose or cake-decorating gel—put between gums and cheek and rub in. ✓ Look for person to wake up ✓ Recheck BS in 10-20 min ✓ *Once alert—* follow actions in Mild column ✓ **(Can use low-dose glucagon, 1 unit per year of age, if very disoriented or out of control)**	✓ Glucagon: *can be given with an insulin syringe, like insulin* Less than 5 years: **30 units** 5-16 years: **50 units** Older than 16 years: **100 units (all of dose)** ✓ If giving 50- or 100-unit doses, may use syringe in box and inject through clothing. ✓ **Check BS every 10-15 min until >80 mg/dL** ✓ **If no response, may need to call 911** ✓ **Check BS every hour for 4-5 hrs** ✓ High risk for more lows for 24 hrs *(need to ↑ food intake and ↓ insulin doses)*
Recovery time	10-20 min	20-45 min	**Call RN/MD and report the episode** Effects can last 2-12 hrs

BS, Blood sugar.

Table 4.5 Sick-Day Management for Diabetes

	Type 1	Type 2
Hydration	8 oz fluid per hour Every third hour, consume the 8 oz fluid as a sodium-rich choice, such as bouillon.	Same as type 1
SMBG	Test every 2 to 4 hours while BG is elevated, or until symptoms subside.	Same as type 1
Ketones	Test every 4 hours or until negative.	Determine for the individual.
Medications	Continue as able. Adjust insulin doses to correct hyperglycemia Hold metformin during serious illness.	Same as type 1
Food and beverages	Guide patients to consume 150 to 200 g of carbohydrates daily, in divided doses. Switch to soft foods or liquids as tolerated. Provide patients a list of foods and beverages in portion sizes containing 15 g of carbohydrates.	Same as type 1
Contact health care professionals	Provide guidelines on conditions that require the patient to call: • Vomiting more than once • Diarrhea more than 5 times or for longer than 6 hours • Blood glucose levels >300 on two consecutive measurements that are not responsive to increased insulin and fluids Moderate or high urine ketones, or blood ketones >0.6 mmol/L	Same as type 1

From Trence DL. Hyperglycemia. In Mensing C, McLaughlin S, Halstenson C, eds. The Art and Science of Diabetes Self-Management Education Desk Reference, 2nd ed. Chicago: American Association of Diabetes Educators, 2011, p 581.

DISORDERS OF GLUCOSE METABOLISM

4

Insulin pumps

GOALS OF THERAPY

- To achieve optimal metabolic control and improve the quality of life for motivated patients and families who meet the selection criteria
- To minimize long-term complications

PATIENT SELECTION CRITERIA

Patient selection criteria should be individualized, taking into account patient/family motivation; commitment; consistent blood glucose monitoring; compliance/follow-up; and financial, behavioral, mental, and physical ability to undertake the intensive diabetes program associated with pump therapy.

ADJUSTMENTS FOR BASAL RATES AND BOLUS RATIOS

- See Box 4.3 for determining insulin pump starting doses.
- Patients/families then monitor glucose levels eight times/day and call for help with management issues daily until the desired glycemic pattern is achieved.
- On average, patients/families will need to call daily for 2-3 weeks, after which weekly contact is maintained for 3 months.
- At 3 months, a follow-up HgbA1c level is obtained to ensure that pump therapy has maintained or improved glycemic outcome. Once it has been validated that continuous subcutaneous insulin infusion is effective, blood glucose is monitored four to six times per day.[13]

SCHOOL PUMP GUIDELINES

Provide the school with a general overview on insulin pump therapy. The school staff must understand that the pump delivers fast-acting insulin continually to the body, is programmed to give additional meal "bolus" doses to cover what is eaten, and may be adjusted to an individual's specific needs. The student and family receive extensive training to use the insulin pump, including changing the pump site, programming, and loading the pump, as well as the ability to self-dose and self-administer care needed to effectively and safely run the insulin pump (depending on age of the child).

SCHOOL NEEDS OF CHILDREN ON INSULIN PUMP

1. A place to store extra supplies
2. Ability to carry meter and testing supplies at all times to test blood sugar throughout the day
3. One trained staff member to remove the insulin pump if student has a severe low blood sugar reaction
4. The pump should be taken off by the student by disconnecting the tubing.
5. Call parent and 911 if student has a severe low blood sugar reaction.
6. Glucagon emergency kit on site to be used in event of a severe low blood sugar reaction
7. High blood sugar levels over 240 mg/dL for two readings in a row will require the student or staff member to contact parent/health care provider.
8. If pump is not working, student can remove pump and must take short-acting insulin for the remainder of the school day.

Continuous Glucose Monitoring

Continuous glucose monitoring (CGM) systems measure the glucose level in the interstitial fluid, not in the blood. Interstitial glucose readings are slightly different from blood glucose readings, but they are usually within 20% of the blood glucose level, unless blood glucose levels are rapidly rising or falling.[14]

CGM is not a replacement for blood sugar monitoring, but it does give additional information to the patient or family about glucose levels and trends. Several CGM systems are approved by the FDA. Please refer to the educational resources and web sites on pages 96-98 for additional information.

DISORDERS OF GLUCOSE METABOLISM ❹

Box 4.3 Starting Pediatric Dosing Calculations

Basal and Bolus Calculations

1. Determine how much insulin to use in the pump by averaging the total units of insulin used per day for 2 weeks. Decrease by 20% for hypoglycemia, by 10% for euglycemia, and make no reduction for hyperglycemia for children.

2. Divide the total dosage in half: 50% for basal and 50% bolus.

3. Divide the portion for bolus by 3. Divide the portion for basal by 24 to determine the hourly basal rate.

4. Check midnight and 3 AM blood glucose levels for 2 weeks before pump placement for evidence of night or early-morning abnormalities of glycemia. For hypoglycemia, reduce the nighttime basal rate by 10%. For hyperglycemia, increase the 3 AM by 10%.

5. Determine the insulin:carbohydrate ratio. (Divide 450 or 500 rule by the total units per day to determine the number of grams of carbohydrate for 1 unit of insulin.)

6. Determine the correction dose for elevated glucose levels. (Divide 1800 for insulin aspart or lispro by the total units of insulin per day to determine the mg/dL that 1 unit of insulin decreases the blood glucose value.)

Childrens Hospital Los Angeles methods. (From Bode BW, Tamborlane WV, Davidson PC. Insulin pump therapy in the 21st century. Strategies for successful use in adults, adolescents, and children with diabetes. Postgrad Med 11:69-78, 2002; Kaufman FR, Halvorson M, Carpenter, et al. Pump therapy for children: weighing the risks and benefits: view 2: insulin pump therapy in young children with diabetes. Diabetes Spectr 14:84-89, 2001.)

OTHER HYPERGLYCEMIA

DIAGNOSIS	CLINICAL FINDINGS	DIAGNOSTIC FINDINGS
Chemotherapy-Induced Diabetes Mellitus Hyperglycemia associated with use of chemotherapy (L-asparaginase)	**Pertinent History** History of acute lymphoblastic leukemia (ALL) or non-Hodgkin's lymphoma (NHL) and treatment with L-asparaginase	Consistent with the established criteria for the diagnosis of diabetes mellitus (see p. 75 for these criteria).
Cystic Fibrosis–Related Diabetes Mellitus Pancreatic fibrosis destroys the islets of Langerhans, resulting in insulin deficiency. In addition, insulin resistance due to factors unique to cystic fibrosis (CF) (i.e., chronic/acute infection, high cortisol levels, or use of corticosteroids) can contribute to the development of diabetes.	**Pertinent History** History of CF with unexplained chronic decline in pulmonary function, failure to gain or maintain weight despite nutritional intervention, weight loss, polydipsia, polyuria, poor growth **Physical Findings** Growth deceleration, delayed pubertal progression, decreased muscle mass	• HgbA1c ≥6.5%* • 2 hr PG ≥200 mg/dL during 75 g OGTT* • Random PG ≥200 with classic symptoms of infection, hyperglycemia • Ketosis rare *In the absence of unequivocal hyperglycemia, this should be confirmed by repeat testing.
Impaired Fasting Glucose (IFG) Metabolic stages of impaired glucose homeostasis	Usually asymptomatic	Fasting plasma glucose 100-125 mg/dL 2 hr PG on the 75 g OGTT 140-199 mg/dL HgbA1c 5.7%-6.4%

4

DISORDERS OF GLUCOSE METABOLISM

DIAGNOSIS	CLINICAL FINDINGS	DIAGNOSTIC FINDINGS
Impaired Glucose Tolerance (IGT) Metabolic stage of impaired glucose homeostasis between normal glucose and diabetes	Usually asymptomatic but may report polydipsia, polyuria, or other mild symptomatology	Fasting plasma glucose 100-125 mg/dL 2 hr PG on the 75 g OGTT 140-199 mg/dL HgbA1c 5.7%-6.4%
Gastroenteritis Inflammation of the stomach and intestinal tract	**Pertinent History** Not usually associated with parental reports of weight loss, polydipsia, or polyuria prior to onset of illness **Physical Findings** Abdominal tenderness, nausea, and vomiting. If prolonged, dehydration may be present.	It is not unusual for a child with gastroenteritis to experience a transient random blood glucose >200 mg/dL. Thus it is essential to review the child's history for indicators of diabetes mellitus before excluding the diagnosis.

EDUCATIONAL RESOURCES

Betschart-Roemer J. Type 2 Diabetes in Teens: Secrets for Success. John Wiley & Sons, 2002.

Chase HP. Understanding Diabetes: A Handbook for People Who Are Living With Diabetes, 11th ed., Denver, CO: Paros Press, 2006. This book can be ordered through the Children's Diabetes Foundation, 777 Grant Street #302, Denver, CO 80203, 1-800-695-2873 (ISBN 0-967-53985-4).

Choose Your Foods: Exchange Lists for Diabetes. American Diabetes Association, The American Dietetic Association, 2008.

Netzer CT. The Complete Book of Food Counts. New York: Bantam Dell, 2009.

Travis LB. An Instructional Aid on Insulin-Dependent Diabetes Mellitus, 12th ed. Austin, TX: Designer's Ink, 2003. This book can be ordered through Designer's Ink, PO Box 200633, Austin, TX 78758; 1-512-832-0611.

Wysocki T. The Ten Keys to Helping Your Child Grow Up With Diabetes, 2nd ed. American Diabetes Association, 2004.

SUPPORT GROUPS

American Diabetes Association (ADA)
1701 N. Beauregard Street
Alexandria, VA 22311
1-800-DIABETES
www.diabetes.org

Cystic Fibrosis Foundation
6931 Arlington Road
Bethesda, MD 20814
1-800-FIGHT CF OR 1-301-951-4422
www.cff.org

International Diabetes Federation (IDF)
Chaussée de la Hulpe 166
B-1170 Brussels, Belgium
+32-2-5385511
FAX +32-2-5385114
www.idf.org

Juvenile Diabetes Foundation International (JDF)
120 Wall Street
New York, NY 10005
1-800-JDF-CURE
www.jdf.org

WEB SITES

Abbott: *www.abbottdiabetescare.com*

American Academy of Pediatrics (AAP): *www.aap.org*

American Association of Diabetes Educators (AADE): *www.diabeteseducator.org*

Animas Corporation: *www.animascorp.com*

Barbara Davis Center for Childhood Diabetes (Denver):
www.barbaradaviscenter.org

Centers for Disease Control's Diabetes and Public Health Resource:
www.cdc.gov/diabetes

Children's Diabetes Foundation at Denver: *www.childrensdiabetesfoundation.org*

Children With Diabetes: *www.childrenwithdiabetes.com*

Dexcom Glucose Sensor: *www.dexcom.com*

DISORDERS OF GLUCOSE METABOLISM

Insulet Corporation (OmniPod insulin management system): *www.myomnipod.com*

Medtronic MiniMed (insulin pumps and CGM): *www.minimed.com*

National Institute of Diabetes & Digestive & Kidney Diseases (NIDDK): *www.diabetes.niddk.nih.gov/*

Roche/Disetronic Medical Systems (Accu-Check Spirit insulin pump system): *www.accu-chekinsulinpumps.com*

❺ OBESITY

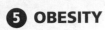

OVERVIEW

The rising incidence of obesity in childhood and adolescence is a major issue today. In 2007-2008, the National Center for Health Statistics estimated that 17% to 19% of children and adolescents were overweight. The percentage of preschool children who are overweight is more than 10%.[1] Treatment of obesity is frustrating and difficult. Early screening for obesity and referral to a pediatric obesity treatment specialist is essential in order to minimize secondary complications. The goal for treating pediatric obesity is regulation of body weight through adequate nutrition for growth and development, thereby preventing interruption of linear growth, minimizing loss of lean body mass, and preventing endocrine disturbances. In addition, ideal treatments should be associated with positive changes in physiologic and psychologic sequelae of obesity. Treatments should modify eating and exercise behaviors along with the factors that regulate these behaviors so that the new, healthier behaviors persist. It is very important to understand that poor nutritional habits or environmental factors are the most common causes of obesity.[2]

SCREENING RECOMMENDATIONS

Since the first publication regarding pediatric obesity in 1998, experts from 15 professional organizations, appointed scientists and clinicians, and three writing groups came together to review the current literature and establish new guidelines for the prevention, assessment, and treatment of childhood obesity in the United States (Fig. 5.1, p. 100). This group of experts, known as the *Expert Committee*, has published new guidelines to help clinicians treat this worldwide epidemic.[3]

The Expert Committee recommends that a child with a BMI ≥85th percentile but <95th percentile or 30 kg/m² now be considered overweight and evaluated further (Table 5.1).[3]

Table 5.1   Terminology for BMI Categories

BMI Category	New Terminology
<5th percentile	Underweight
5th-84th percentile	Healthy weight
85th-94th percentile	Overweight[4]
≥95th percentile	Obesity[4,5]

Adapted from Barlow SE; Expert Committee. Expert committee recommendations regarding the prevention, assessment and treatment of child and adolescent overweight and obesity: summary report. Pediatrics 120(Suppl 4):S164-S192, 2007.

Identification, Assessment, and Prevention of Childhood Obesity

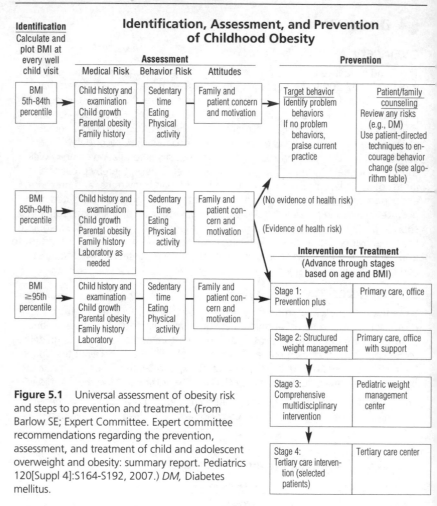

Figure 5.1 Universal assessment of obesity risk and steps to prevention and treatment. (From Barlow SE; Expert Committee. Expert committee recommendations regarding the prevention, assessment, and treatment of child and adolescent overweight and obesity: summary report. Pediatrics 120[Suppl 4]:S164-S192, 2007.) *DM*, Diabetes mellitus.

Children and adolescents with obesity should be screened for complications such as hypertension, dyslipidemias, orthopedic disorders, sleep disorders, gallbladder disease, insulin resistance, type 2 diabetes mellitus, and nonalcoholic fatty liver disease (NAFLD). Other conditions that may require consultation include pseudotumor cerebri, obesity-related sleep disorders, orthopedic problems, massive obesity, and obesity in children under 2 years.[6,7]

HISTORY

HPI/ROS Developmental delay, sudden weight gain within 6 to 12 months, poor linear growth, headaches, nighttime breathing problems, daytime somnolence, abdominal pain, knee or hip pain, oligomenorrhea or amenorrhea.

Medical history Current medications, acute or recent illness, surgical history, hospitalization history, history of chronic disease.

Family history Obesity, non-insulin-dependent diabetes mellitus, cardiovascular disease, hypertension, dyslipidemias, and gallbladder disease.

Social history Tobacco use, depression, eating disorders, ease of making friends, academic history, behavioral problems.

PHYSICAL EXAMINATION (Tables 5.2 through 5.4)

Height, weight, body mass index (BMI)*	Hirsutism, violaceous striae
Waist circumference†	Optic disks, tonsils, abdominal
Truncal obesity	tenderness
Blood pressure	Undescended testicle(s)
Dysmorphic features	Limited hip range of motion
Acanthosis nigricans	Lower leg bowing
Triceps skinfold measurement‡§	

*BMI calculation = Weight (kg)/height (m²)

†Provides a better estimate of accumulated visceral adipose tissue that is linked to increased health risks in adults.[7]

‡The midpoint between the acromion and the olecranon process on the posterior surface of the right arm is determined and marked. While the patient's arm is relaxed, the skinfold is grasped approximately 1 cm above the midpoint (excluding muscle from the grasp). The skinfold thickness is measured with calipers at the midpoint two to three times, and the average is recorded.[8]

§Expert Committee on childhood obesity no longer recommends clinical use of skinfold thickness measurements because of the lack of readily available reference data.

Table 5.2 Cutoff Points for 99th Percentile BMI According to Age and Sex

Age in Years*	99th Percentile BMI Cutoff Point (kg/m²)	
	Boys	Girls
5	20.1	21.5
6	21.6	23.0
7	23.6	24.6
8	25.6	26.4
9	27.6	28.8
10	29.3	29.9
11	30.7	31.5
12	31.8	33.1
13	32.6	34.6
14	33.2	36.0
15	33.6	37.5
16	33.9	39.1
17	34.4	40.8

Adapted from Freedman DS, Mei Z, Srinivasan SR, et al. Cardiovascular risk factors and excess adiposity among overweight children and adolescents: the Bogalusa Heart Study. J Pediatr 150:12-17, 2007.
*The cutoff points are at the midpoint of the child's age.

Table 5.4 International Classification and National BMI Percentages

Overweight and Obesity Prevalence for Children (International Classification and National BMI Percentiles), by Age and Sex

Aged 2-15 With a Valid BMI Measurement

BMI Status	Age (yr)						
	2	3	4	5	6	7	8
International classification							
Males							
Overweight (%)*	19.3	11.6	16.5	14.0	13.1	12.4	17.1
Obese (%)*	5.3	5.5	4.6	4.9	4.3	4.4	5.6
Overweight including obese (%)	24.6	17.1	21.0	18.9	17.4	16.8	22.7

From the International Obesity Task Force (IOTF) 2008. Reproduced under terms of the Click-Use License. Available at http://www.archive2.official-documents.co.uk/document/deps/doh/survey02/hcyp/tables/hcypt159.htm.
*Categories are independent, i.e., overweight does not include those who are obese.
†Overweight was defined as ≥85th-<95th BMI percentile; obese was defined as ≥95th BMI percentile.

Table 5.3   Smoothed 95th Percentiles of Triceps Skinfold Thickness for NHANES I Subjects

Age (yr)	Males (mm)	Females (mm)
6-6.9	14	16
7-7.9	16	18
8-8.9	17	20
9-9.9	19	22
10-10.9	21	24
11-11.9	22	26
12-12.9	23	28
13-13.9	24	30
14-14.9	23	31
15-15.9	22	32
16-16.9	22	33
17-17.9	22	34
18-18.9	22	34
19-19.9	22	35

Adapted from Barlow SE, Dietz WH. Obesity evaluation and treatment: expert committee recommendations. Pediatrics 102:1-11, 1998.

OBESITY 5

							2001-2002 Total
9	10	11	12	13	14	15	2-15
16.8	16.6	19.7	18.4	20.4	14.2	18.0	16.3
5.9	6.4	8.1	5.5	5.1	5.2	5.6	5.5
22.6	23.0	27.8	23.8	25.5	19.4	23.6	21.8

(continued)

Table 5.4 International Classification and National BMI Percentages—cont'd

Overweight and Obesity Prevalence for Children (International Classification and National BMI Percentiles), by Age and Sex

Aged 2-15 With a Valid BMI Measurement

	Age (yr)						
BMI Status	2	3	4	5	6	7	8
International classification—cont'd							
Females							
Overweight (%)*	20.2	18.1	15.5	14.2	19.3	18.3	22.1
Obese (%)*	1.8	5.9	7.3	7.2	7.6	7.3	7.9
Overweight including obese (%)	21.9	24.0	22.8	21.5	26.9	25.5	29.9
National BMI percentiles†							
Males							
Overweight (%)*	15.9	13.6	17.8	14.6	11.8	14.9	12.1
Obese (%)*	13.9	13.4	13.8	13.9	12.0	11.1	17.7
Overweight including obese (%)	29.9	27.0	31.7	28.5	23.7	26.0	29.9
Females							
Overweight (%)*	19.0	18.4	13.2	12.1	13.8	11.0	13.6
Obese (%)*	10.4	11.2	11.8	10.4	13.1	14.7	16.5
Overweight including obese (%)	29.4	29.6	25.0	22.5	26.9	25.6	30.2
Bases (weighted)							
Males	*265*	*330*	*382*	*381*	*404*	*426*	*410*
Females	*297*	*324*	*358*	*400*	*384*	*405*	*431*
Bases (unweighted)							
Males	*236*	*282*	*337*	*322*	*348*	*359*	*352*
Females	*265*	*285*	*318*	*345*	*319*	*347*	*351*

*Categories are independent, i.e., overweight does not include those who are obese.
†*Overweight* was defined as ≥85th-<95th BMI percentile; *obese* was defined as ≥95th BMI percentile.

OBESITY ⑤

9	10	11	12	13	14	15	2001-2002 Total 2-15
21.4	26.6	24.0	20.6	19.7	23.1	19.4	20.3
10.8	6.6	7.4	6.3	8.4	7.3	7.3	7.2
32.2	33.2	31.4	26.9	28.1	30.4	26.7	27.5
15.0	12.5	16.0	18.1	14.0	11.8	11.6	14.3
17.7	17.9	22.0	17.5	18.7	15.4	17.9	16.0
32.7	30.4	38.0	35.6	32.7	27.2	29.5	30.3
11.5	16.3	16.7	13.5	14.4	16.6	18.6	14.8
21.9	18.4	18.1	19.3	19.8	18.7	15.6	15.9
33.4	34.7	34.8	32.8	34.2	35.3	34.2	30.7
408	*420*	*427*	*427*	*397*	*386*	*378*	*5542*
412	*403*	*435*	*390*	*402*	*368*	*371*	*5381*
352	*361*	*377*	*363*	*357*	*349*	*345*	*4740*
350	*348*	*376*	*336*	*364*	*323*	*345*	*4672*

DIAGNOSTIC TESTING

Thyroid function
HgbA1c
AM and PM cortisol
Lipid profile
C-peptide
Triglycerides
Cholesterol
Karyotype

Insulin
Fasting blood glucose
Growth hormone
Calcium and phosphorus
DNA methylation testing
Liver function tests (ALT, AST, ALP, bilirubin) to rule out nonalcoholic fatty liver disease (DAFLD)

DIAGNOSIS	CLINICAL FINDINGS	DIAGNOSTIC FINDINGS
ENDOCRINE		
Cushing's Syndrome	Moon faced, truncal obesity, abdominal striae, centripetal fat distribution, muscle wasting, poor wound healing, poor growth, possibly adrenarche	Hypercortisolism; ↑urinary 17OH-CS and 17OH-KS; normal or ↑AM/PM serum cortisol, abnormal dexamethasone suppression test
Hypothyroidism	Delay in linear growth, recent weight gain, lethargy, dry skin, constipation, family history of thyroid disorders, edema, irregular menses	↓T4, T3 ↑TSH
Polycystic Ovarian Syndrome (PCOS)	Acne, seborrhea, alopecia, hyperhidrosis, acanthosis nigricans, anovulation, hirsutism	↑Androgen levels, polycystic ovaries per pelvic ultrasound, ↓sex hormone binding globulin, ↑insulin level

MANAGEMENT/EDUCATION	EVALUATION
See pp. 40-43. MRI to rule out adenoma	See pp. 40-43.
See p. 185. Thyroid replacement therapy	See p. 185.
See pp. 211-213.	See pp. 211-213.

DIAGNOSIS	CLINICAL FINDINGS	DIAGNOSTIC FINDINGS
ENDOCRINE— cont'd		
Type 2 Diabetes Mellitus	Acanthosis nigricans, hirsutism, hyperglycemia, features of PCOS, strong genetic disposition of ethnic groups such as Pima Indians, Pacific Islanders, and African Americans	Hyperinsulinism
PSYCHOLOGIC		
Bulimia	Persistent overconcern with body shape and weight, binge eating, evidence of self-induced vomiting, chronic esophagitis, parotitis, dental caries, chronic sore throat, distinctive hand lesions, persistent weight fluctuation	Fluid and electrolyte imbalance, dehydration, abdominal cramping, cardiac arrhythmias
Depression	Irritability, moodiness, social withdrawal, low self-esteem, depressed affect, tearfulness, anxiety, suicidal/morbid thoughts, enuresis/ encopresis	History of depression, traumatic event, loss of family member/pet, absence of eye contact, history of social withdrawal, poor grades

MANAGEMENT/EDUCATION	EVALUATION
See pp. 77-78.	See pp. 77-78.
DXA, SEE, METs, BIA, or RQ may be ordered if baseline information is needed to determine percent of obesity.	
Medications:	
Glucophage® (metformin hydrochloride tablets) is indicated for children ages 10 years and older with type 2 diabetes mellitus.[10]	
Glucophage XR (metformin hydrochloride extended-release tablets) is indicated for patients 17 years and older with type 2 diabetes mellitus.[10]	
Hospitalization for fluid maintenance, psychologic evaluation, and behavior modification, EKG	Outpatient psychologic counseling with patient and family members
Laboratory testing to include Na, K, Cl, CO_2, and CBC	Referral to gastroenterology and cardiology
Nutritional evaluation	Outpatient nutritional services as needed
Indirect calorimetry	
Psychologic evaluation, behavior modification	Psychologic counseling on outpatient basis for patient and family members
Medications: antidepressants	

OBESITY

5

DIAGNOSIS	CLINICAL FINDINGS	DIAGNOSTIC FINDINGS
GENETIC		
Prader-Willi Syndrome	Delayed growth, undescended testicles, developmental delay, dysmorphic features	Chromosome analysis indicative of syndrome DNA analysis with methylation may detect 98% of affected individuals.

GENERAL APPROACHES TO THE MANAGEMENT OF OBESITY[2,3,11,12] (Table 5.5)

1. Intervention should begin early.
2. The family must be ready for change.
3. Clinicians should educate families about medical complications of obesity.
4. Clinicians should involve the family and all caregivers in the treatment program.
5. Treatment programs should institute permanent changes, not short-term diets or exercise programs aimed at rapid weight loss.

MANAGEMENT/EDUCATION	EVALUATION
Growth hormone therapy may be used in conjunction with a weight management program to optimize therapy benefits. (See Chapter 11, pp. 289, 291.)	Weight maintenance by decreasing caloric intake to 70% of normal requirements. • Strict 24-hour caloric intake supervision • Hypocaloric, well-balanced diet

5 OBESITY

6. As part of the treatment program, a family should learn to monitor eating and activity.
7. The treatment program should help the family make small, gradual changes.
8. Clinicians should encourage and empathize and not criticize.
9. Staged intervention is recommended by the Expert Committee:
   a. Prevention plus
   b. Structured weight management
   c. Comprehensive multidisciplinary intervention
   d. Tertiary care intervention

Table 5.5　Stages for Managing Childhood Obesity

STAGE 1	STAGE 2
Prevention Plus	**Weight Management**
Focus on exercise, eating behaviors, and healthy lifestyle changes.	Dietary evaluation from dietician
Minimize sugar-sweetened drinks.	Planned diet or daily eating plan, portion control, and scheduled snacks
Decrease television and computer (screen) viewing time.	Additional reduction of TV (screen) viewing time recommended to <1 hr/day
Increase physical activity to ≥1 hr/day.	Planned physical activity to 60 minutes/day
Prepare more meals at home and eat at table with the family 5-6 times per week.	Monitoring behaviors with logs and diaries is recommended.
Involve the entire family in the lifestyle changes.	
Help families tailor new behaviors to their cultural values.	
After 3-6 months, monitor progress. If progressing with improvement, may move to next stage.	

Adapted from Barlow SE; Expert Committee. Expert committee recommendations regarding the prevention, assessment, and treatment of child and adolescent overweight and obesity: summary report. Pediatrics 120(Suppl 4):S164-S192, 2007.

STAGE 3	TERTIARY CARE
Multidisciplinary Intervention	**INTERVENTION**
A structured program of monitoring food intake, short-term diet, physical activity, goal setting, and contingency management	Intensive interventions under this stage apply to some severely obese youths that go beyond the goal of balanced healthy eating and physical activity. These interventions include medications for weight loss, very low caloric diets, and weight control surgery.
Parental participation and behavior modification techniques	
Systemic evaluation of body measurements, diet, and physical activity should be performed at baseline and throughout the program.	
Maximize use of the multidisciplinary team.	
Frequent office visits: weekly for 8-12 weeks recommended, then monthly	
May utilize group sessions	
Commercial weight management programs may be used, but the primary care physician's office personnel need to screen the programs before usage.	

OBESITY

CURRENT DRUG TREATMENTS

Glucophage (metformin hydrochloride tablets) is indicated for children 10 years and older with type 2 diabetes mellitus.[10,13]

Glucophage XR (metformin hydrochloride extended-release tablets) is indicated for patients 17 years and older with type 2 diabetes mellitus.[10,13]

EMERGING THERAPIES

The following current drugs are under investigation for pediatric usage:
- Xenical (orlistat)[14]
- Alli (over the counter)[15]

ADDITIONAL RESOURCES

- BMI tables and calculators
  www.nhlbisupport.com/bmi/bmicalc.htm
  http://pediatrics.about.com/cs/growthcharts2/l/bl_bmi_tables.htm
  www.cdc.gov/nccdphp/dnpa/healthyweight/assessing/bmi/00binaries/bmi-checkbook.pdf

- Body mass index for age percentiles growth charts: *www.cdc.gov/growthcharts*

- Weight and Dietary Assessment Tools

  Weight, Activity, Variety, and Excess (WAVE) (child version)
  http://med.brown.edu/nutrition/acrobat/wave.pdf

  Rapid Eating Assessment for Parents (REAP)
  http://med.brown.edu/nutrition/acrobat/REAP%206.pdf

  RateYour Plate (RYP): *http://med.brown.edu/nutrition/acrobat/RYP.pdf*

  ChooseMyPlate.gov: *www.choosemyplate.gov*

  Healthy Eating Index (HEI)
  www.cnpp.usda.gov/Publications/HEI/healthyeatingindex2005factsheet.pdf

  SHAPEDOWN: *www.shapedown.com*

⑥ HYPERLIPIDEMIA

OVERVIEW

In the United States, cardiovascular disease is the leading cause of death. Studies have shown that with the increasing numbers of obese children and children with genetic forms of hyperlipidemia and secondary conditions causing lipid abnormalities, children should be screened and possibly treated for lipid abnormalities in childhood (Table 6.1). This chapter presents an overview of lipid disorders in children, screening recommendations, and diagnostic and therapeutic management recommendations.

Table 6.1 NCEP and NHANES Laboratory Cut Points for Lipids and Lipoproteins in Children and Adolescents

Cut Points for Borderline-High LDL-C, mmol/L (mg/dL)			Cut Points for High LDL-C, mmol/L (mg/dL)		
NCEP	2.85-3.34 (110-129)		>3.37 (>130)		
NHANES	**Males**	**Females**	**Males**	**Females**	
Age (yr)					
12	3.24 (125)	2.96 (114)	3.98 (154)	3.52 (136)	
13	3.15 (122)	2.98 (115)	3.86 (154)	3.55 (137)	
14	3.08 (119)	3.00 (116)	3.76 (145)	3.57 (138)	
15	3.06 (118)	3.03 (117)	3.74 (145)	3.61 (140)	
16	3.11 (120)	3.07 (119)	3.81 (147)	3.68 (142)	
17	3.18 (123)	3.13 (121)	3.91 (151)	3.77 (146)	
18	3.25 (126)	3.22 (125)	4.00 (155)	3.9 (151)	
19	3.32 (128)	3.32 (128)	4.09 (158)	4.06 (157)	
20	3.37 (130)	3.37 (130)	4.14 (160)	4.14 (160)	

From Kwiterovich PO. Cut points for lipids and lipoproteins in children and adolescents: should they be reassessed? Clin Chem 54:1113-1115, 2008.

IDENTIFICATION OF HIGH-RISK PEDIATRIC DISEASE GROUPS

According to the American Heart Association's Expert Panel on Population and Prevention Science and the Council on Cardiovascular Disease in the Young,[2] there are eight major disease groups that place a child at high risk for the development of cardiovascular events in childhood and/or early adulthood. These eight groups are listed below:

1. Familial hypercholesterolemia
2. Diabetes mellitus, type 1 and type 2
3. Chronic kidney disease
4. Heart transplantation
5. Kawasaki disease
6. Congenital heart disease
7. Chronic inflammatory disease
8. Childhood cancer

Multiple research studies of patient cardiovascular events in childhood and early adulthood in each of these high-risk groups led to the development of a stratification protocol by the Expert Panel (Fig. 6.1; see Table 6.2, p. 118; Box 6.1, p. 119-121; and Box 6.2, pp. 122-123).

STEPS FOR DETERMINING RISK STRATIFICATION AND TREATMENT

1. Risk stratification by disease process (see Table 6.2, p. 118).
2. Assess all cardiovascular risk factors. If there are ≥2 comorbidities, assign patient to the next-higher risk tier for subsequent management.
3. Tier-specific treatment goals/intervention cut points defined.
4. Initial therapy: For tier I, initial management is therapeutic lifestyle change (see Box 6.1, pp. 119-121) PLUS disease-specific management (see Box 6.2, p. 118). For tiers II and III, initial management is therapeutic lifestyle change (see Box 6.1, pp. 119-121).
5. For tiers II and III, if goals are not met, consider medication as outlined in Box 6.2.

High-Risk Pediatric Populations: Risk Stratification and Treatment

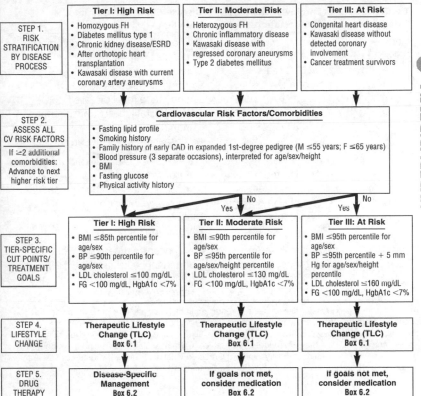

Figure 6.1 Risk-stratification and treatment algorithm for high-risk pediatric populations. (Reprinted with permission. Circulation, 2006;114:2710-2738. ©2006 American Heart Association, Inc.) *BP*, Blood pressure percentile; *CAD*, coronary artery disease; *CV*, cardiovascular; *ESRD*, end-stage renal disease; *FG*, fasting glucose; *HgbA1c*, hemoglobin A1c.

Table 6.2   Stratification of Disease and Associated Risk

Tier/Risk Category	Cardiovascular Manifestations	Disease/Condition Associated With Risk
Tier I— High Risk (see Boxes 6.1, 6.2)	Clinical evidence of CAD <30 years of age	Homozygous familial hypercholesterolemia (FH) Diabetes mellitus type 1 Chronic kidney disease (CKD)/ end-stage renal disease (ESRD) Postorthostatic heart transplantation (OHT) Kawasaki disease with current coronary aneurysms
Tier II— Moderate Risk (see Box 6.1)	Accelerated atherosclerosis: pathophysiologic evidence	Heterozygous FH Kawasaki disease with regressed coronary aneurysms Diabetes mellitus type 2 Chronic inflammatory disease
Tier III— At Risk (see Box 6.1)	High-risk setting for accelerated atherosclerosis	Postcancer treatment survivors Congenital heart disease (CHD) Kawasaki disease without detected coronary involvement

Adapted from Kavey et al. Cardiovascular risk reduction in high-risk pediatric patients: a scientific statement from the American Heart Association Expert Panel on Population and Prevention Science; the Councils on Cardiovascular Disease in the Young, Epidemiology and Prevention, Nutrition, Physical Activity and Metabolism, High Blood Pressure Research, Cardiovascular Nursing, and the Kidney in Heart Disease; and the Interdisciplinary Working Group on Quality of Care and Outcomes Research: endorsed by the American Academy of Pediatrics. Circulation 114:2710-2738, 2006.

Box 6.1 Treatment Recommendations for Diseases/Conditions in Table 6.2

GROWTH/DIET

- Nutritionist evaluation, diet education for all: total fat <30% of calories, saturated fat <10% of calories, cholesterol <300 mg/dL, avoid *trans* fats; adequate calories for growth
- Calculate BMI percentile for gender/height
  If initial BMI >95th percentile:

⇨ **Step 1:**
- Age-appropriate, reduced-calorie training for child and family
- Specific diet/weight follow-up every 2 to 4 weeks for 6 months; repeat BMI calculation at 6 months
- Activity counseling (see below)

If follow-up BMI >85th percentile for tier I, >90th percentile for tier II, or >95th percentile for tier III:

⇨ **Step 2:**
- Weight-loss program referral plus exercise training program appropriate for cardiac status

BLOOD PRESSURE (Tiers I, II, and III)

- BP measurement/interpretation for age/gender/height
  - If SBP and/or DBP ≥90th to 95th percentile or BP >120/80 mm Hg (three separate occasions within 1 month):

⇨ **Step 1:** Decreased calorie intake, increased activity for 6 months
  - If initial SBP and/or DBP >95th percentile (confirmed within 1 week) *OR* 6-month follow-up SBP and/or DBP >95th percentile:

⇨ **Step 2:** Initiate pharmacologic therapy per Fourth Task Force recommendations

(continued)

BP, Blood pressure; *DBP,* diastolic blood pressure; *LDL-C,* LDL cholesterol; *SBP,* systolic blood pressure; *TG,* triglycerides.

HYPERLIPIDEMIA

⑥

Box 6.1   Treatment Recommendations for Diseases/Conditions in Table 6.2—cont'd

LIPIDS

- LDL-C (tiers II and III)
  - See Box 6.2 for recommendations for LDL-C for tier I.
  - If initial LDL-C ≥130 mg/dL (tier II) or >160 mg/dL (tier III):

  ⇨ **Step 1:** Nutritionist training for diet with ≥30% of calories from fat, <7% of calories from saturated fat, cholesterol <200 mg/dL, avoidance of *trans* fats for 6 months
  - If repeat LDL-C >130 mg/dL in tier II or >160 mg/dL in tier III and child older than 10 years:

  ⇨ **Step 2:** Initiate statin therapy with LDL goal of 130 mg/dL
- Triglycerides
  - If initial TG = 150 to 400 mg/dL:

  ⇨ **Step 1:**
  - Nutritionist training for low, simple carbohydrate, low-fat diet
  - If elevated TGs are associated with excess weight, nutritionist referral for weight loss management: energy balance training plus activity recommendations (see pp. 121-122)
  - If TG >700 to 1000 mg/dL, initial or follow-up:

  ⇨ **Step 2:**
  - Consider fibrate or niacin if older than 10 years.
  - Weight loss recommended when TG elevation is associated with overweight/obesity.

GLUCOSE (Tiers I, II, and III, except for patients with diabetes mellitus)

- If fasting glucose = 100 to 126 mg/dL:

  ⇨ **Step 1:** Reduced-calorie diet, increased activity aimed at 5% to 10% decrease in weight over 6 months

- If repeat fasting glucose = 100 to 126 mg/dL:

  ⇨ **Step 2:** Insulin-sensitizing medication per endocrinologist

- Casual glucose >200 mg/dL or fasting glucose >126 mg/dL = Diabetes mellitus → Endocrine referral for evaluation and management

- Maintain HgbA1c <7%

SMOKING (Tiers I, II, and III)

⇨ **Step 1:** Parental smoking history at every visit; child smoking history beginning at age 10. Active antismoking counseling for all; smoke-free home strongly recommended at each encounter

⇨ **Step 2:** Smoking cessation referral for any history of cigarette smoking

ACTIVITY (Tiers I, II and III)

- For children in all tiers, participation in activity is at the discretion of the physician(s) directing care. For specific cardiac diagnoses such as Kawasaki disease and congenital heart disease, activity guidelines are referenced.

  ⇨ **Step 1:** Specific activity history for each child, focusing on time spent in active play and screen time (television + computer + video games). Goal is ≥1 hour of active play/day; screen time limited to ≤2 hour/day.

- Encourage activity at every encounter.

  ⇨ **Step 2:** After 6 months, if goals not met, consider referral for exercise testing, recommendations from exercise specialist.

6

HYPERLIPIDEMIA

Box 6.2   Specific Treatment Recommendations for Tier I Conditions

- Rigorous age-appropriate education in diet, activity, and smoking cessation for all
- Specific therapy as needed to achieve BP, LDL-C, glucose, and HgbA1c goals as indicated for each tier, as outlined in Fig. 6.1; timing individualized for each patient and diagnosis. Step 1 and Step 2 therapy for all outlined in Box 6.1.
- For diagnosis-specific guidelines, references are provided.

HOMOZYGOUS FH

- LDL management: Scheduled apheresis every 1 to 2 weeks beginning at diagnosis to maximally lower LDL-C, plus statin and cholesterol absorption inhibitor
- Treatment per cardiologist/lipid specialist. (Specific therapeutic goals for LDL-C are not meaningful with this diagnosis.)
- Assess BMI, BP, and FG: Step 1 management for 6 months
- If tier I goals not achieved, proceed to Step 2

DIABETES MELLITUS, TYPE 1

- Intensive glucose management per endocrinologist, with frequent glucose monitoring/insulin titration to maintain PG <200 mg/dL, HgbA1c <7%
- Assess BMI, fasting lipids: Step 1 management of weight, lipids for 6 months
- If goals not achieved, proceed to Step 2; statin therapy if older than 10 years to achieve tier I treatment goals
- Initial BP >90th percentile: Step 1 management plus no added salt, increased activity for 6 months
- BP consistently >95th percentile for age/sex/height: Initiate ACE inhibitor therapy with BP goal <90th percentile or <130/80 mm Hg, whichever is lower.

CKD/ESRD

- Optimization of renal failure management with dialysis/transplantation per nephrology
- Assess BMI, BP, lipids, FG: Step 1 management for 6 months
- If goals not achieved, proceed to Step 2; statin therapy if older than 10 years to achieve tier I treatment goals

AFTER HEART TRANSPLANTATION

- Optimization of antirejection therapy, treatment for CMV, routine evaluation by angiography/perfusion imaging per transplant physician
- Assess BMI, BP, lipids, FG: Initiate Step 2 therapy, including statins, immediately in all patients older than 10 years to achieve tier I treatment goals

KAWASAKI DISEASE WITH CORONARY ANEURYSMS

- Antithrombotic therapy, activity restriction, ongoing myocardial perfusion evaluation per cardiologist
- Assess BMI, BP, lipids, FG: Step 1 management for 6 months
- If goals not achieved, proceed to Step 2; statin therapy if older than 10 years to achieve tier I treatment goals

ACE, Angiotensin-converting enzyme; *BMI*, body mass index: *BP*, blood pressure; *CKD*, chronic kidney disease; *CMV*, cytomegalovirus; *ESRD*, end-stage renal disease; *FG*, fasting glucose; *FH*, familial hypercholesterolemia; *LDL-C*, LDL cholesterol; *PG*, plasma glucose.

HYPERLIPIDEMIA ⑥

PRIMARY LIPIDEMIAS

DIAGNOSIS	CLINICAL FINDINGS	DIAGNOSTIC FINDINGS
Familial Hyper-cholesterolemia[2-4] • Autosomal dominant monogenic condition • Homozygous (rare) (1:1000,000) • Heterozygous (1:500)	**Homozygous FH** Presents within first decade of life. Physical findings: Cholesterol deposition (tendon xanthomata, cutaneous xanthelasma, corneal arcus); symptoms of atherosclerotic CV disease **Heterozygous FH** Typically asymptomatic with no physical findings on examination.	Diagnostic findings are typically found while screening child for hyperlipidemia in families. Other findings may occur with examination, blood screening, or as clinical manifestations of early CV disease. **Homozygous FH** LDL levels vary from 15-25 mmol/L (500-1000 mg/dL) with HDL levels reduced from 0.5-1.0 mmol/L (20-40 mg/dL). **Heterozygous FH** LDL levels at or above the 95th percentile

SECONDARY LIPIDEMIAS

DIAGNOSIS	CLINICAL FINDINGS	DIAGNOSTIC FINDINGS
Type 1 Diabetes Mellitus	See Chapter 4, Disorders of Glucose Metabolism	See Chapter 4, Disorders of Glucose Metabolism

MANAGEMENT/EDUCATION	EVALUATION
Homozygous FH	Evaluate after disease-specific management, then if goals are not obtained, consider medications to lower LDL levels.
Requires intensive therapy to reduce LDL levels.	
Interventions to prevent or reduce risk factors are also important.	
Low-dose anticoagulation may also be indicated.	
Complete cardiovascular assessment.	
Heterozygous FH	
Referral to lipid specialist.	
Reduction of LDL levels with pharmacologic treatments.	
For both types of hyperlipidemia, dietary lifestyle changes plus exercise are also indicated.	

HYPERLIPIDEMIA 6

MANAGEMENT/EDUCATION	EVALUATION
See Chapter 4, Disorders of Glucose Metabolism	See Chapter 4, Disorders of Glucose Metabolism

DIAGNOSIS	CLINICAL FINDINGS	DIAGNOSTIC FINDINGS
Chronic Kidney Disease (CKD)[5]	Recommendations are directed toward children with CKD stage 5 with glomerular filtration rates (GFR) <15 ml/min^{-1}, 1.73 m^{-2}. Other recommendations include children undergoing dialysis and renal transplant recipients.	Identify any underlying cardiac risk factors by complete cardiovascular workup to include echo-cardiography; rule out end-organ injury, left ventricular mass, or coronary calcium. Refer to the cardio-vascular risk management recommendations from the National Kidney Foundation's Kidney Dialysis Outcomes and Quality Initiative.
Pediatric Heart Transplantation[2,6]	Posttransplantation coronary heart disease such as congestive heart failure (CHF), hypertension related to chronic steroid use and/or immunosuppressants, allograft dysfunction or rejection, hyperlipidemia	Abnormalities of allograft function by evaluation of echocardiographic shortening fraction Abnormalities in hemodynamic studies Posttransplantation coronary artery disease as evidenced by coronary angiography Coronary intimal thickening

MANAGEMENT/EDUCATION	EVALUATION
See Fig. 6.1, p. 117; Box 6.1, pp. 119-121; and Box 6.2, pp. 122-123.	See Fig. 6.1, p. 117; Box 6.1, pp. 119-121; and Box 6.2, pp. 122-123.
See Fig. 6.1, p. 117; Box 6.1, pp. 119-121; and Box 6.2, pp. 122-123.	See Fig. 6.1, p. 117; Box 6.1, pp. 119-121; and Box 6.2, pp. 122-123.

⑥

HYPERLIPIDEMIA

DIAGNOSIS	CLINICAL FINDINGS	DIAGNOSTIC FINDINGS
Kawasaki Disease[5]	Characterized by fever, bilateral nonexudative conjunctivitis, erythema of the lips and oral mucosa, changes in the extremities, rash, and cervical adenopathy Likely to be caused by infectious agent(s) that produce clinical signs of the disease in genetically predisposed individuals	Currently there are no diagnostic tests or pathognomonic clinical feature that can confirm diagnosis early in the illness. Early in the illness, coronary arteries demonstrate edema and infiltration of the arterial wall by neutrophils that rapidly transition to mononuclear cells, primarily CD8+ cells, monocytes, macrophages, and IgA plasma cells. Coronary artery stenosis and aneurysms may also occur.
Chronic Inflammatory Disease[5]	Patients with highest risk are those exhibiting systemic lupus erythematosus (SLE) and rheumatoid arthritis (RA).	Increased intima-media thickness. Inflammation markers such as C-reactive protein (CRP), cytokines, and serum amyloid-A may be present. Antiphospholipid antibodies may develop.

MANAGEMENT/EDUCATION	EVALUATION
See Fig. 6.1, p. 117; Box 6.1, pp. 119-121; and Box 6.2, pp. 122-123.	See Fig. 6.1, p. 117; Box 6.1, pp. 119-121; and Box 6.2, pp. 122-123.
See Fig. 6.1, p. 117; Box 6.1, pp. 119-121; and Box 6.2, pp. 122-123.	See Fig. 6.1, p. 117; Box 6.1, pp. 119-121; and Box 6.2, pp. 122-123.

6

HYPERLIPIDEMIA

DIAGNOSIS	CLINICAL FINDINGS	DIAGNOSTIC FINDINGS
Congenital Heart Disease (CHD)[5]	Lesions with coronary artery abnormalities and obstructive lesions of the left ventricle and aorta, hypertrophic cardiomyopathy, and congenital heart disease.	See Box 6.1, pp. 119-121.
Childhood Cancer Survivors[5]	Any child with a childhood cancer who has undergone chemotherapy treatment is at risk for the development of CHD.	Diagnostic findings may vary depending on the type of therapeutic agents used to treat cancer.

CURRENT DRUG TREATMENTS[3,5,7-12]

- Bile acid sequestrates: Cholestyramine and colestipol may be used in children 10 years or older.
- Nicotinic acid: Safety and effectiveness in children have not been established.
- Gemfibrozil (Lopid): Safety and effectiveness in children have not been established.
- Atorvastatin (Lipitor) may be prescribed in children 10 years or older if diet and physical exercise therapy have not lowered cholesterol levels.
- Pravastatin (Pravachol) may be used in children 8 years or older.
- Rosuvastatin (Crestor): Safety and effectiveness in children have not been established.
- Ezetimibe/simvastatin (Vytorin): Pharmacokinetic data in the pediatric population younger than 10 years are not available.
- Fluvastatin sodium (Lescol): Safety and effectiveness in children have not been established.

MANAGEMENT/EDUCATION	EVALUATION
See Fig. 6.1, p. 117; Box 6.1, pp. 119-121; and Box 6.2, pp. 122-123.	See Fig. 6.1, p. 117; Box 6.1, pp. 119-121; and Box 6.2, pp. 122-123.
See Fig. 6.1, p. 117; Box 6.1, pp. 119-121; and Box 6.2, pp. 122-123.	See Fig. 6.1, p. 117; Box 6.1, pp. 119-121; and Box 6.2, pp. 122-123.

6

HYPERLIPIDEMIA

CURRENT DIAGNOSTIC RESEARCH[13-16]

- Low-density lipoprotein apheresis in children with familial hypercholesterolemia
- High-sensitivity C-reactive protein as a cardiovascular marker
- Oxidative stress effects on arterial dysfunction and enhanced intima-media thickness
- Alanine aminotranferase and high-sensitivity C-reactive protein as a cardiovascular marker and correlates with cardiovascular risk in youth

7 PITUITARY DISORDERS

OVERVIEW

The pituitary gland is located in a saddle-shaped cavity in the sphenoid bone called the *sella turcica*. It is composed of two lobes, called the anterior and posterior pituitary lobes.

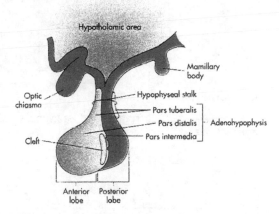

Figure 7.1 The pituitary gland. (This figure was published in Endocrine Physiology, 2nd edition, Porterfield SP, p 21, Copyright Elsevier, 2001.)

ANTERIOR PITUITARY (Adenohypophysis)

Synthesis and secretion of anterior pituitary hormones are regulated by releasing and inhibiting hormones that originate in the hypothalamus and are carried to the anterior pituitary by the hypophyseal portal system secretion. All hypothalamic-releasing hormones and all anterior pituitary hormones have pulsatile episodic secretion—short, regular quantal bursts of hormone release.

Endocrine Feedback Systems

- Long loop system: The anterior pituitary hormone acts on the target organ to increase the production of hormone; the hormone exerts a negative feedback on the anterior pituitary.
- Short loop system: The anterior pituitary hormone itself feeds back on the hypothalamus, exerting a negative feedback.
- Ultrashort loop system: The releasing hormone acts directly on the hypothalamus to control its own secretion.

ANTERIOR PITUITARY HORMONES

HORMONE	HYPOTHALAMIC REGULATION
Luteinizing Hormone (LH) Synthesized by the gonadotrope	Gonadotropin-releasing hormone (GnRH) Transported via hypophyseal portal system
Follicle-Stimulating Hormone (FSH) Synthesized by the gonadotrope	GnRH Transported via hypophyseal portal system
Thyroid-Stimulating Hormone (TSH) Synthesized by the thyrotropes	Thyrotropin-releasing hormone (TRH) Growth hormone–inhibiting hormone (GHIH) Acts by the phosphatidylinositol pathway
Pro-opiomelanocortin (POMC) Synthesized by the corticotropes	

Adapted from Porterfield SP, ed. Endocrine Physiology. St Louis: Mosby–Year Book, 1997.

FUNCTION

Male
Works on Leydig's cells of the testis

Regulator of testicular steroidogenesis

Stimulates growth of testis and production of testicular androgens

Female
Stimulates conversion of ovarian follicle to corpus luteum

Stimulates estrogen and progesterone secretion

Male
Acts on Sertoli's cells to stimulate estrogen formation from androgens

Works with testosterone to produce androgen-binding protein

Female
Acts on ovarian follicle to stimulate follicular growth

Stimulates aromatilzation of thecal androgens to estrogens

Regulates growth and metabolism of thyroid gland

Stimulates synthesis and secretion of thyroid hormones T4 (thyroxine) and T3, which function to maintain normal body metabolism necessary for normal growth and brain development in infants and children

Forms N-terminal peptide, beta-lipotropic pituitary hormone, and ACTH

HORMONE	HYPOTHALAMIC REGULATION
Adrenocorticotropic Hormone (ACTH)	Corticotropin-releasing hormone (CRH)
Growth Hormone (GH) Synthesized by the somatotropes	Growth hormone–releasing hormone (GHRH) Somatostatin

FUNCTION

Peaks in early morning and late afternoon; pulsatile

Signals adrenal glands to produce cortisol

> **NOTE** A lack of ACTH results in a cortisol deficiency. Cortisol is necessary in maintaining normal blood sugar, salt and water balance, and protection of the body during periods of physical stress.

Stimulates growth and steroid production in the adrenal cortex

Increases skin pigmentation

Stimulates lipolysis

Stimulated by stress, hyperglycemia, surgery, trauma, infection, hypoxia, hypoglycemia, adrenal hypoplasia, anxiety, depression

Inhibited by cortisol

Peaks in early morning just before awakening; pulsatile

Stimulates skeletal and visceral growth

Regulates IGF-1 production

Inhibits somatostatin release

Metabolic actions (carbohydrate):
- Increases blood glucose
- Decreases peripheral insulin sensitivity
- Increases hepatic output of glucose

Proteins:
- Increases tissue amino acid uptake
- Increases incorporation into proteins
- Decreases urea production
- Produces positive nitrogen balance

Lipids:
- Is lipolytic
- Can be ketogenic

HORMONE	HYPOTHALAMIC REGULATION
Prolactin (PRL) Synthesized in the lactotropes	Prolactin-releasing factor (PRF) Prolactin-inhibiting hormone (PIH)

POSTERIOR PITUITARY HORMONES

HORMONE	HYPOTHALAMIC REGULATION
Vasopressin (ADH)	Synthesized in the hypothalamus and secreted from the posterior pituitary

FUNCTION

Initiates and maintains lactation, which involves mammogenesis, lactogenesis, and galactopoiesis:

- *Mammogenesis:* Growth and development of the mammary gland
- *Lactogenesis:* Initiation of lactation, stimulated by PRL
- *Galactopoiesis:* Maintenance of milk production, requires PRL and oxytocin

Can have reproductive actions

Can decrease GnRH release, resulting in decreased LH release

Excessive PRL secretion inhibits reproductive function.

Hyperprolactinemia produces glucose intolerance and hyperinsulinemia.

Human placento lactogen (hPL) is a major cause of diabetes in pregnancy.

Stimulated by stress, sleep, nursing and breast stimulation, hormones (estrogen, TRH, glucagon), dopamine antagonists (chlorpromazine, antihypertensives, tricyclic antidepressives)

Inhibited by dopamine agonists, hormones (somatostatin, dopamine)

TRH can stimulate PRL release, which is why patients with longstanding hypothyroidism have elevated prolactin levels.

FUNCTION

Renal actions (primarily on kidney)
↑ Water and urea permeability controlling urine and osmolality

Stimulates mesangial cell contraction

↓ Glomerular filtration rate

Inhibits renin release

(continued)

HORMONE	HYPOTHALAMIC REGULATION
Vasopressin (ADH)—cont'd	
Oxytocin	Produced in paraventricular nuclei

FUNCTION

Cardiovascular actions
Stimulates arteriolar constriction

Adrenal-pituitary axis
Stimulates ACTH secretion by ↑ sensitivity to CRH and by direct effect on ADH receptor

Released in response to stress

Released in response to ↑ extracellular fluid osmolality

Stimulated by drop in effective blood volume

Alcohol is suppressor of ADH secretion, leading to dehydration.

Stimulates myoepithelial cell contraction as part of milk ejection reflex and uterine motility

Magnitude of action dependent on phase of menstrual cycle (estrogens ↑ response, progestogens ↓ response)

May be blocked by pain, fear, or stress

Stimulates sodium retention and antidiuresis

HISTORY
Newborn Period

HPI/ROS Hypoglycemia in the neonate, which can be manifested as apnea, cyanosis, pallor, lethargy, jitteriness, seizures; poor feeding, hyperbilirubinemia

Medical history Complications in the neonatal period in a full-term infant, including evaluations for sepsis, temperature instability, unexplained apnea; hyponatremia

Older Infants/Childhood

HPI/ROS Growth failure, headaches, visual disturbances, and other neurologic complaints; polyuria and polydipsia associated with short stature; lack of puberty or pubertal arrest, constipation, lethargy, weakness; in females, amenorrhea; in males, impotence, loss of libido

Medical history Breech delivery with complications in the perinatal period, hypoglycemia in a child with failure to thrive, short stature, or slow growth; craniopharyngiomas and other tumors in the hypothalamic region; cranial radiation, trauma, or infection in the central nervous system

Family history Familial pattern of growth, including height and onset of puberty, midparental heights, growth hormone deficiency

Social history Development, evidence of psychosocial problems in the home

PHYSICAL EXAMINATION

Complete endocrine examination with careful attention to the following:

Growth Height, weight, head circumference, growth velocity, arm span, upper/lower segment ratio

General Appearance, dysmorphology

HEENT Funduscopic exam, visual fields, dentition

Thyroid Palpation for size

Genitourinary Tanner staging—breast development, pubic/axillary hair, stretched penile length, testicular volume, clitoral length

Neurologic Mental status, cranial nerves, deep tendon reflexes

Musculoskeletal Muscle weakness, symmetry

Skin Color, temperature

DIAGNOSTIC TESTING

Perform a complete pituitary evaluation of the function of each hormone to determine extent of pituitary insufficiency. See pp. 301-311 for specific tests.

HYPOPITUITARISM/PANHYPOPITUITARISM

- Deficiency of one, some, or all of the six major hormones (LH, FSH, GH, thyrotropin, corticotropin, and prolactin) secreted by the pituitary gland
- The most common sequence of loss of pituitary hormones is GH, gonadotropin (FSH, LH), thyrotropin, corticotropin.
- In children, the most common manifestation is growth failure and delayed puberty.
- Can occur as a result of trauma at delivery or later in life resulting in damage to the pituitary or hypothalamus, tumors of the hypothalamus or pituitary (craniopharyngioma—most common), infectious processes in the CNS, chemotherapy, radiation, surgical resection, disorders that destroy normal tissues (hemochromatosis, sarcoidosis, histiocytosis X), congenital syndromes

Table 7.1   Growth Hormone

	Factors Stimulating Growth Hormone	Factors Inhibiting Growth Hormone
Metabolic	↓ Blood glucose, ↑ amino acids (arginine, leucine)	↑ Blood glucose
Hormonal	GHRH, glucagon, dopamine, uncontrolled diabetes	Somatostatin, IGF-1, hypothyroidism
Drugs	Dopamine agonists	Dopamine antagonists
Other	Exercise, sleep (stages 3, 4), stress, puberty	Emotional deprivation, aging, obesity

Clinical presentations of pituitary dysfunction vary with age and specific hormone deficiency. Refer to each individual pituitary hormone section for clinical presentation, diagnostic testing, management, and evaluation.

7

PITUITARY DISORDERS

GROWTH FAILURE

- Growth occurs at differing rates throughout life.
- Any deviation from the normal growth pattern may be the first manifestation of a variety of disorders.
- Since the pituitary plays a central role in the regulation of growth, it may be necessary to perform a complete pituitary evaluation in a child with growth failure to distinguish an isolated hormone deficiency from multiple hormone deficiencies and a possible functional or anatomic defect involving the pituitary gland and/or hypothalamus.

Classification of Growth Retardation

Endocrine causes	Nonendocrine causes
Hypothyroidism	Osteochondrodysplasias
Cushing's syndrome	Chromosomal abnormalities
Pseudohypoparathyroidism	Intrauterine growth retardation
Rickets	Malnutrition
IGF deficiency	Chronic disease
Hypothalamic dysfunction	Constitutional delay of growth and puberty
GH deficiency	Genetic short stature
GH resistance	Idiopathic short stature
Insulin deficiency	Psychosocial short stature

Adapted from Reiter EO, Rosenfeld RG. Normal and aberrant growth. In Wilson JD, Foster DW, Kronenberg HM, et al, eds. Williams Textbook of Endocrinology, 9th ed. Philadelphia: WB Saunders, 1998. With permission from Elsevier.

Adults with growth hormone deficiency (GHD) can be grouped into three categories:
- History of prior childhood GHD
- Acquired GHD secondary to structural lesions or trauma
- Idiopathic GHD. See Box 7.1 for causes of GHD.

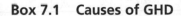

Box 7.1   Causes of GHD

Congenital

Transcription factor defects (PIT-1, PROP-1, LHX3/4, HESX-1, PITX-2)

  GHRH receptor gene defects

  GH secretagogue receptor gene defects

  Prader-Willi syndrome

Associated with brain structural defects

  Agenesis of corpus callosum

  Septo-optic dysplasia

  Empty sella syndrome

  Holoprosencephaly

  Encephalocele

  Hydrocephalus

  Arachnoid cyst

Associated with midline facial defects

  Single central incisor

  Cleft lip-palate

Acquired

Trauma

  Perinatal

  Postnatal

Central nervous system infection

Tumors of hypothalamus or pituitary

  Pituitary adenoma

  Craniopharyngioma

  Rathke's cleft cyst

  Glioma/astrocytoma

  Germinoma

  Metastatic

  Other

Infiltrative/granulomatous disease

  Langerhans cell histiocytosis

  Sarcoidosis

  Tuberculosis

  Hypophysitis

  Other

Cranial irradiation

Surgery

Idiopathic

From Molitch ME, Clemmons DR, Maolzowsk S, et al. Evaluation and treatment of adult growth hormone deficiency: an endocrine society clinical practice guideline. J Clin Endocrinol Metab 91:1621-1634, 2006.

7

PITUITARY DISORDERS

DIAGNOSIS	CLINICAL FINDINGS	DIAGNOSTIC FINDINGS
Idiopathic Short Stature Non–growth hormone deficient short stature May or may not have short parents Height ≤−2.25 SD Diagnosis of exclusion	**Pertinent History** Normal size at birth No history of systemic disease, malnutrition, or other endocrine disorders **Physical Findings** Height ≤−2.25 SD, associated with growth rates, unlikely to permit attainment of normal adult height No dysmorphology	Normal CBC, sedimentation rate Normal electrolytes, including calcium, phosphorus, prealbumin, iron-binding protein Normal thyroid function tests (TSH, T4, free T4) Normal ACTH, cortisol FSH, LH, testosterone, estradiol appropriate for age and pubertal stage IgA or IgG tissue transglutaminase (ttG) antibodies Chromosome analysis: • Normal 46 XX, female or 46 XY, male • 1%-2% may have mutations in SHOX gene • IGF-1, IGFBP-3 normal for age • Normal GH secretion (>10 ng/mL) Bone age: • Open epiphysis • Presence of absence of bone age delay

MANAGEMENT/EDUCATION	EVALUATION

GH therapy as indicated

If diagnostic findings indicated systemic disease, refer to specialist for further evaluation.

If +IgA or IgG tissue transglutaminase antibodies, refer to pediatric gastroenterologist.

Provide reassurance to child and family.

Psychosocial intervention when appropriate

Encourage children's participation in activities they like and perform well to boost self-esteem and positive self-worth.

Medical therapy alternatives:
- *Anabolic steroids:* Oxandrolone may ↑ height velocity in short term without significant ↑ in adult height.[4]
- *GnRH analogs:* Monotherapy in both sexes has shown small and variable effect on adult height gain. Combination therapy with GnRHa and GH may ↑ adult height gain.[5]
- *Aromatase inhibitors:* Slow tempo of bone age and have ↑ predicted adult height in males with ISS/GHD who have been treated for at least 2 years.[6] Aromatase inhibitors should not be used in girls; long-term effects of treatment are not known.

Monitor height, weight, growth velocity, and sexual development every 3-6 months.

If on treatment, monitor for adverse events every 3-6 months.

Assess child's and parents' perception of problem and level of concern.

Obtain bone age periodically to reassess height prediction.

Reevaluate response to therapy at 1 year; refer to GH response curves in ISS.[7]

7

PITUITARY DISORDERS

DIAGNOSIS	CLINICAL FINDINGS	DIAGNOSTIC FINDINGS
Constitutional Delay of Growth and Puberty (CDGP)	**Pertinent History** Strong family history of delayed growth and maturation. Referred to as "late bloomers" May have history of familial short stature No history of systemic illness Normal predicted adult heights: • Males >163 cm • Females >150 cm **Physical Findings** Short stature, retarded linear growth beginning in the first 3 years of life, then following a normal growth pattern paralleling a normal curve until puberty with catch-up growth at time of pubertal growth spurt Normal body proportions No phenotypic abnormalities Delayed puberty	**Laboratory Tests** Normal thyroid function tests Normal CBC, sedimentation rate, electrolytes, BUN IGF-1, IGFBP-3 may be normal for bone age but may be ↓ for chronologic age. GH levels may be ↓ at time of delayed pubertal growth spurt. If pretreated with gonadal steroids, would be expected to have normal GH provocative test results **Radiologic Studies** Bone age delayed as much as 4 years

MANAGEMENT/EDUCATION	EVALUATION

Medications

May use testosterone therapy in males with a bone age >12 years (less risk of advancing the bone age and compromising adult height)

Education

Reinforce that this pattern of growth is normal.

Positive family history offers reassurance.

Consider psychological therapy for patients with poor self-image and social involvement associated with short stature and delayed puberty.

Height, weight, growth velocity, and sexual development

Consider GH testing if no growth spurt at onset of puberty.

Follow-up for patients receiving testosterone therapy: monthly for injections

Monitor for signs of puberty:
- ↑ Testicular volume
- Testosterone level in pubertal range

DIAGNOSIS	CLINICAL FINDINGS	DIAGNOSTIC FINDINGS
Familial Short Stature (FSS) Also called *genetic short stature*	**Pertinent History** Short parental height Height is within normal in relation to parental heights. May or may not have constitutional growth delay Rule out history of environmental factors: • Nutrition • Use of drugs • Illness Consider medical history of parents. **Physical Findings** ↓ Growth rate from 6 to 18 months of age then follows steady growth channel <5th percentile for height for 2 to 3 years Normal growth velocity Tubular bone alterations: • Fifth metacarpal bone shortening • Rhizomelia • Disproportionate limb shortening more prevalent in FSS	Predicted height is normal for midparental height (short). **Radiologic Studies** Consider radiologic studies in presence of disproportionate limb shortening to rule out hypochondroplasia. **Laboratory Tests** Normal laboratory findings

MANAGEMENT/EDUCATION	EVALUATION
Provide reassurance to child and family. Encourage children's participation in activities they like and perform well to promote self-esteem and positive self-worth.	Ongoing assessment of height, weight, growth velocity and psychosocial adaptation

PITUITARY DISORDERS

DIAGNOSIS	CLINICAL FINDINGS	DIAGNOSTIC FINDINGS

Psychosocial Short Stature (PSS)

Diagnosis of exclusion in infancy, childhood, and adolescence

Patient presents with growth failure and/or delayed puberty in association with emotional deprivation.

Pertinent History

Failure to thrive (nutritional deficiency)

Multiple siblings

Overburdened mother

Poor maternal/infant attachment

May have bizarre behaviors (eating from garbage, stealing food, prowling at night)

May have enuresis, encopresis, temper tantrums, sleep disorders

Retarded speech

Emotional deprivation

Depression

Physical Findings

May be underweight for height

Short stature

Delayed puberty

May have protuberant abdomen

Laboratory Tests

Includes testing as above for child with short stature, which is negative for an organic cause

GH secretion most often normal, but may be ↓ in some cases. This may be associated with the sleep disorders.

May have ↓ corticotropin levels in response to metyrapone

May have abnormal thyroid function

Steatorrhea may be present.

MANAGEMENT/EDUCATION	EVALUATION

Assess daily caloric intake.

Goal of treatment is to change the child's psychologic environment.

In severe cases, physical removal from the home is a treatment option.

Hospital admission may be necessary to perform a complete evaluation.

A team approach including social workers and legal authorities is needed to handle these cases efficiently.

Education

Provide education regarding nutrition and adequate caloric intake.

Assess parenting skills and provide referrals for psychosocial support services as needed.

Follow-up includes height, weight, nutritional status, psychosocial assessment.

In severe cases, patients removed from the home (even temporarily for evaluation) will show immediate improvement in growth response.

Prognosis for growth and emotional stability and cognitive development is good if diagnosis is made early and physical removal from the adverse environment is achieved.

GH abnormalities usually reverse when patient removed from adverse environment.

PITUITARY DISORDERS 7

DIAGNOSIS	CLINICAL FINDINGS	DIAGNOSTIC FINDINGS
Small for Gestational Age (SGA) Birth weight and/or length <-2 SD Intrauterine growth retardation (IUGR) identifies slow fetal growth based on two ultrasound measurements. ~10% of SGA children fail to show catch-up growth by 2 years of age.	**Pertinent History** Maternal factors: • Maternal size, age (>38 years and young maternal age) • Poor maternal weight gain • Chronic under-nutrition maternal illness • Cardiac sickle cell diagnosis • Asthma • Infections (TORCH) • Maternal smoking • Drug/alcohol use • Multiple fetuses • Failure to thrive • "Picky eaters" May have emotional conduct disorders ADHD **Physical Findings** *Growth:* Typical infant born SGA has accelerated linear growth during 1st year of life, with catch-up growth by 2 years of age (90%). Premature infants and infants with more severe growth retardation are less likely to reach normal stature. Untreated children, compromised height *(continued)*	GH provocative tests not part of routine care unless signs of GHD, hypopituitarism, or persistent poor growth velocity Low to normal IGF-1 and IGFBP-3 May have genetic abnormalities of GH/IGF-1 axis: IGF-1 and IGF-1 receptor gene deletions, point muta-tions, or polymorphisms Bone age—delayed May not be predictor of pubertal timing or adult height May have reduced BMD BP, BMI, fasting glucose, lipids may indicate insulin resistance

MANAGEMENT/EDUCATION	EVALUATION

rhGH therapy indicated for SGA children who fail to demonstrate catch-up growth by age 2 years.

Defined as weight and/or length persisting below −2 SD

Higher doses of GH used, especially in most severe growth retardation.

(See dosing information, pp. 416-417.)

Appropriate nutritional intake

Early neurodevelopmental evaluation and intervention are warranted in at-risk children.

Nursing Considerations

Adverse events for GH treatment not more common in this population. (See Nursing Considerations for GHD, p. 159.)

Children born SGA may have risk for metabolic disorders especially in presence of other risk factors for metabolic disorders: weight gain, ethnicity, family history.

Early identification and intervention utilizing general pediatric guidelines for obesity and lifestyle intervention

1st year of life, measure length, weight, HC every 3 months then every 6 months for early identification of patients without adequate catch-up growth.

+GH response to treatment

Height velocity >+0.5 SD for first year

Monitor IGF-1 level for dose optimization.

If GH treatment stopped early, will have catch-down growth d/c in adolescence—growth rate <2 cm/year.

If inadequate response, reevaluation needed:
- Consider compliance, GH dose, diagnosis, and decision to d/c treatment.
- Monitor fasting glucose; insulin may ↑ transiently on GH.
- Monitor BMI and rapid weight gain during childhood.
- ↑BMI (17 kg/m^2) at risk of abnormal glucose metabolism in adulthood

(continued)

PITUITARY DISORDERS ⑦

DIAGNOSIS	CLINICAL FINDINGS	DIAGNOSTIC FINDINGS
(Small for Gestational Age)	*Puberty:* • May have early puberty • Rapid progression through puberty, leading to loss of adult height Boys: • Hypospadias • Cryptorchidism more common If rapid weight gain, girls may develop premature adrenarche May have dysmorphic features of Russell-Silver syndrome (see pp. 294-296) Body composition: • ↓ Lean mass • May have ↑ central adiposity • Rapid weight gain in infancy associated with obesity later in life Neurologic: • Cognitive impairment • Worse outcome in patients without catch-up in height or head circumference for gestational age • ↓ Cognition in math or reading comprehension	

MANAGEMENT/EDUCATION	EVALUATION
	Monitor for development of insulin resistance, type 2 diabetes mellitus, and cerebrovascular disease.

DIAGNOSIS	CLINICAL FINDINGS	DIAGNOSTIC FINDINGS

Growth Hormone Deficiency (GHD)

4 : 1 male to female ratio, which may be due to selection bias based on who is referred for short stature evaluation

May be permanent or transient

May be isolated or occur with other pituitary deficiencies

May be acquired or genetic

Pertinent History

In the newborn period, hypoglycemia in the absence of hyper-insulinemia

In the older child, hypo-glycemia accompanied with short stature, usually seen if other pituitary deficiencies present

May have lower than normal energy levels

Emotional immaturity and/or poor school performance

Physical Findings

Severe short stature (height >3 SD below mean, depending on age at diagnosis)

Height disproportion-ately short relative to the mid-parental height

Growth velocity <5% for chronologic age

Growth plot crosses channels on the longitudinal growth curves

"Cherubic" appearance = short, normal, or infantile proportions

(continued)

Laboratory Tests

Normal CBC, sedimen-tation rate, total protein, prealbumin, iron binding protein, electrolytes (including calcium, phosphorus, urinalysis)

IGF-1 low or normal, IGFBP-3 low or normal

In males, testosterone low or normal

GH stimulation testing
Peak GH levels on 2 stimulation tests <10 ng/mL. (See section on stimulation testing for use of agents.)

Hypothyroidism must be corrected prior to screening for GHD because it can decrease GH production.

In the first week of life, serum GH levels are higher than later in life, therefore a random low sample (<10 ng/mL) is suggestive for GH deficiency.

(continued)

MANAGEMENT/EDUCATION	EVALUATION

Medications

Growth Hormone Therapy (GHT)
(See medication section for dosing considerations.)

In panhypopituitarism, GHT treatment is usually lifelong.

GnRH analogues in conjunction with GH have been used to arrest adolescent development and allow for prolonged responsiveness to GH.

In patients with hypopituitarism and ACTH deficiency, cortisol must be replaced first; with TSH deficiency and GH deficiency, replace thyroxine prior to starting GH.

Emergency use in newborn with hypoglycemia and ACTH deficiency requiring cortisol and GHT. Adjust dose according to blood glucose, growth patterns, and presence or absence of cushingoid appearance.

Nursing Considerations

Assess appropriateness of medication delivery system.

Verify correct dilution, dosing, and administration technique with patient and caregiver.

In patients with sudden onset hip/knee pain, limp, obtain X-ray of femoral head.

If signs/symptoms of ↑ICP, immediate referral to ophthalmologist

In cases of pseudotumor cerebri, discontinuation of GH usually resolves signs/symptoms. Subsequent restart of therapy at lower dose has been tolerated.

Education

Instruct patient/family to report side effects: ↑ICP, hip/knee pain, limp, hypothyroidism.

Reinforce importance of medication compliance to maximize response.

EVALUATION

Follow-up every 3 months on GH therapy

Include height, weight, sexual development, injection sites, side effects from therapy.

Increase dosage based on ↑weight and responsiveness to treatment.

Thyrotropin deficiency may be revealed during initial phase of GHT.

Obtain baseline TSH, T4, free T4, then in first 3 months of therapy and annually.

Assess glucose and insulin levels every 12 months.

If GnRH analogs are used, LH suppression on GnRH stimulation testing should be achieved.

Assessment of IGF 1 level may be helpful in determining response, calculating correct dose (especially during puberty), assessing compliance, and indicating GHD in adulthood.

(continued)

(continued)

PITUITARY DISORDERS ⑦

DIAGNOSIS	CLINICAL FINDINGS	DIAGNOSTIC FINDINGS
(Growth Hormone Deficiency)	Pudgy child who appears younger than his/her age Delayed eruption of primary and secondary teeth May have midline defects in the head or face (e.g., cleft lip/palate) Delayed sexual development	***Hypopituitarism*** ↓ GH, ↓ cortisol, ↓ glucose, ↓ insulin in newborn period GH <10 ng/mL, cortisol <21 μg/dL in the presence of glucose levels <40 mg/dL during insulin-induced or spontaneous hypoglycemia *May have decreased secretion of insulin antagonists, GH, and cortisol, making the individual more sensitive to actions of insulin* **Radiologic Studies** Bone age delayed MRI of the brain and pituitary gland normal or may show any of the following: • Ectopic neurohypophysis • Pituitary stalk dysgenesis • Hypoplasia or aplasia of the anterior pituitary gland • Empty sella syndrome • Pituitary or hypothalamic tumor If pituitary stalk abnormalities, ↑ risk of developing other hormone deficits

MANAGEMENT/EDUCATION	EVALUATION

Hypopituitarism
Stress importance of continuing daily injections in times of intercurrent illness as well as increasing dosage of oral glucocorticoids during illness.

Patients with panhypopituitarism should wear a medical alert bracelet at all times.

Bone age evaluation every 6-12 months once puberty begins in order to assess epiphyseal closure.

Transition to Adult

Children with idiopathic GHD with isolated/MPHD: evaluate GHD by provocative testing

Discontinue GH 1 month before reevaluation of GH/IGF-1 axis.

(See diagnostic testing, management, and evaluation for AGHD, pp. 162-163.)

DXA scan for BMD

Benefit of ↑ BMD by continuing GH treatment after epiphyseal closure

Evaluate pituitary function (T4, cortisol, and/or testing of adrenal reserve) and gonadal function if symptoms of deficiency occur.

In isolated GH deficiency, evaluate need for GH as adult with IGF-1 levels, bone density scan, and lipid profile.

Assess for biologic changes and psychosocial problems that occur as a part of adult GH deficiency.

PITUITARY DISORDERS

7

DIAGNOSIS	CLINICAL FINDINGS	DIAGNOSTIC FINDINGS
Adult Growth Hormone Deficiency (AGHD)	**Pertinent History** May have history of childhood GHD related to genetic mutations. Congenital malformations of the pituitary region or structures of the brain, pituitary tumors (adenomas and craniopharyngiomas most common), infiltrative diseases Reduced exercise capacity May have reduced quality of life associated with depression, anxiety, reduced energy, impairment of memory and concentration, and social isolation **Physical Findings** Reduced lean body mass and musculature ↑ Body fat (abdominal and visceral) Truncal obesity May have hypertension Impairment in cardiac function	**Laboratory Tests** GH stimulation testing, arginine-GHRH, and ITT have good sensitivity and specificity—peak response <5 ng/mL In MPHD, probability of GHD is high IGF-1 and IGFBP-3 low If IGF-1 normal, stimulation testing needed for diagnosis Alterations in lipid profile (↑ serum cholesterol) Presence of insulin resistance Bone mineral density normal to low ↑ Osteopenia—most severe in patients <30 years of age Severity of GHD correlates with severity of osteopenia Echocardiography: ↓ LV, posterior wall, and interventricular thickness

Medications

GHT:
- Dosing is lower than in childhood-onset, since normal GH levels are reduced in adults.
- Dosing should be individualized and not weight based, starting at low doses and titrating up
- Need to take age, sex, and estrogen status into consideration.
- See medication section for dosing, pp. 416-417.

Replacement of other deficient hormones when clinically indicated:
- Estrogen
- Testosterone
- Levothyroxine
- Cortisol

Hypothalamic-pituitary adrenal axis should be reassessed during GH treatment.

Education

Adults are more susceptible than children to side effects of GH.

Instruct patients on adverse effects:
- Fluid retention
- Joint and muscle stiffness/pain
- Swelling of extremities
- Paresthesias
- Carpal tunnel syndrome

Instruct patients that clinical benefits may not become apparent until 6 months of therapy.

Counseling and assessment of support systems are essential, since GHD adults are at risk for social isolation, depression, and poor self-perception.

Follow-up every 1-2 months initially until maintenance doses achieved, then every 6 months.

Assess for side effects: most common are edema of hands and feet, arthralgias, myalgias, muscle stiffness, paresthesias.

Measure IGF-1 level.

Dosage is titrated according to clinical response, IGF-1 level, and side effects.

Most adverse effects resolve with dose reduction or temporary discontinuation of GH.

Monitor lipid profile, fasting glucose annually.

Monitor thyroid function, cortisol levels.

Baseline DXA scan: If abnormal, repeat every 1 to 2 years to evaluate need for additional treatment modalities.

(continued)

DIAGNOSIS	CLINICAL FINDINGS	DIAGNOSTIC FINDINGS
(Adult Growth Hormone Deficiency)		
Organic Growth Hormone Deficiency (Acquired GHD)	**Pertinent History** Craniopharyngioma, head trauma, infection of the CNS, infiltrative diseases of hypothalamus, irradiation to the CNS, nasopharyngeal or intracranial tumors Major and minor midline defects (holoprosencephaly, anencephaly, septic optic dysplasia) Headaches, symptoms of ↑intracranial pressure Signs of diabetes insipidus **Physical Findings** Growth: an abrupt slowing or deviation of normal pattern Deficit in visual fields or signs of ↑intracranial pressure *(continued)*	**Laboratory Tests** In congenital malformations of hypothalamus, neonatal plasma GH levels are low. In acquired GHD, GH levels ,10 ng/mL on stimulation testing; may also have normal response to stimulation with blunted response on spontaneous GH secretion **Radiologic Studies** MRI findings range from complete absence of anterior pituitary gland to malformations of the gland, empty sella syndrome, craniopharyngioma, Rathke or arachnoid cleft cyst, pituitary adenoma. *(continued)*

MANAGEMENT/EDUCATION	EVALUATION

Nursing Considerations

GH therapy is contraindicated in presence of active malignancy.

In patients with diabetes mellitus, antidiabetic medications may require adjustments.

Hypopituitary patients on thyroid hormone may need dose adjustments based on free T4 levels.

GH therapy

Treat other hormone deficiencies.

In complete absence of anterior pituitary gland, early diagnosis and treatment of adrenal insufficiency and pituitary function necessary to prevent neonatal mortality

Education

Instruct patient and family that hormone replacement therapy (HRT) is life-sustaining and should not be interrupted.

(See section on GH management, pp. 158-161.)

(Refer to GH evaluation section, pp. 158-161.)

Transition to Adult

↑Likelihood of permanent GHD—MPHD, low IGF-1 with one or more:
- Congenital defect in sellar/suprasellar region
- Genetic mutation
- Known hypothalamic/pituitary disease
- Previous surgery
- Irradiation
- Genetic/molecular mutation

Congenital and genetic do not revert to normal GH status.

If IGH-1 is low after 1 month off GH, no provocative testing is needed for documentation of continued deficiency.

Discontinue GH therapy for 1 month before reevaluation.

PITUITARY DISORDERS

DIAGNOSIS	CLINICAL FINDINGS	DIAGNOSTIC FINDINGS
(Organic Growth Hormone Deficiency)	Presence of facial dysmorphism as in holoprosencephaly; cyclopia to hyper-telorism; cleft lip/palate; single, central incisor	If MRI shows defects, higher risk for developing multiple hormone deficiencies
Severe Primary Insulin-like Growth Factor-1 Deficiency (IGFD) (growth hormone insensitivity [GHI] syndrome) GHI caused by: • GH receptor defect • Abnormalities of GH-GHR signal transduction • GHR signaling defects (JAK/STAT) • IGF-1 gene deletions or mutations • Defects of IGF-1 synthesis • Defects of ALS synthesis • Inactivating mutations of the IGF-1 gene (bioactive IGF-1)	**Pertinent History** Growth failure from birth No previous history of malnutrition, chronic disease, pituitary tumors History of hypoglycemia History of chronic pulmonary infections History of recurrent herpes zoster, chronic eczema, hemorrhagic varicella (Stat5B gene deletion) **Clinical Findings** Represents a spectrum of phenotypes depending on biochemical and genetic defects Normal or small at birth with progressive post-natal growth failure, range <-2 to -12 SD[8] Small head circumference Small jaw *(continued)*	**Laboratory Tests** Normal or elevated GH levels to stimulation testing IGF-1 ≤ -3 SD May have ↑ prolactin (Stat5B gene deletion) May have presence of GH antibodies (GH gene deletion) IGFBP-3, ALS very low; GHBP low or normal Absent to minimal increase in IGF-1 after GH administration Genetic testing for gene defects in the GH/IGF-1 axis **Radiologic Studies** Bone age delayed

MANAGEMENT/EDUCATION	EVALUATION

Medications

rhIGF-1 treatment

(See medication section for dosing, p. 398.)

rhIGF-1 must be given with snack and/or meals.

Cannot be expected to respond adequately to exogenous GH treatment

Nursing Considerations

Verify correct dosing and administration technique with patient/caregiver.

In patients with sudden onset of hip/knee pain or limp, obtain x-ray of femoral head to rule out SCFE.

If signs/symptoms of ↑ ICP, immediate referral to ophthalmologist

Education

Instruct patient and family to report possible adverse events:
- Hypoglycemia
- Headache
- Tonsillar hypertrophy
- Site reactions
- Lipohypertrophy or pain
- Redness or bruising
- Limping
- Hip or knee pain

Monitor height, weight, growth response every 3 months.

Maintain appropriate dose for weight at each visit to maximize growth response.

Important to increase rhIGF-1 dose initially to maintenance dose, because growth response is dose dependent.

Preprandial glucose monitoring can be considered at initiation of treatment until well tolerated dose reached

If hypoglycemia occurs despite adequate food intake, ↓ dose.

(continued)

DIAGNOSIS	CLINICAL FINDINGS	DIAGNOSTIC FINDINGS
(Severe Primary Insulin-like Growth Factor-1 Deficiency)	Prominent forehead, frontal bossing Hypoplastic nasal bridge May have intellectual impairment (IGF-1 gene deletion) Hypoglycemia (30% or more of patients) Microphallus Sensorineural hearing loss (IGF-1 gene deletion)	
Septo-optic Dysplasia (DeMorsier's Syndrome)	Extent of anatomic and functional abnormalities varies. **Pertinent History** Decreased maternal age **Physical Findings** Growth failure, eye anomalies (pendular nystagmus, coloboma of the iris, hypoplastic optic disks), impaired vision, blind (severe cases), micropenis, delayed puberty, although true precocious puberty may also occur.	Hypoglycemia in the newborn period GH testing shows GHD. May or may not have accompanying ACTH, TSH, FSH/LH deficiencies, diabetes insipidus MRI of the brain and pituitary gland shows an absence or hypoplasia of the septum pellucidum or corpus callosum, and absence or hypoplasia of the optic chiasm or optic nerves.

MANAGEMENT/EDUCATION	EVALUATION
Instruct parents on signs/symptoms of hypoglycemia.	
Instruct patients/parents on importance of taking only with meals and not to take more than one dose at a time to make up for missed doses.	
Reinforce importance of medication compliance to maximize growth response.	
In presence of other pituitary hormone deficiencies, cortisol should be replaced first; thyroxine should also be replaced prior to the start of GH therapy to obtain proper growth and avoid adrenal crisis.	
(See GH, ACTH, TSH, FSH/LH, and DI sections for management and evaluation, pp. 158-161, 180-190.)	

7

PITUITARY DISORDERS

OVERGROWTH/TALL STATURE: GROWTH HORMONE EXCESS

DIAGNOSIS	CLINICAL FINDINGS	DIAGNOSTIC FINDINGS
## Sotos' Syndrome Cerebral gigantism Mutation of the nuclear reception SET domain-containing protein 1 (NSD1) in the majority of patients Mostly sporadic occurrence, some familial (autosomal dominant) cases reported	### Pertinent History Feeding problems and irritability in neonatal period Delay in developmental milestones Intellectual impairment, IQ 70-75 History of consanguinity In utero and postnatal overgrowth ### Physical Findings Birth length exceeds +2 SD in 85% of neonates. Birth weights do not exceed +2 SD. Rapid linear growth in first year of childhood; HC, height, and weight are increased compared with norms. In adults, HC remains enlarged, height/weight move toward mean or upper normal. Abnormal body proportions, arm span > height by 5 cm or less Facies: • Sparse frontotemporal hair • Prominent forehead *(continued)*	### Laboratory Tests Diagnosis is made on the clinical presentation. There are no definitive laboratory findings. GH and IGF-1 levels are normal. ### Radiologic Studies Bone age: • Advanced by 1 to 2 years • Premature epiphyseal fusion CT scan: Mild dilation of cerebral ventricles

MANAGEMENT/EDUCATION	EVALUATION
Medical management to modify final height may be considered in extreme cases.	Monitor growth and body proportions.
Management focuses on treatment of behavioral and developmental disabilities.	Final height exceeds target height in males by 11 cm and in females by 6 cm.
Early intervention to improve level of motor and intellectual function	Poor prognosis for normal adult intellectual development.
	No specific tumor screening has been developed, but need to monitor for development of tumors.
	Assess for associated anomalies.

PITUITARY DISORDERS

7

DIAGNOSIS	CLINICAL FINDINGS	DIAGNOSTIC FINDINGS
(Sotos' Syndrome)	• Downward-slanting palpebral fissures • Pointed mandible • Dolichocephaly • Macrocephaly • High, arched palate • Hypertelorism • Prominent ears, jaw, chin Neurologic: • Mental retardation • Motor incoordination May have early puberty May exhibit aggressive behavior Anomalies of CV: • PDA • ASD Anomalies of GU and CNS: • Ventricular dilation • Hypoplasia of the corpus callosum • Septo-optic dysplasia (SOD) • Enlarged extracerebral fluid spaces, which can be associated with seizures 2%-4% risk for tumor development: • Teratoma • Wilms tumor • Neuroblastoma hepatocellular carcinoma	

MANAGEMENT/EDUCATION	EVALUATION

DIAGNOSIS	CLINICAL FINDINGS	DIAGNOSTIC FINDINGS
Growth Hormone Excess (acromegaly or pituitary gigantism) A rare syndrome in childhood Takes 15-20 years to diagnose in many cases	**Pertinent History** History of oligomenorrhea/amenorrhea, sleep apnea, sleep disturbances McCune-Albright syndrome Headaches History of excessive sweating, glucose intolerance, diabetes, arthritis **Physical Findings** Rapid rate of linear growth, with stature >midparental height, and continued growth when deceleration is expected; occurs before epiphyseal fusion Hypertension Clinical signs of acromegaly occur with increasing GH hypersecretion duration: Skin: • Thickening of subcutaneous tissue (cutis verticis gyrata) resulting in enlarged hands and feet • Heel pad thickening • Prominent nasolabial fold	**Laboratory Tests** GH levels may be normal or ↑ (20 × normal). ↑IGF-1, IGFBP-3 for age and gender Prolactin may be normal or ↑ (if cosecreting tumor). ↑GHRH in patients with extopic secretion, normally not found in peripheral blood OGTT—inability to suppress GH to <1 ng/mL Evaluate pituitary hormone function. Assess visual fields. **Radiologic Studies** MRI of the pituitary in 99% of cases reveals pituitary adenomas. MRI of the body may be necessary if no pituitary abnormality, to exclude the possibility of an ectopic GHRH-producing tumor of pancreas or elsewhere (1% of cases).

(continued)

Primary Management

Transsphenoidal surgery for removal of tumor

Refer to pituitary center for neurosurgical consult and management.

If procedure is unsuccessful or cannot be attempted, radiation can be considered.

Medical Therapy

Somatostatin analogs

Dopamine agonists

GHR antagonist

Nursing Considerations

Provide counseling and offer support services to those with physical deformities and psychologic problems associated with untreated and partially treated patients.

Long-term therapy and follow-up is necessary.

Instruct patients on expected side effects of medications.

Monitor BP each visit since Na$^+$ retention from excess GH levels may lead to hypertension.

Tumor should be followed by serial MRI.

Monitor IGF-1, GH levels periodically to assess effectiveness of medical treatment since mortality rate is related to control GH/IGF-1 hypersecretion

Monitor insulin, glucose levels, and signs of insulin resistance (10% of acromegalics develop type 2 diabetes).

Evaluate for respiratory problems, the leading cause of death.

DIAGNOSIS	CLINICAL FINDINGS	DIAGNOSTIC FINDINGS
(Growth Hormone Excess)	• Coarse facial features • May have increase in birthmarks or skin tags Vision: • Loss of visual acuity • Narrowing of visual fields Bone: • Prominence of jaw resulting in malocclusion • Large frontal sinus resulting in frontal bossing • Increased spine with barrel chest • Complaints of joint pain Respiratory difficulties from obstruction from thickened subcutaneous tissue leading to sleep apnea Cardiovascular changes include cardiomyopathy with thickening of the left ventricle. • Visceromegaly	

MANAGEMENT/EDUCATION	EVALUATION

DIAGNOSIS	CLINICAL FINDINGS	DIAGNOSTIC FINDINGS
Familial Tall Stature	**Pertinent History** Family history of tall stature Onset of puberty tends to follow family pattern. **Physical Findings** Height >2 SD above the mean Length may be normal at birth, tall stature evident by 3 to 4 years of age. Normal body proportions	**Laboratory Tests** GH, IGF-1, IGFBP-3 levels in upper range of normal **Radiologic Studies** Bone age: varies, may be advanced or equivalent to chronologic age

MANAGEMENT/EDUCATION	EVALUATION

Medications

Therapy reserved for extreme cases due to its potential risks

Goal to accelerate puberty and cause early epiphyseal closure

Optimal to start prior to onset of puberty

In females, estrogen with added progesterone therapy until evidence of epiphyseal fusion

In males, testosterone has been used in reducing final height.

Recommendations for therapy include final height predictions in boys >198 cm and in girls >183 cm.

Must rule out the diagnosis of obesity, which is associated with rapid skeletal growth and an early onset of puberty

Nursing Considerations

In some cases, individual or family psychotherapy is needed.

Education

With family history of tall stature, provide reassurance and support.

Estrogen treatment: Discuss with patient and family adverse effects of therapy (nausea, weight gain, edema, hypertension).

In the initial phases of treatment, will have accelerated growth

Final height attainment consistent with height attained by family members

Expected outcome in prepubertal girls on estrogen therapy: 5 to 6 cm less than predicted adult height

7

PITUITARY DISORDERS

ADRENOCORTICOTROPIC HORMONE (ACTH)

DIAGNOSIS	CLINICAL FINDINGS	DIAGNOSTIC FINDINGS
Idiopathic Isolated ACTH Deficiency	**Pertinent History** Congenital malformation of the pituitary gland Head trauma at birth or later in life that resulted in hypopituitarism Hypothalamic tumors Craniopharyngiomas Irradiation of a brain tumor Congenital malformations of the brain such as midline defects that result in a CRH deficiency Hemochromatosis, sarcoidosis CNS infections Prolonged high-dose corticosteroid use **Physical Findings** Hypoglycemia Girls with isolated ACTH deficiency may have scant pubic hair at puberty.	**Laboratory Tests** Includes plasma ACTH, cortisol performed simultaneously, 24-hour urine free cortisol, stimulation testing for ACTH reserve ↓ Corticotropin (ACTH) (See lab section for handling and processing ACTH.) Hypoglycemia may be present Low to low-normal Cortisol (8 AM): >20 μg/dL excludes adrenal insufficiency, does not assess ACTH reserve. 24-hour urine free cortisol Stimulation testing for ACTH reserve Cosyntropin 1 μg test is helpful in diagnosing mild adrenal insufficiency. Insulin-induced hypoglycemia (also used for GH reserve): cortisol levels >20 μg/dL in presence of glucose level <40 μg/dL indicate normal response. If levels ↓, corticotropin deficiency is present. (See Chapter 12 for further stimulation testing.) *(continued)*

Medications

Glucocorticoid replacement

If basal cortisol levels are low, maintenance and stress glucocorticoid therapy is required. When basal cortisol levels are normal, only stress therapy may be needed.

Patients with panhypopituitarism most likely require stress oral glucocorticoid therapy.

In ACTH and GH deficiency, the lowest dose of hydrocortisone (max 10 mg/m^2) should be used to avoid impairment of GHT response.

In patients with deficiency of both TSH and ACTH, cortisol replacement should be initiated prior to thyroxine replacement to avoid precipitation of adrenal crisis.

In patients receiving glucocorticoid therapy at a greater than replacement dose for longer than 4 weeks, suppression of CRH and ACTH is expected. Oral, topical, ophthalmologic, and inhaled gluco-corticoids can cause partial or complete suppression. This may be diagnosed if there is hypoglycemia with a 1 μg ACTH stimulation test. Suppression may last up to 6 months in 90% of patients.

Treatment during times of stress may be required at doses of two to three times replacement level.

Education

(Refer to the adrenal section on pp. 38-39 for further management.)

(See Secondary Adrenocortical Deficiency, p. 39, for evaluation.)

It is important to check the function of all pituitary hormones.

7

PITUITARY DISORDERS

DIAGNOSIS	CLINICAL FINDINGS	DIAGNOSTIC FINDINGS
(Idiopathic Isolated ACTH Deficiency)		MRI of the head may show cause of hypopituitarism

GONADOTROPINS

Gonadotropin Deficiency

Familial or sporadic

Isolated or with multiple hormone deficiencies (Kallman's syndrome: see Syndromes chapter for further discussion.)

May be difficult to predict the gonadotropin status before the individual has reached a skeletal age of 13-14 years

Pertinent History

Males more commonly affected

Midline defects

Hyperprolactinemia

Anorexia nervosa

Infertility, menstrual disorders, or amenorrhea

GH, ACTH, TSH deficiencies

Physical Findings

Growth: appropriate height for age, eunuch-oid body proportions

Impaired olfaction (Kallman's syndrome)

Genitalia:
- Small
- May have unde-scended testes
- Small phallus
- Microphallus in newborn period

Absence of sexual characteristics

May have normal adrenarche

Laboratory Tests

FSH/LH levels same as prepubertal children with exception of absent nocturnal gonadotropin pulse

Low estradiol (similar to follicular phase of menstrual cycle)

Testosterone levels in prepubertal range

Skeletal age: 13-14 years—basal FSH/LH levels <1.0 IU/L

Suspect pubertal-aged GHD patients who show minimal or no LH and/or FSH response to GnRH.

Radiologic Studies

MRI of brain and pituitary gland

Medications

Testosterone replacement therapy in males and estrogen-progestin therapy in females (See pp. 386-387, 420-421.)

Initiation of therapy: Microphallus—testosterone therapy during infancy
- *In boys:* bone age of 13 years or no change in bone age for 1 year
- *In girls:* bone age between 11.5 and 12.5 years or growth rate <3 cm/year

Nursing Considerations

Consider the child's psychologic need to develop sexually at same time as peers and the effects of sex hormones on bone maturation and final height.

Follow-up every month

Evaluate height, weight, sexual development.

May see every 2 weeks for testosterone injections

Clinical exam is usually evidence of sexual development and response to treatment.

May check testosterone/ estradiol annually

PITUITARY DISORDERS

DIAGNOSIS	CLINICAL FINDINGS	DIAGNOSTIC FINDINGS
TSH—Thyroid/ Secondary Deficiency Occurs late in course of hypopituitarism	**Pertinent History** Malaise, lack of energy, increased sleeping, constipation Gonadotropin, ACTH deficiency **Physical Findings** Poor growth; weight gain; cool, dry skin; coarse, dry hair	**Laboratory Tests** ↓T4 and TSH TRH stimulation test: ↓TSH and ↓T4 response In hypothalamic hypothyroidism, a delayed, exaggerated peak of TSH is demonstrated with TRH stimulation.

PROLACTIN

Hyperprolactin- emia	**Pertinent History** In females, menstrual dysfunction and infertility Males may have impotence and decreased sexual libido. Increased estrogens as in pregnancy, oral contraceptives, brain infections or tumors Use of drugs that effect action or release of dopamine (Risperdal, Reglan, Prozac) *(continued)*	**Laboratory Tests** ↑Prolactin: >200-250 μg/L, prolactinoma Mildly ↑(25 μg/L) indicative of stress response and should be repeated Cortisol, testosterone, estrogens **Radiologic Studies** MRI may reveal prolactinomas or other tumors of the pituitary gland.

MANAGEMENT/EDUCATION	EVALUATION

Medications

Levothyroxine replacement therapy

Adjust dose according to clinical response, maintaining T4, free T4, T3 levels in the middle to upper range of normal.

Nursing Considerations

Patients should be evaluated for ACTH deficiency before start of levothyroxine therapy to avoid precipitation of adrenal crisis.

In accompanied GH deficiency, replace thyroxine before start of GH.

(See pp. 218-222 for further evaluation and management.)

Monitor T4, free T4

TSH not useful once diagnosis of TSH deficiency is made

Follow-up depends on age at diagnosis:
- <12 months: see initially at 1 week, 1 month, then every 3-4 months until age 3 years.
- 1-3 years: see initially at 1-2 months, then every 3-4 months until age 3 years.
- 3-18 years: see initially at 1-3 months, then every 4-6 months.

Medications

Bromocriptine, cabergoline (to inhibit prolactin production)

Surgery may be necessary if tumor present.

Radiation therapy if medication or surgery is not effective

Replace with thyroxine in cases of primary hypothyroidism.

In medical management, normal to low level of prolactin should be achieved.

Persistent abnormal prolactin levels after surgical removal of microadenoma could be due to incomplete removal of tumor, abnormal function of pituitary gland, hypothalamic abnormalities.

DIAGNOSIS	CLINICAL FINDINGS	DIAGNOSTIC FINDINGS
(Hyperprolactinemia)	May be associated with multiple ovarian cysts, weight gain, acne, primary hypothyroidism, and hirsutism Exercise—female avid runners with amenorrhea Galactorrhea may or may not be present. Tactile stimulus **Physical Findings** Delayed puberty or lack of pubertal development Galactorrhea may or may not be present.	

POSTERIOR PITUITARY (Neurohypophysis)

The posterior pituitary is composed of the median eminence, the pituitary stalk, and the posterior pituitary lobe; it is highly vascularized, thus facilitating diffusion of hormones. The posterior pituitary acts as the site of the hypophyseal portal system, which transports releasing hormones to the anterior pituitary. Hypophysectomy may not affect secretion of these hormones, which will decrease for a time but may return to normal.

ADH/AVP—VASOPRESSIN

DIAGNOSIS	CLINICAL FINDINGS	DIAGNOSTIC FINDINGS
Diabetes Insipidus (DI) ADH deficiency Excretes large volume of urine Increased thirst	**Pertinent History** Most commonly seen with: • Vasopressin deficiency or resistance • Primary renal disease • Head injury *(continued)*	*Symptoms of polyuria and polydipsia:* Perform fasting urine (second morning void, NPO after 2400); obtain serum sample immediately after urine. *(continued)*

MANAGEMENT/EDUCATION	EVALUATION

MANAGEMENT/EDUCATION	EVALUATION

Medications

Vasopressin (PO or intranasal) or chlorpropamide
(if anterior pituitary intact)

During acute phase:
- Hospitalization with frequent monitoring of urine specific gravity
- IV fluids (400-600 mL/m²/day + urine output)

(continued)

Monitor electrolytes

Assess neurologic status; watch for lethargy or ↑ sleep

Strict intake/output during acute phase

(continued)

DIAGNOSIS	CLINICAL FINDINGS	DIAGNOSTIC FINDINGS
(Diabetes Insipidus)	• Neurosurgery • CNS tumor • History of histiocytosis • Congenital malformations (septo-optic dysplasia) • Infection • Idiopathic **Physical Findings** *Infants:* • Failure to thrive • Unexplained fevers • Vomiting • Constipation • Poor growth • Hypertonicity • Poor nutrition *Older children:* • Recent onset excessive thirst • Nocturia • New onset enuresis • Distended bladder • Polyuria (often >2 L/d) • Lethargy • Sleepiness With history of headache, watch for ocular signs (visual field restriction, optic atrophy, strabismus, nystagmus, papilledema).	Send urine for osmolality, creatinine, calcium, potassium. Send serum for osmolality, sodium, creatinine, calcium, potassium, and vasopressin. Serum osmolality >287 mOsm/L and a simultaneous urine osmolity <200 mOsm/L Urine osmolality of 200-400 mOsm/kg suggests primary or secondary renal disease. If urine dilute (<200 mOsm/kg) and hypertonic and hypernatremic, obtain plasma vasopressin level and the urine and serum osmolality response to exogenous vasopressin. ***Urine*** Hypotonic Polyuria not seen if due to hypothalamic disease ↓ Specific gravity

(continued)

MANAGEMENT/EDUCATION	EVALUATION
• Strict intake/output • Twice-daily weights	Check urine for glucose (not present in DI).

Nursing Considerations

Remember to adjust therapy for times of high fluid intake (newborn period, early infancy, or with IV fluids).

Fluids as needed for thirst, with extra water during night (ice water preferred)

Dehydration occurs quickly if access to water is denied.

Avoid diets high in protein and salt.

Children in school need access to water and toilet facilities, including ability to leave classroom.

Educate family on measuring intake/output and specific gravity and on administering medication.

Daily or twice-daily weights

Specific gravity every void

May need daily office visit initially to monitor hydration status

Thereafter, follow up every 6 months to monitor weight gain and linear growth.

With acquired DI, need MRI at regular intervals to assess hypothalamic tumors and infiltrative processes.

7

PITUITARY DISORDERS

DIAGNOSIS	CLINICAL FINDINGS	DIAGNOSTIC FINDINGS
(Diabetes Insipidus)		**Blood (electrolytes, glucose, calcium, urea, creatinine)** Hypertonicity and hypernatremia **Neurohypophyseal disease** If symptoms relieved by vasopressin **Nephrogenic DI** If no response to vasopressin ↓K, ↑Ca consider diagnosis other than primary vasopressin deficiency May need formal water deprivation test (see p. 279) MRI, skull films, biopsy of maculopapular skin rash if present to confirm etiology May need to test primary relatives

MANAGEMENT/EDUCATION	EVALUATION

PITUITARY DISORDERS

DIAGNOSIS	CLINICAL FINDINGS	DIAGNOSTIC FINDINGS
Nephrogenic DI Normal or ↑ADH production but lacks normal renal ADH response High morbidity and mortality	**Pertinent History** Usually familial: • X-linked trait • Receptors nonfunctional • History of maternal polyuria, and with males, polyhydramnios Newborn males: • Okay until weaning begun or solids added **Physical Findings** Infection; rapid deterioration Slow failure to thrive Initially, unexplained fever, severity of dehydration often underestimated due to high urine output Mental impairment due to ischemic injury from dehydration End-stage renal insufficiency due to ↑intravesical pressure	Urine flow will not ↓ with ADH. ↑ Na >160 mmol/L ↓ Urine osmolality ↑ Urine volume If ADH administered, ↓ urine volume and ↑ osmolality
Psychogenic DI Compulsive water drinkers		Will respond to ADH administration

MANAGEMENT/EDUCATION	EVALUATION
Excretion of solute residue amounting to ≤600 mOsm/m/day requires 6 L water and at least another L/m/day to cover extra renal water losses.	Monitor electrolytes closely.
Infants and children become rapidly dehydrated if unable to drink or denied access to water.	Daily weights
Breast-feeding is ideal.	Specific gravity
If breast-feeding is not possible, dilute cow's milk with water and add carbohydrates and fat, or use low renal solute residue formula alternately with plain water or 2% glucose water with ↑ frequency of feedings.	May need to be seen in clinic every day until stable

Medications

Thiazide diuretics (also furosemide and amiloride) have paradoxic action and improve water economy.

Prostaglandin synthetase inhibitors (indomethacin, acetylsalicylic acid, or tolmetin) used with a thiazide will help reduce water turnover.

If fluids withheld, still produce excessive urine volume and dilution

If fluids withheld, ↑ ADH secretion; ↓ urinary flow; ↑ osmolality

PITUITARY DISORDERS 7

DIAGNOSIS	CLINICAL FINDINGS	DIAGNOSTIC FINDINGS
Syndrome of Inappropriate Secretion of Antidiuretic Hormone (SIADH) ↑ ADH concentrations relative to plasma osmolality	**Pertinent History** Usually caused by trauma, IV therapy, infections, CNS tumors, surgery near hypothalamus or pituitary gland May have pulmonary etiology **Physical Findings** ↓ Urine output ↑ Specific gravity Normal water consumption Hypervolemia, water retention, weight gain, nausea, vomiting, headaches, malaise Brain edema due to rapid changes in systemic osmolality Severe signs: disorientation, confusion, coma, and seizures	**Laboratory Tests** ↓ Na ↓ Serum osmolality ↑ Urine osmolality If water restricted, serum Na and osmolality will return to normal. If serum Na falls acutely to 130 mOsm/kg during inappropriately rapid infusion of hypotonic solutions, seizures may occur. Acutely presenting neurologic signs require rapid intervention and will be successful if hyponatremia is only partially corrected.

MANAGEMENT/EDUCATION	EVALUATION

Management

Fluid restriction is safest and most efficient therapy.

Correct hyponatremia and hypernatremia slowly and cautiously over 48 hours.

Long-standing hyponatremia: may be as low as 115 mOsm/kg or below and patient relatively asymptomatic; correct very slowly.

Chronic SIADH
Demeclocycline therapy:
• Effective after at least 24 hours of administration
• Dose requires titration
• Urea has also been highly successful.

Acute SIADH
With symptoms of brain swelling, immediate medical attention needed with hospitalization

Anticonvulsants are used to treat seizures if they occur.

Strict intake/output

Daily or twice-daily weights

Monitor serum sodium levels every 4-6 hours.

Vital signs and neurologic status every 2 hours

PITUITARY DISORDERS

RESOURCES

Human Growth Foundation
997 Glen Cove Ave.
Glen Head, NY 11545
1-800-451-6434
http://hgfound.org

Magic Foundation
6645 W. North Ave.
Oak Park, IL 60302
1-800-3-MAGIC-3 OR 1-708-383-0808
FAX 1-708-383-0899
www.magicfoundation.org

Pituitary Foundation
PO Box 1944
Bristol, BS99 2UB, United Kingdom
(0845) 450-0377
www.pituitary.org.uk
E-MAIL *helpline@pituitary.org.uk*

Sotos Syndrome Support Association
PO Box 4626
Wheaton, IL 60189
888-246-7772
www.sotossyndrome.org

Health Facts for You: Hypopituitarism
University of Wisconsin Hospital and Clinics
Patient and Family Education, Suite 300
3330 University Ave.
Madison, WI 53705
1-608-623-8734
FAX 1-608-265-5444
www.uwhealth.org/healthfacts/B_EXTRANET_HEALTH_INFORMATION-FlexMember-Show_Public_HFFY_1126651622794.html

Pituitary Network Association
16350 Ventura Blvd., Suite 231
Encino, CA 91436
1-805-499-2262
FAX 1-805-499-1523
www.pituitary.org

Septo-Optic Dysplasia/Optic Nerve Hypoplasia Support Group
PO Box 1958
Thousand Oaks, CA 91358
1-805-499-9973
FAX 1-805-480-0633
www.focusfamilies.org/focus

8 DISORDERS OF SEXUAL DEVELOPMENT

OVERVIEW

Puberty is the developmental stage during which sexual maturity is completed and reproduction is possible. Disorders of puberty usually refer to the development of secondary sex characteristics either before or after the normal timing of puberty. Normal breast development begins for girls between 7 and 13 years. African American girls can begin breast development as early as 6 years. Menses begins between 12 and 13 years. Testicular development begins for boys between 9 and 14 years of age. During the initial stages of puberty, LH and FSH levels rise. As puberty progresses, LH becomes predominant. Pubertal delay is the absence of onset of puberty by age 14 in girls and age 15 in boys.

HISTORY

HPI/ROS Age of onset of breast development, penile/testicular enlargement or pubic hair; rate of linear growth; (>5 cm/yr); rate/tempo of pubertal progression (rapid or arrested); onset of menses, occurrence of nocturnal emissions, bone age advanced or delayed relative to chronologic age; excessive weight gain; pregnancy and birth (maternal drug ingestion) history; access to exogenous estrogen, testosterone, androgens (oral contraceptive pill [OCP], topical creams), smelling abnormalities

Medical history Hypothyroidism, hyperthyroidism, adrenal insufficiency, diabetes insipidus, congenital adrenal hyperplasia, midline defects, cancer diagnosis followed by irradiation or chemotherapy, head trauma, genetic syndromes, seizure disorders, McCune-Albright syndrome, or testotoxicosis

Family history Age of onset of puberty in parents, siblings; age of menarche of mother; height increase after age 16, father or mother

Social history Abusive or deprived home environment; emotional concerns/teasing due to precocious/delayed development; vulnerability to sexual advances by older peers, family members

PHYSICAL EXAMINATION

Growth Height/weight plotted on growth curve, over past 5 years if available; plot growth velocity

HEENT Midline abnormalities present, dental development ahead or delayed, thyroid enlarged, papilledema of optic nerves

Chest Tanner stage of breast (see p. 200), development/maturity of areola, galactorrhea, presence of gynecomastia in boys

Genitourinary Tanner stage of pubic hair (see p. 200), clitoromegaly, color of vaginal mucosa, character of vaginal discharge, testicular volume and penile size, color and texture of scrotum

Skin Acne; axillary body odor; sebaceous activity; body hair on axilla, chest, abdomen; hyperpigmentation; café au lait spots; dry/cool skin

Neurologic Possible CNS disorders

DIAGNOSIS	CLINICAL FINDINGS	DIAGNOSTIC FINDINGS
Precocious Puberty Puberty that is progressive and occurs earlier than normal for age and race More common in girls (10:1) More common in children adopted from foreign countries	**Pertinent History** Menses <9.5 years Brain abscess or inflammation Hydrocephalus Cancer threapy: chemotherapy, radiation Surgery Trauma (head) **Physical Findings** Accelerated linear growth Increased weight for age *(continued)*	**Laboratory Tests** GnRH stimulation test: LH response dominant over FSH response: LH >10 IU/L Leuprolide acetate stimulation test: LH >8 IU/L IFMA: Basal LH >0.6 IU/L[1] **Radiologic Studies** Bone age shows advancement over chronologic age. Large ovarian cyst or tumor on pelvic ultrasound *(continued)*

DIAGNOSTIC TESTING

Stimulation testing for gonadotropin-releasing hormone (GnRH) (formerly called luteinizing hormone–releasing hormone [LHRH])
Leuprolide stimulation testing
Adrenocorticotropic (ACTH) stimulation testing
Bone age X-ray
Chest X-ray
MRI of brain
Pelvic ultrasound: ovaries, testes, adrenals
Serum T4, free T4, thyroid-stimulating hormone (TSH)
Plasma dehydroepiandrosterone sulfate (DHEA-S), DHEA
Luteinizing hormone (LH), third generation LH assay, follicle-stimulating hormone (FSH), estradiol, testosterone
Prolactin, human chorionic gonadotropin (HCG), sex hormone–binding globulin (SHBG)
Insulin
Chromosomes
DNA methylation testing
IGF-1, IGF-BP3

MANAGEMENT/EDUCATION	EVALUATION
Medications *GnRH agonist therapy options* • Lupron Depot-Ped (intramuscular injection) • Histrelin acetate (subcutaneous injection) • Synarel (nasal spray) • Zoladex (goserelin acetate implant) *McCune-Albright syndrome* Testolactone, ketoconazole, tamoxifen, aromatase inhibitors **Other Treatment** Implant **Nursing Considerations** Final height with and without treatment usually influences family decision for treatment. Once medication is started, the rate of pubertal arrest and linear deceleration is gradual, over 6-12 months. *(continued)*	Determine if pubertal development has stabilized or progressed. May see regression of puberty to earlier stage Repeat GnRH or leuprolide acetate stimulation test during first 1-3 months on therapy and every 6 months thereafter. For boys, plasma testosterone in prepubertal range after 1 month of therapy can indicate adequate suppression. *(continued)*

⑧

DIAGNOSIS	CLINICAL FINDINGS	DIAGNOSTIC FINDINGS
(Precocious Puberty)	Tanner 2 or greater breast development <7-8 years	Possible hypothalamic hamartoma brain tumor/cyst or malformation on MRI scans
	Tanner 2 or greater testicular development/ penile growth <9 years	Possible testicular tumor, adrenal tumor, neurofibromatosis; needs MRI scan to rule out
	Scrotum is reddened and thinner	
	Tanner 2 or greater pubic hair	Rule out McCune-Albright syndrome.
	Vaginal mucosa pink and thicker; secretions clear or whitish	Rule out congenital adrenal hyperplasia, long-term hypothyroid-ism (primary)
	Sebaceous activity on face, comedones, acne	
	Café au lait spots, bone lesions on X-ray show polycystic fibrous dysplasia along with precocious puberty	

MANAGEMENT/EDUCATION	EVALUATION

If treatment shows the potential for significantly limiting final height, may consider adding growth hormone therapy.

No known complications with fertility

Bone mineral density may be checked if long-term therapy is required.

Education

Since risk for sexual advances by others is higher, anticipatory guidance should be offered.

Advise on age-appropriate clothing.

Girls may experience vaginal bleeding (estrogen withdrawal) first 4 weeks of treatment; bleeding after this period is abnormal.

If signs of adrenarche are present, they can remain and possibly progress.

Moodiness and emotional lability should improve.

Masturbation, if present, should decrease.

Compliance with therapy is necessary to keep puberty suppressed

Sterile abscesses are possible side effect of Lupron Depot. Alternative medication should be considered if this occurs.

When treatment is discontinued, generally at normal age for puberty: 12-12.5 yr (bone age) girls, 13-13.5 yr (bone age) boys,[1] puberty should commence within 6-12 months and proceed normally, though tempo may be hastened.

Adequate calcium intake, at least, should be encouraged.

LH can be checked 30-60 minutes after GnRH agonist therapy is administered.

Possible to check suppression with a random LH; expect result to be low

Perform stimulation test just prior to next dose of Lupron Depot.

LH result <2 IU/L. If LH not suppressed, increase LHRH analog dose and/or frequency.

Estradiol <5.0

Testosterone <10.0

Bone age every 6-12 months

Continue treatment until 11 to 11.5 years for girls and until 12 to 12.5 years for boys.

DISORDERS OF SEXUAL DEVELOPMENT

8

DIAGNOSIS	CLINICAL FINDINGS	DIAGNOSTIC FINDINGS
Benign Precocious Thelarche Isolated breast development that occurs earlier than normal in girls Most common <2 years, >6 years	**Pertinent History** Exposure to estrogen preparation No increase in growth velocity **Physical Findings** Unilateral/bilateral breast development without areolar maturation No estrogenization of vaginal mucosa: vagina is red, clear secretions No other signs of puberty present	**Laboratory Tests** Prepubertal GnRH stimulation test: LH <5-10 IU/L FSH > LH Estradiol <5 ng/mL Testosterone <10 ng/mL **Radiologic Studies** Bone age correlates with chronologic age. Bone age should be <+2 SD. Pelvic ultrasound may or may not show ovarian cyst(s).
Benign Precocious Adrenarche Isolated early development of pubic hair in girls <8 years, boys <9 years[1] Rare before age 6 years	**Pertinent History** Usually no increase in growth velocity, although can be greater **Physical Findings** Tanner 2 or greater pubic hair Can be accompanied by axillary hair, body odor, mild acne, and oily skin Tanner 1 breast/phallus No vaginal maturation No virilization: no clitoromegaly; no change in size, color, texture of scrotum Testes 3 cc or less Overweight	**Laboratory Tests** Plasma DHEA or DHEA-S level correlates with stage of pubic hair. **Radiologic Studies** Bone age correlates with chronologic age, or slightly advanced.

MANAGEMENT/EDUCATION	EVALUATION
Watchful waiting every 2-6 months Repeat pelvic ultrasound if ovarian cysts noted. **Education** Reassure family that thelarche is usually self-limiting. Advise on use of loose-fitting clothing. Educate parents on signs of progressing puberty for return to clinic. Reassure that balance of pubertal stages should occur at normal age.	No progression of puberty over time, reassess in 2 months No skeletal advancement by bone age Ovarian cysts resolved
Watchful waiting every 3-6 months; reassess growth velocity and pubertal status each visit. **Education** Reassure family that adrenarche is usually self-limiting. Address privacy concerns for undressing in school, childcare, and locker rooms. Educate parents on signs of progressing puberty for return to clinic. Reassure that balance of pubertal stages should occur at normal age. Educate on increased risk of developing polycystic ovary syndrome later in life.	No progression of pubic hair or puberty over time No skeletal advancement over chronologic age No increase in growth velocity Reassess growth and puberty in 3-6 months.

DISORDERS OF SEXUAL DEVELOPMENT

DIAGNOSIS	CLINICAL FINDINGS	DIAGNOSTIC FINDINGS

Delayed Puberty

No signs of puberty >13 years 11 months in girls, >14 years 11 months in boys

Arrest of pubertal progression at Tanner 2 or 3 for more than 2 years

Female: No menses after 4 years from initiation of puberty or ≥15 years of age

Male: Lack of testicular growth completion after 4 years from onset of puberty

Pertinent History

Prepubertal growth velocity

Growth delay in the family

History of constitutional growth delay

Possibly arrested pubertal progression

Chronic illness such as cystic fibrosis, irritable bowel syndrome, Crohn's disease, undiagnosed type 1 diabetes, cancer diagnosis (pelvic irradiation, chemotherapy) or renal disease; or as result of undernutrition, anorexia, or long-term glucocorticoid therapy

Physical Findings

Tanner 1 breast and pubic hair in girls

Tanner 1 phallus and pubic hair in boys, testes ≤3 cc bilaterally

No maturation of vaginal mucosa or scrotum

No acne, sebaceous activity

No facial hair, little muscle development

Longer limb length due to longer time interval prior to puberty[2]

Short stature for age

Weight possibly less than average for age

Normal breast tissue with scant pubic hair may indicate androgen insensitivity syndrome.

Laboratory Tests

Prepubertal LH values, baseline and stimulated with GnRH stimulation test

Elevated LH, FSH indicates gonadal failure.

A rise in LH over time suggests that delayed puberty is constitutional.

Persistently low LH values over time suggest a hypothalamic or pituitary problem; consider MRI scan.

Hypothyroid (low T4, low free T4, high or low TSH) adolescents will have delayed puberty and poor growth prior to replacement with thyroid hormone.

GHD can cause delayed puberty (stimulated GH values <10 ng/mL)

DNA methylation testing: to diagnose Prader-Willi syndrome

Chromosomal analysis will diagnose Turner syndrome, 45X, Klinefelter syndrome diagnosed 47XXY.

Elevated prolactin level is suggestive of hyperprolactinemia: need MRI scan to rule out microadenoma.

(continued)

(continued)

MANAGEMENT/EDUCATION	EVALUATION

Medications

If boy's chronologic age is 12.5-13 years and bone age is at least 11-12 years, can give low-dose testosterone enanthate or cypionate every 4 weeks, or testosterone gel at low doses; treat for 3-6 months. If girl's chronologic age is 10-12 years and bone age is at least 10-10.5 years, can give low-dose estrogen/ethinyl estradiol/transdermal estrogen for 3-6 months.

Children with Kallmann's syndrome, Prader-Willi syndrome, Klinefelter syndrome, or primary testicular failure require lifelong testosterone or estrogen replacement. Slowly work up to adult replacement of 200 mg intramuscularly every 2 weeks, or equivalent in gel or patch form. Start on small dose of 50-70 mg when bone age is at least 11 years.

Prader-Willi syndrome patients need growth hormone therapy.

Females with primary ovarian failure and Turner syndrome require estrogen replacement: low-dose (0.3 mg every other day conjugated estrogen), or ethinyl estradiol 5 μg daily, or transdermal estrogen (0.025 mg 2/week). Start cycling after 1 year with progesterone 5 mg/day for 10 days each month.[3] Work up to adult dose. Turner syndrome will also need growth hormone therapy.

Hypothyroid adolescents when dosed with thyroid hormone can accelerate puberty and bone age quickly; need to monitor carefully and frequently.

Hyperprolactinemia: bromocriptine, cabergoline, or dopamine agonist

Education

Encourage parents and family to have age-appropriate expectations.

Reassure that linear growth and sexual development will occur, but later than peers.

Encourage sports that do not depend on size or muscle development in patients with delayed puberty.

(continued)

After 3-4 doses of testosterone, assess pubertal stage and testosterone level. If at least Tanner 2, increased growth velocity: most probably constitutional growth delay. Recheck in 6 months.

For adolescent girls, assess breast development/pubic hair and increased growth velocity after 4-6 months of low-dose estrogen.

For long-term replacement, check growth velocity, pubertal progression, LH, estradiol/testosterone level, IGF-1, and bone age to determine when to increase sex steroid dose.

For growth hormone therapy, need to check the same parameters and labs as for long-term replacement above (see also p. 159).

Hypothyroid adolescents receiving thyroid hormone replacement therapy will need thyroid profile 4-6 weeks after start of therapy and after each dose adjustment (dose: 50-75 μg/m^2/day).

Assess pubertal status, growth velocity every 3 months.

Bone age X-ray every 6-12 months

(continued)

DIAGNOSIS	CLINICAL FINDINGS	DIAGNOSTIC FINDINGS
(Delayed Puberty)	Smell test results within normal unless adolescent has Kallmann's syndrome: anosmia; cleft lip, cleft palate, and other midline defects have higher incidence of Kallmann's syndrome If adolescent overweight and has microphallus, almond-shaped eyes, small hands and feet: rule out Prader-Willi syndrome Short stature with poor growth velocity, webbed neck, trident hairline, pigmented nevi, increased carrying angle of arms, low-set posteriorly rotated ears, history of chronic otitis media, high-arched palate, hypoplastic nails Tanner 1-2 breast development and pubic hair, delayed bone age suggestive of Turner syndrome If onset of puberty not delayed but incomplete virilization noted, tall stature, long legs, decreased upper-to-lower segment, low IQ, poor gross motor control, behavior problems, gynecomastia suggest Klinefelter syndrome Short stature, delayed puberty, cardiomyopathy, webbing of neck, low hairline, chest deformity, and valvular pulmonic stenosis suggest Noonan's syndrome.	**Radiologic Studies** Delayed bone age If bone age is <10.5-11 years for girls or <12.5-13 years for boys, it is not possible to assess if LH is delayed or problematic; need to wait until bone age is in pubertal range. May need MRI scan to rule out microadenoma, hyperprolactinoma, anatomic abnormality of the pituitary or hypothalamus

MANAGEMENT/EDUCATION	EVALUATION

Potential side effects of estrogen: blood clots, hypertension, glucose intolerance, moodiness

Hormonal treatment of constitutional delay of puberty is rarely necessary in girls. However, it may be considered for boys or girls in the presence of significant psychologic distress.

Reassure that fertility should not be affected.

Testosterone gel comes in 75 mg pumps; multidosage pump for titration of dose.

Application sites: shoulders, abdomen, upper arms. Only patients should apply.

Testosterone patches 2.5 mg, 5 mg strength; apply in evening.

If puberty progresses too quickly, may need to suppress with GnRH agonist.

Prolactin levels decreasing

Periodic MRI scan: microadenoma stable or decreasing in size, resolving galactorrhea

DISORDERS OF SEXUAL DEVELOPMENT

DIAGNOSIS	CLINICAL FINDINGS	DIAGNOSTIC FINDINGS

Pubertal Gynecomastia

Glandular enlargement >0.5 cm of male breast, unilateral or bilateral

Common, occurs in up to two thirds of boys in puberty[4]

Most common between ages 13-14 years, resolves by age 17 years

Caused by high estrogen-to-free testosterone ratio

Pertinent History

Medications associated with gynecomastia[5,6]:
ACE inhibitors
Amphetamines
  Vasotec
Bicalutamide
Chemotherapy agents
Cimetidine
Digitalis
Estrogens
Finasteride
Flutamide
Growth hormones
Ketoconazole
Marijuana
Methyldopa
Metoclopramide
Penicillamine
Risperidone
Spironolactone
Tricyclic antidepressants

Physical Findings

Tanner 2 or greater breast tissue (palpated as rubbery or firm); may be tender to palpation

Obesity

Normal male external genitalia exam, rule out testicular tumor

No adrenal masses on abdominal exam

Laboratory Tests

Elevated SHGB

Can check HCG, prolactin, estradiol, and LH if gynecomastia worsens

If HCG and/or estradiol elevated, need testicular ultrasound to rule out testicular tumor

If LH elevated, adolescent may have primary hypogonadism, Klinefelter syndrome, or testicular damage

If LH not elevated, may have secondary hypogonadism

Radiologic Studies

If prolactin elevated, obtain brain MRI

If testicular ultrasound negative, obtain chest X-ray looking for germ cell tumor outside testes or may need MRI of adrenal gland to rule out tumor

(continued)

Medications

Medical management for emotionally distraught boys:

- Clomiphene citrate[7]
- Tamoxifen[7]
- Testolactone[7]

Surgery

Surgical removal (using small incision around areolae) of persistent gynecomastia for adolescents who have completed puberty

Nursing Considerations

If history uncovers offending medication or drug, then recommend adolescent stop using or refer to drug rehab.

If no abnormalities found on exam, adolescent should be reassured of resolution within 18-36 months.

If adolescent extremely self-conscious, can recommend psychotherapy or drug therapy

Education

If no abnormalities found on exam, adolescent should be reassured of resolution within 18-36 months.

Recheck adolescent in 6 months.

Reassess emotional distress related to gynecomastia.

Check on patient/family follow-through/ compliance with recommended therapy

If adolescent on medication, need to follow progress every 4-6 months

DISORDERS OF SEXUAL DEVELOPMENT 8

DIAGNOSIS	CLINICAL FINDINGS	DIAGNOSTIC FINDINGS
(Pubertal Gynecomastia)	Assess for signs of feminization, discharge from breast, spider hemangioma, or palmar erythema. Rule out secondary hypogonadism, Klinefelter syndrome, true hermaphroditism, testosterone enzyme defect	
Polycystic Ovary Syndrome Caused by androgen excess from the ovary or adrenals Anovulation/irregular menses	**Pertinent History** Abnormal menstrual patterns Birth history of SGA Hyperinsulinism Previous premature adrenarche increases risk. Type 2 diabetes **Physical Findings** Hirsutism on face, chest, and/or abdomen Acne Obesity Acanthosis nigricans Virilization	**Laboratory Tests** Increased DHEA, DHEA-S Decreased sex steroid-binding globulin (SSBG) Increased testosterone, free testosterone Increased LH (basal) Increased basal LH : FSH ratio Increased LH-to-GnRH stimulation test Increased insulin level Can have elevated glucose, elevated cholesterol, low HDL, elevated LDL, elevated triglycerides[8] Blood pressure may be elevated.

(continued)

MANAGEMENT/EDUCATION	EVALUATION

Medications

Oral contraceptive pills (OCPs) will help to decrease ovarian androgen secretion, decrease free testosterone level. Need to choose low androgen pill and dose (e.g., Ovcon 35, Ortho-Cyclen, or Desogen)

Spironolactone either alone or in combination with OCPs[14]

GnRH analog along with OCPs for 6-12 months[9]

Ortho-Tri-Cyclen for treatment of acne and menstrual cycle regulation

Metformin may be appropriate for type 2 diabetes.

Education

Recommend weight loss to reduce hirsutism and improve insulin level. Refer to dietician for weight reduction planning. Recommend exercise.

Reassure that therapy will take up to 6 months to reduce new hair growth. Present hair growth can be treated with laser therapy, depilatories, electrolysis, or bleaching.

(continued)

Monitor degree of hirsutism and acne.

Recheck DHEA, androstenedione, DHEA-S, SSBG, testosterone, free testosterone, LH, FSH, insulin level in 3 months.

If obese, measure fasting glucose level, lipids, total cholesterol, HDL, LDL, triglycerides.

Monitor degree of weight loss and evaluate weight maintenance.

Insulin level should improve with weight loss.

(continued)

DIAGNOSIS	CLINICAL FINDINGS	DIAGNOSTIC FINDINGS
(Polycystic Ovary Syndrome)	Adrenal disorders, for 3B-HSD deficiency, late onset 21-hydroxylase deficiency Elevated blood pressure	**Radiologic Studies** Pelvic ultrasound may show ovarian cysts.

PATIENT EDUCATION RESOURCES

Benign Premature Adrenarche
www.fpnotebook.com
Choose: Endocrinology → Sexual Development Chapter → Benign Premature Adrenarche
www.medhelp.org
Enter *premature adrenarche* in Search box and click on *Search*

Delayed Puberty
www.childrensnyp.org/mschony
Choose: Health Library → D → Delayed Puberty

Polycystic Ovary Syndrome
www.asrm.org
Choose: Topics Index → Hirsutism → Hirsutism and Polycystic Ovary Syndrome/ Fact Sheets and Info Booklets

emedicine.medscape.com/refarticle/924698-overview

www.pcosupport.org

Gynecomastia
www.livestrong.com/article/107526-gynecomastia-its-treatment/

Turner Syndrome
www.turnersyndrome.org
www.hgfound.org

MANAGEMENT/EDUCATION	EVALUATION

Reassure that menstrual periods should become more regular.

Will need to be followed by an adult endocrinologist for insulin and lipid levels and weight monitoring

Advise overweight patients on risk of developing type 2 diabetes.

Advise on high risk of developing metabolic syndrome, infertility, possibly endometrial cancer.[10]

Transition to Adulthood

Recommend long-term follow-up by an adult endocrinologist for insulin and lipid levels and weight monitoring.

DISORDERS OF SEXUAL DEVELOPMENT

⑨ THYROID DISORDERS

OVERVIEW

Thyroid disease can present through laboratory tests, physical examination, and/or medical history. The thyroid gland produces hormones thyroxine (T4) and triiodothyronine (T3), which stimulate metabolism in all body tissues and promote growth. Function of the thyroid gland is regulated through a negative feedback system. Thyroid-stimulating hormone (TSH) is stored in the pituitary and can be released by stimulation from the hypothalamus hormone, thyrotropin-releasing hormone (TRH).

Signs and symptoms of thyroid disease vary with each patient. It is important to record a detailed subjective history at each visit. An assessment and evaluation of administration of drug therapy should be elicited from the patient and family. Diagnosis of thyroid disease is frequently made not from specific symptoms, but from a combination of individual manifestations.

HISTORY

HPI/ROS Recent changes in weight (gain/loss), appetite changes, goiter, anterior neck tenderness, eye changes, dry skin, diaphoresis, hair loss, tachycardia, palpitations, cold/heat intolerance, changes in sleep patterns, fatigue, restlessness, tremors, constipation, diarrhea, onset of menarche, menstrual irregularities, weakness, inability to concentrate, tremor, nervousness

Medical history Current medications (prescription and OTC), recent viral illness

Family history Thyroid disorders, autoimmune disorders, radiation exposure

Social history Development/school performance

PHYSICAL EXAMINATION

Growth Height, weight: plot on growth chart, note changes in linear growth and weight; head circumference (<2 years of age): plot and compare with previous measurements.

HEENT Fontanelles (anterior and posterior open/closed, size), cranial sutures (infant), presence of exophthalmos/proptosis, eyelid lag, lymph nodes, voice quality, dentition, facial edema, hearing loss

Thyroid gland Size, shape, consistency (full, firm, soft, nodular), symmetry, tenderness

> **NOTE** Palpation can be done in one of two ways. Stand facing or stand behind the patient to palpate the isthmus, main body, and lateral lobes. Palpate and record size, shape, consistency, configuration, tenderness, and any nodules (size). Water may be given to a child unable to swallow on request. Swallowing will elevate and depress the gland. The right lobe is usually greater in size than the left.

Cardiovascular Rate, rhythm, S1, S2, palpate precordium, peripheral pulses, blood pressure, pulse pressure

Pulmonary Routine

Gastrointestinal Umbilical hernia, abdominal distention

Genitourinary Tanner staging

Neurologic Deep tendon reflexes (delayed/brisk), tremors

Musculoskeletal Muscle strength/tone

Skin Dry, smooth, mottled, color (pale, mottled, jaundiced, flushed), hair texture, hand edema

Development Milestones, school performance

SCANNING TECHNIQUES

Radioactive iodine uptake (RAIU)

I-131 utilized for thyroid cancer imaging and treatment and for hyperthyroidism treatment

I-123 utilized for routine thyroid RAIU and scans; has a short half-life and delivers low radiation dose to patient

PATIENT PREPARATION Extensive if on thyroid medications (consultation regarding specific preparation required); none if patient receiving no thyroid medication or iodine-containing agents

> **NOTE** Adolescent females should receive a serum human chorionic gonadotropin (HCG) test prior to scan (refer to institution guidelines for timing of HCG test).

Technetium

Measures uptake of technetium (Tc 99m-pertechnetate) by thyroid gland

Tc 99m-pertechnetate is actively concentrated by the thyroid gland. It is given as a single IV bolus with imaging performed about 20-30 minutes later. Technetium has a short half-life and negligible organic binding. Due to its transient stay in the thyroid, the amount of radiation delivered is very low.

PATIENT PREPARATION None

Increased uptake in hyperthyroidism

Decreased uptake in hypothyroidism (except in dyshormonogenesis, in which it may be increased), thyroxine-binding globulin (TBG) deficiency

I-123 and Tc 99m scans determine thyroid location and uptake. Iodine scans can determine iodine uptake and organification of iodine. Ultrasonography determines location of the thyroid gland and if it is bilobed or hypertrophied. If hypertrophied, may suggest dyshormonogenesis or iodine deficiency.

THYROID DISORDERS

DIAGNOSIS	CLINICAL FINDINGS	DIAGNOSTIC FINDINGS

Congenital Hypothyroidism

Permanent primary congenital hypothyroidism (PPCH)

Occurs in 1 of 2500-4000 newborns[1]

Pertinent History

Advanced gestational age (42 weeks)

Maternal factors
- History of abdominal irradiation during pregnancy
- Ingestion of iodides, propylthiouracil (PTU), Tapazole
- Administration of radioactive iodide during pregnancy (may cause transient form of hypothyroidism, not true congenital hypothyroidism)

Family history of autoimmune diseases[2,3]

Physical Findings

Most infants are asymptomatic; about 10% have symptoms usually developing in weeks to months after birth, which may include hypotonia, lethargy, open posterior fontanelle (>0.5-1.0 cm), open cranial sutures, umbilical hernia, prolonged jaundice, pallor, enlarged tongue, hoarse cry, constipation, dry skin, respiratory difficulties, poor weight gain, edema, goiter (hyperextend neck to examine for goiter), abdominal distention, increased birth weight.[2-5]

Laboratory Tests[3]

↑ TSH
↓ T4
↓ Free T4

Radiologic Studies

Thyroid scan shows underdeveloped, ectopic (lingual), absent (athyreosis) tissue, or poor uptake

Delayed bone age[1,2,6]

Treatment to be initiated in the first 4 weeks of life

Medications

Levothyroxine sodium replacement

Adjust levothyroxine dose to normalize TSH and *maintain T4 and/or Free T4 in upper half of normal range as rapidly as possible.*[2,4]

Education

Crush and mix medication with small amount of water, breast milk, formula, or baby food.[3,7]

Synthroid does not dissolve well in water.

Do not mix with soy formula; consider avoiding soy formula as formula of choice in infants with hypothyroidism.

Initial Diagnosis

Newborn screening of T4 and/or TSH performed in all 50 states

Follow-up assessment at: 2 and 4 weeks after levothyroxine treatment started; 1-2 months in first 6 months of age; every 3-4 months (6 months-3 years of age); every 6-12 months until growth completed[4]

Monitor T4, Free T4, and TSH at these same intervals and 4 weeks after any change in levothyroxine dose.[1]

Depending on initial diagnostic testing and if permanent hypothyroidism has not been established, may stop T4 treatment for 4 weeks after 3 years of age, and check Free T4, T4, and TSH. If thyroid function tests are normal, may presume it was transient hypothyroidism.[4]

80%-90% of cases of PPCH result from developmental defects of thyroid gland.[1]

Athyreosis or ectopic thyroid indicates need for lifelong thyroxine treatment and trials of thyroxine are not necessary.[5]

Transition to Adulthood

Counsel regarding lifelong treatment with thyroxine.

THYROID DISORDERS 9

DIAGNOSIS	CLINICAL FINDINGS	DIAGNOSTIC FINDINGS

Acquired Hypothyroidism

May occur as a result of:
- Acute lymphocytic thyroiditis
- Chronic autoimmune thyroiditis (Hashimoto's disease)
- TSH deficiency
- Thyroidectomy or radioactive iodine thyroid therapy
- Subacute thyroiditis[8]

Pertinent History

Family history of autoimmune diseases

Pituitary disorders secondary to tumors, trauma, infection, congenital anomalies, irradiation/chemotherapy, thyroidectomy, radioactive iodine treatment, ingestion of goitrogens or thioamides

Goiter, anterior neck fullness/tenderness

Weakness, lethargy, fatigue, decreased appetite, cold intolerance, constipation, weight gain, poor linear growth/retardation, irregular menses, changes in school performance, unexplained hypoglycemia in insulin-dependent diabetes mellitus (IDDM) patients[2,8,9]

Physical Findings

Goiter or fullness and mild tenderness in anterior neck; poor growth; weight gain; dry skin; coarse hair; delayed pubertal development (rarely precocious); delayed dentition; edema of face, hands, and eyes; delayed deep tendon reflexes; decreased heart rate and blood pressure[8,9]

Laboratory Tests

↓T4
↓Free T4
↓T3
↑TSH
± Antithyroid peroxidase (anti-TPO; most sensitive screen for chronic autoimmune thyroiditis) and/or thyroglobulin antibodies[3]

MANAGEMENT/EDUCATION	EVALUATION

Medications

Levothyroxine replacement[2,3,8]

Monitor TSH, free T4, T4, T3.

Follow-up depends on age at diagnosis:
- Less than 12 months: see initially at 1 week, 2 weeks, and 1 month of age, then every 1-3 months during first 12 months of age.
- 1-3 years: see initially at 1-2 months and then every 3-4 months until 3 years of age.
- 3-18 years: see initially at 1-3 months, then every 4-6 months.[4,8]

Transition to Adulthood

***Acquired hypothyroidism* (TSH deficiency, thyroidectomy)**
Counsel regarding lifelong treatment with thyroxine.[1]

Hashimoto's thyroiditis

Counsel regarding possibility of lifelong treatment; may have trial of treatment to determine thyroid function[8]

Women: Euthyroid state necessary for pregnancy[8]

THYROID DISORDERS ⑨

DIAGNOSIS	CLINICAL FINDINGS	DIAGNOSTIC FINDINGS
TSH Deficient Hypothyroidism (See Pituitary Disorders, pp. 184-185.)	Hypothalamic/ hypopituitary disorders (insufficient TSH to stimulate thyroid gland)	

Thyrotoxicosis Refers to manifestations of excessive quantities of circulating thyroid hormones[5]	**Pertinent History** See Hyperthyroidism (Graves' disease), p. 224. Less common pertinent history: exogenous source hormone from environment, inflammatory disease (e.g., hashitoxicosis), iodine excess, drug-induced thyroiditis, subacute thyroiditis, transient thyroiditis, thyroid adenoma, toxic multinodular goiter, TSH-secreting pituitary adenoma Typical symptoms of hyperthyroidism in history and on physical examination Patient may have known goiter or Graves' disease. Usually a hypermetabolic picture, but presentation can be subclinical Subclinical disease may be associated with fever, thyroid gland pain and/or tenderness, and may be without palpable goiter. *(continued)*	**Laboratory Tests** ↑ Serum T4 ↑ Free T4 ↓ TSH ↑ T3 (often elevated to a greater degree than T4 and free T4)[6,9,10] In subclinical states, may have normal free T4 and T3 with low TSH If ↑ T4 and ↑ T3 in the presence of a normal or elevated TSH and ↑ free alpha subunit, consider MRI to rule out a TSH-secreting pituitary adenoma.

MANAGEMENT/EDUCATION	EVALUATION
Management is challenging in childhood.	Close follow-up is necessary after interpreting lab values to maintain euthyroidism and prevent cardio-vascular and neurologic complications.[10]
Decrease the dose of thyroid hormone.	
Remove exogenous supply in environment.	
Adjust thyroid medication for hyperthyroidism and monitor for side effects of medications.	
Emergency management of thyrotoxicosis (thyroid storm) if necessary, with PTU, SSKI	
Propranolol and hydrocortisone[10]	

DIAGNOSIS	CLINICAL FINDINGS	DIAGNOSTIC FINDINGS
(Thyrotoxicosis)	**Physical Findings** Thyroid gland can become 3-4 times its normal size, feels warm to touch, and may be tender. Texture is frequently soft and fleshy. Less often and usually associated with coexisting Hashimoto's thyroiditis, the gland may be firm and asymmetrically enlarged.[6,9,10]	
Hyperthyroidism (Graves' Disease)	**Pertinent History** Family history of autoimmune diseases, hyperactivity, increased appetite, sleep disturbance, irritability, nervousness, headache, inability to concentrate, decreased school performance Weight loss, heat intolerance, sweating, restlessness, tachycardia, palpitations, increased frequency of bowel movements[3,9,10] **Physical FIndings** Tachycardia, hypertension, increased pulse pressure, exophthalmos, proptosis, *(continued)*	**Laboratory Tests** ↑T4 ↑T3 ↓TSH ↑TSH receptor antibodies Anti-TPO and anti-thyroglobulin antibodies may also be positive. **Radiologic Studies** Radioactive thyroid uptake scan generally not used to diagnose Graves' disease (high uptake) in children; however, it may be used to differentiate painless (silent) thyroiditis (low uptake) or the toxic phase of subacute thyroiditis.[3,9,10]

MANAGEMENT/EDUCATION	EVALUATION

Medications

To treat overstimulation of cardiovascular system:
Propanolol

To suppress hypersecretion of thyroid hormones

Potassium iodide or methimazole

Suppression therapy may induce a hypo-thyroid state; consider decreasing suppression therapy and/or adding levothyroxine sodium to maintain a euthyroid state.[2,9,10]

> NOTE PTU is no longer recommended for antithyroid therapy in children due to PTU-induced liver failure.[11]

Close follow-up necessary to maintain euthyroidism, prevent cardiovascular and neurologic complications

Monitor total and free T4, T3, TSH, TSH receptor antibodies.

When antibodies and goiter have decreased, may begin trial off medications; follow closely. Remission may occur within the first 2 years.

May need to consider radio-ablation of gland or surgery if not responsive to medical therapy[2,10]

(continued)

(continued)

THYROID DISORDERS 9

DIAGNOSIS	CLINICAL FINDINGS	DIAGNOSTIC FINDINGS
(Hyperthyroidism [Graves' Disease])	tremors, bruit over thyroid gland, hypertonia, goiter characterized by diffuse enlargement (smooth, firm, nontender), restlessness. Accelerated bone maturation and accelerated linear growth associated with prolonged hyperthyroidism.[6,9,10,12]	
Neonatal Hyperthyroidism Most commonly transient or, less commonly, protracted Estimated 1 of 25,000 births in mothers with Graves' disease[1]	**Pertinent History** Maternal hyperthyroidism (only small percentage of infants born to mothers with Graves' disease are affected)—0.6% **Physical Findings** Tachycardia, hypertension, irritability, diaphoresis, goiter, tremors, closed or small fontanelles, premature craniosynostosis, respiratory distress, hypertonia, diarrhea, poor feeding, poor weight gain	**Laboratory Tests** ↑ Free T4 ↑ T3 ↓ TSH ↑ TSH receptor antibodies

MANAGEMENT/EDUCATION	EVALUATION

Education

Medication administration

Side effects of medication: Immediately report symptoms of fever, infection, irritability/lethargy, poor appetite, or rash.

> **NOTE** T3 may be a more accurate indicator of thyroxine replacement in this state, since T4 is more rapidly converted to T3, and T4 may be low.[2,9,10,13]

Transition to Adulthood

Counsel regarding the possibility of recurrence after remission (if initially achieved).

Counsel regarding regular follow-up and immediate follow-up if symptoms of hyperthyroidism recur.[6,10,13]

Medications

To treat overstimulation of cardiovascular system:
Propanolol

To suppress hypersecretion of thyroid hormones: Potassium iodide, propylthiouracil, or methimazole

Above treatment may cause a hypothyroid state; may need to add L-thyroxine to maintain a euthyroid state.

Treatment usually temporary. As antibodies clear from infant, symptoms resolve (usually 3-12 weeks).[1,2,9]

Close follow-up necessary to maintain euthyroidism, prevent cardiovascular and neurologic complications

Monitor total and free T4, T3, TSH, and TSH receptor antibodies.[1,2]

Education

Medication administration

Side effects of medication: Immediately report symptoms of fever, infection, irritability/lethargy, poor feeding, or rash.

Condition is usually temporary and symptoms will resolve as antibodies clear from infant.[1,2,9]

THYROID DISORDERS 9

DIAGNOSIS	CLINICAL FINDINGS	DIAGNOSTIC FINDINGS
Congenital Thyroxine-Binding Globulin (TBG) Deficiency Inherited X-linked dominant traits affecting 1 of 5000 to 12,000 live births[6]	**Pertinent History** Not significant for other thyroid disorders **Physical Findings** If no clinical signs or symptoms of hypothyroidism or panhypopituitarism, congenital TBG deficiency should be suspected.[6]	**Laboratory Tests** N Free T4 N TSH ↓T4 ↓TBG level (definitive for diagnosis) ↑T3 resin uptake[6]
Thyroid Carcinoma	**Pertinent History** <20 years of age, >70 years of age Male External neck irradiation in childhood/adolescence Radiation exposure Previous thyroid cancer Family thyroid cancer Hoarseness, dysphagia, rapid growth of nodule Family history of multiple endocrine neoplasia type 2[14-17] **Physical Findings** Firm consistency of nodule Irregular-shaped nodule Nodule affixed to tissue Possible regional adenopathy (cervical lymphadenopathy) Asymptomatic mass, difficulty in swallowing, hoarseness, or symptoms of hypothyroidism or hyperthyroidism[6,14-17]	**Laboratory Tests** TSH, free T4, T3, antithyroid peroxidase, and antithyroglobulin antibodies (likely normal) Thyroglobulin (TG) level may be elevated (not diagnostic, since it may be elevated with other thyroid conditions such as thyroiditis). Calcitonin level elevated in medullary carcinoma Screen for gene responsible for multiple endocrine neoplasia (MEN) II. **Radiologic Studies** Thyroid scan (radioiodine or technetium) to evaluate thyroid nodule to determine if nodule is "hot" or "cold." A hypofunctioning ("cold") area may lead to suspicion of malignancy, but is not diagnostic. *(continued)*

MANAGEMENT/EDUCATION	EVALUATION
Failure to diagnose TBG deficiency may lead to a false diagnosis of congenital hypothyroidism and unnecessary treatment.	These infants are considered normal; no further workup or follow-up is necessary.[6]

Education

Inform parents that for future lab tests with a different medical provider, a free T4 should be checked instead of a total T4.[6]

Surgery

Risk of vocal cord paralysis and temporary/permanent hypocalcemia depending on the extent of thyroid resection

Radioiodine treatment

Medications

Thyroxine replacement[14-17]

Frequent follow-up for first 2 years after treatment

Laboratory evaluation: free T4, T3, TSH, and TG

Palpation of neck lymph nodes[14-17]

DIAGNOSIS	CLINICAL FINDINGS	DIAGNOSTIC FINDINGS
(Thyroid Carcinoma)		Ultrasound to differentiate cystic from solid nodules; cystic nodules are less likely to be malignant.
		X-rays of neck to determine the presence of calcifications
		Chest X-ray to evaluate the presence of metastases[15-17]
		Medical Procedures
		Fine needle aspiration/ biopsy to determine type of nodule
		Subject to technique and interpretation[15-17]
Nodular Thyroid Disease	**Pertinent History**	**Laboratory Tests**
	See above for workup for malignancy.	Same as above with serum thyroid antibodies
	A firm, palpable, localized thyroid mass (nodule) must be carefully evaluated.[13]	Identify nature of the nodule (hypofunctioning vs. hyperfunctioning).
	In children, can be confused with other neck masses	TSH can be normal, elevated, or low.[15,17]
	Evaluation includes same history and physical examination as in the thyroid carcinoma section above.	**Radiologic Studies**
		Ultrasound to determine nature and size of the nodule (cystic vs. solid)
		Thyroid radioisotope scan to determine if nodule is hot versus cold (see Thyroid Carcinoma section above)
		Hot nodules are rarely malignant.[6,10,13,15]
		(continued)

MANAGEMENT/EDUCATION	EVALUATION

Medications

May need thyroid medication if thyroid function lab tests reveal an autonomously functioning adenoma

Treatment for a minimum of 3 months, then reassessed

If suppression is not achieved through medication and nodule size does not change, then surgical intervention may be considered.

Education

Patient should have regular follow-up physical examination, including measurement of the nodule by consistent examiner.

May need to be rebiopsied

Unless the nodule decreases in size, may need to repeat fine needle aspiration

Ultrasound is helpful to assess changes in size of nodule.

Lifelong follow-up one or two times per year

Teach family and patient self-examination to monitor nodule for any changes.

DIAGNOSIS	CLINICAL FINDINGS	DIAGNOSTIC FINDINGS
(Nodular Thyroid Disease)		**Medical Procedures** Fine needle aspiration (FNA) to evaluate type of nodule through biopsy; not always conclusive Nodules ≥1 cm should be biopsied by FNA. Excisional biopsy[15-17]
Sick Euthyroid (Low T3 Syndrome or Nonthyroidal Illness)	**Pertinent History** Premature infants Patients with protein calorie malnutrition or anorexia nervosa, diabetic ketoacidosis, severe trauma, burns, cirrhosis, renal failure Fasting patients Postoperative patients Febrile states Thyroid gland is functioning normally, although due to a severe nonthyroid illness the peripheral metabolism of the thyroid hormones is impaired.[6]	**Laboratory Tests** ↓T3 ↑or N rT3 ↑or ↓ or N T4 ↑or N free T4 N TSH ↓ or N TBG[6]

MANAGEMENT/EDUCATION	EVALUATION

Thyroxine replacement is not indicated.

Treatment directed toward primary systemic illness[6]

PATIENT EDUCATION RESOURCES

Family Resource Library
British Columbia's Children's Hospital
Ambulatory Care Building
4480 Oak Street, Rm K2-126
Vancouver, B.C. Canada
V6H 3V4
1-800-331-1533, ext. 2
or 1-604-875-2345, local 5102
FAX 1-604-875-3455
www.bcchildrens.ca/KidsTeensFam/FamilyResourceLibrary

Magic Foundation
6645 W. North Avenue
Oak Park, IL 60302
1-708-383-0808
PARENT HELPLINE 1-800-3MAGIC3 or 1-800-362-4423
www.magicfoundation.org

Contact state organizations responsible for newborn screening of congenital hypothyroidism.

⑩ EFFECTS OF CANCER THERAPY AND CHRONIC ILLNESS

OVERVIEW

Many chronic childhood illnesses or their treatments cause deficits within the endocrine system. As many as 40% of childhood cancer survivors have endocrine disturbances from their malignancy, surgery, radiation therapy, or chemotherapy.[1,2] These disturbances affect growth, sexual development, and thyroid, adrenal function, obesity, hyperlipidemia, metabolic syndrome and hyperprolactinemia. The age at which treatment occurred, length of time since treatment and gender have impacts as well. Many of these effects are not recognized immediately after treatment. Early and ongoing screening should occur to identify deficiencies quickly and provide treatment. Some deficiencies may not show up for many years after treatment. Cancer therapies are changing; thus late effects may also continue to evolve, with future treatment revisions. Other illnesses or their treatments, such as Crohn's disease, celiac disease, cystic fibrosis, asthma, cardiac defects, HIV infection, sickle cell disease, and chronic renal failure, affect growth hormones and other endocrine hormones. These diseases should be considered and appropriate hormone replacement initiated to optimize health.

RADIATION THERAPY	VARIABLES RELATING TO SKELETAL EFFECT ON GROWTH	HORMONE SENSITIVITY
Wait at least 1-2 years after treatment to initiate growth hormone. Cranial irradiation and total body irradiation affect the endocrine system the most.	**Variables Relating to Effect on Growth** Age at time of treatment Type of radiation, dose per fraction, and total dose Volume irradiated Growth potential of the treated site Individual genetic and familial factors Coexisting therapy: surgery and chemotherapy	**Hypothalamus** Usual site affected **Growth Hormone** Most sensitive even to doses of 18 Gy irradiation **Gonadotropins and Adrenocorticotropin** Intermediate **Thyroid-Stimulating Hormone** Least sensitive to radiation **Prolactin** At doses >40 Gy irradiation **Posterior Pituitary** No damage has been reported.

TYPE	EFFECT

IRRADIATION

Cranial Irradiation

Acute lymphocytic leukemia (ALL)

Brain tumors:
- Medulloblastoma
- Astrocytoma
- Craniopharyngioma
- Primitive neuroecto-dermal tumor (PNET)
- Optic glioma

Varies based on involved field, total dose, and schedule

Young children may have more effects from irradiation.

Growth

18 Gy irradiation or more: growth hormone axis may be affected[3]

Puberty

>18 Gy: Possibly precocious puberty, early puberty, or normally timed puberty with rapid progression

>40 Gy: May delay puberty with gonadotropin deficiency, infertility, hyperprolactinemia[3]

(continued)

IMPLICATIONS

Monitor growth velocity closely, watching for signs of sexual precocity.

Monitor bone age, IGF-1 and IGFBP-3 levels.

Monitor standing and sitting height.

Repeated provocative testing may be necessary in some cases before GHD is diagnosed; 24-hour sleep study stimulation may be needed.

May not require provocative testing, depending on other growth parameters or other hormone deficiencies.

Bone age is delayed and typical features of GHD may appear in prepubertal patients.[4]

Females are affected more than males.[5]

If pubertal during treatment, may be at greater risk for pubertal problems

Females are more at risk than males.

Girls:
- Youngest girls at age of irradiation have earliest onset of puberty.[6]
- Some girls will have menstrual irregularities, delayed puberty, premature menopause, infertility or gonadotropin deficiency.
- Monitor LH, FSH, estradiol levels, bone age, and pubertal development. May need DXA scan. Ask about pubertal onset and tempo, sexual function, menstrual and pregnancy history.

Boys:
- Pubertal onset is earliest in those irradiated between 3 and 6 years of age.[6]
- Some boys will have gonadotropin deficiency, delayed puberty, or infertility.
- Monitor LH, FSH, testosterone levels, bone age, and pubertal development. May need DXA scan
- May need treatment with GnRH agonist analog with precocious puberty.
- May need replacement of estrogen/progesterone for girls and testosterone for boys with gonadal failure.

(continued)

EFFECTS OF CANCER THERAPY AND CHRONIC ILLNESS ⑩

TYPE	EFFECT
(Cranial Irradiation)	**Thyroid** Assess thyroid function regularly—may see primary or hypothalamic dysfunction, hyperthyroidism, thyroiditis, and benign or malignant tumors, with peak incidence 2-5 years after treatment.[7,8] Direct thyroid irradiation may cause hypothyroidism, hyperthyroidism, thyroid nodules, or thyroid cancer. Thyroid deficiencies may not be evident for many years after treatment. **Adrenal** May see central adrenal insufficiency, usually over 40 Gy of irradiation.

(continued)

IMPLICATIONS

Hypothyroid symptoms:
- Fatigue
- Weight gain
- Cold intolerance
- Constipation
- Dry skin
- Brittle hair, hair loss
- Depressed mood

Hyperthyroid symptoms:
- Heat intolerance
- Tachycardia, palpitations
- Weight loss
- Emotional lability
- Muscular weakness
- Hyperphagia

Monitor free T4 and TSH at baseline, and annually.

Will often see low total or free thyroxine with low TSH

Careful palpation of thyroid gland for nodules; may need thyroid ultrasound or biopsy

May need TRH stimulation test (see p. 306; will see low TSH with anterior pituitary damage and high TSH with hypothalamus damage[9])

If you use prolonged and elevated TSH response to TRH stimulation testing as criterion of TSH dysfunction, the rate is much higher.[4]

Untreated hypothyroidism may ↑ risk of accelerated atherosclerosis.[6]

Obtain early morning plasma cortisol yearly for 15 years after treatment.

Monitor for failure to thrive, anorexia, dehydration, hypoglycemia, unexplained lethargy, hypotension.

May need corticosteroid replacement therapy

(continued)

TYPE	EFFECT
(Cranial Irradiation)	**Prolactin** May see hyperprolactinemia Monitor for galactorrhea Females: Assess menstrual history Males: Decreased libido **Bones** May see low bone mineral density **Obesity/Metabolic Syndrome** May occur from cranial radiation, may be exacerbated by growth hormone deficiency or hypothyroidism Females and children less than 4 years of age at time of treatment and those with hypothalamic irradiation >18 Gy are most at risk **Dyslipidemia** May be seen, but most common with obesity and with some chemotherapy
Cranial/Spinal Irradiation	>2400 cGy axial skeletal radiation: loss of height, especially for children <age 6 and between ages 11 and 13[4] Short upper body segment seen due to loss of spinal growth Watch for scoliosis. Watch for radiation-induced necrosis. Monitor for cranial effects as described on pp. 236-240. Watch for thyroid and pubertal issues as described above.

IMPLICATIONS

Monitor prolactin levels.

Tumors in the hypothalamic-pituitary region may lead to ADH deficiency prior to surgery or after surgery (neurogenic diabetes insipidus [DI])—increased urination and thirst and dilute urine.[8] See treatment for DI, pp. 186-190.

Monitor height, weight, BMI, blood pressure.

Assess fasting blood glucose, fasting insulin level, fasting lipid profile every 2 years if overweight and every 5 years if normal weight (BMI below 85th percentile).

Monitor fasting lipid profile.

Younger children have a greater worsening of spinal growth than older children.

Primary ovarian failure may result in premature menopause.[4]

TYPE	EFFECT
Total Body Irradiation (TBI)	Effects of TBI are the same as those listed for cranial and craniospinal radiation. May see growth hormone deficiency, primary hypothyroidism, thyroid nodules, thyroid cancer, and primary hypogonadism. May also see increased risk for metabolic syndrome, even at normal weights.
Abdominal and Pelvic Irradiation (Wilms tumor, Hodgkin's disease, pelvic and genital tumors, etc.)	**Gonadal Deficiency** Compromised ovarian function can be seen in postpubertal females. May see increased risk for premature menopause Females that were pubertal at treatment and given 10 Gy or more of radiation, and those treated with high-dose alkylating agents, are at most risk. Males have more germ cell damage at lower doses of radiation than Leydig cell damage. 1-3 Gy: Azoospermia may be reversible. 3-6 Gy: Azoospermia reversal is less likely. >6 Gy: Permanent azoospermia is likely. >20 Gy: Leydig cell damage is likely and may affect production of testosterone.

IMPLICATIONS

Regimens with cyclophosphamide (Cytoxan) only will have minimal effect on growth.

Other factors that affect growth include prolonged corticosteroid therapy, renal failure, and chronic GVHD.

Consider sperm banking or cryopreservation of oocytes prior to bone marrow transplant.

Monitor for growth, thyroid function, adrenal function, pubertal function, and metabolic syndrome, as described under Cranial irradiation, pp. 236-241.

Monitor for pubertal changes, as described in Cranial irradiation section.

May need to perform GnRH stimulation test (see pp. 270-271.)

Monitor for erectile dysfunction (i.e., morning erections and nocturnal ejaculations) and decreased libido.

If uterine atrophy is present (seen by reduced uterine length and endometrial thickness on ultrasound), will be unlikely to benefit from in vitro fertilization with donor oocytes[4]

May see breast atrophy with whole abdominal or flank irradiation performed before puberty and may need cosmetic surgery.[4]

TYPE	EFFECT
Thyroid Irradiation	>10 Gy: May see hypothyroidism and rarely hyperthyroidism
	>25 Gy: Increased risk for thyroid nodules
	Increased risk for thyroid cancer: Increasing risk for doses up to 30 Gy; decreasing risk at higher doses

CHEMOTHERAPY

Heavy Metals Cisplatin, carboplatin	May cause dyslipidemia.
	High-risk patients are those with family history of lipid disorders or those who are overweight.
	Counsel for dietary modifications, exercise, and weight loss. May need pharmacologic management.
	Also monitor those with growth hormone deficiency.
	Monitor for gonadal toxicity.
Alkylating Agents Cyclophosphamide, busulfan, procarbazine, mechlorethamine	Cause high levels of gonadal toxicity
	Males: • Cyclophosphamide >7.5 g/m² causes highest risk for gonadal toxicity. • Germ cell function is impaired at lower doses than Leydig cell function. • Combination chemotherapy and testicular, pelvic, or total body irradiation significantly increases risk of gonadal dysfunction.[9]
	Females: • Watch for delayed or arrested puberty, premature menopause, or infertility. • Increased risk of gonadal dysfunction with combined therapy and chemotherapy with radiation.

IMPLICATIONS

Monitor thyroid function regularly with careful palpation for nodules, as described in cranial irradiation section.

Boys achieve normal adult sexual characteristics and normal testosterone secretion; reproductive capacity varies.[4]

Girls' ovarian function, estrogen secretion, and fertility may be impaired.[4]

May see ↑ FSH at puberty consistent with germ cell damage[4]

May see primary testicular dysfunction[4]

See treatment of SIADH, pp. 194-195.

TYPE	EFFECT
Miscellaneous L-asparaginase	May see hyperglycemia requiring treatment with insulin
Antimetabolite Agents Methotrexate Corticosteroids: prednisone and dexamethasone	Altered bone metabolism may not allow peak bone mass and increases risk of premature osteopenia and more severe osteopenia later in life. Increased risk of decreased bone mineral density with combination of methotrexate and corticosteroids, or with prolonged use of corticosteroids (i.e., graft-versus-host disease) Also at increased risk are patients with GHD, hypogonadism, hyperthyroidism; those who smoke, use alcohol; and those with history of decreased weight-bearing exercise or low calcium intake.
Miscellaneous— Corticosteroids	May see cushingoid appearance, hypertension, obesity May develop hyperglycemia and transient diabetes during treatment May see growth retardation with long-term high-dose use[10]

See treatment of diabetes, pp. 76-96.

Obtain DXA or quantitative CT 2 years after therapy to monitor for decreased bone mass.

Maximize calcium and vitamin D intake.

Encourage weight-bearing exercises.

Decrease salt intake.

Observe for hyperglycemia; patient may need insulin therapy.

EFFECTS OF CANCER THERAPY AND CHRONIC ILLNESS

TYPE	EFFECT
Antitumor Antibiotics (anthracyclines) Daunorubicin, doxorubicin, bleomycin, dactinomycin	At this time these seem to have no late endocrine effects.[3]
Enzymes L-asparaginase	
Plant Alkaloids Vincristine Vinblastine	
Epipodophyllo-toxins Etoposide, teniposide	

TYPE	EFFECT

GASTROINTESTINAL DISEASE

Celiac Disease (Gluten-induced enteropathy)	Monitor for celiac in short stature, Turner syndrome, and thyroid disease, or other autoimmune states May have history of diarrhea and/or steatorrhea May have iron deficiency anemia May have dermatitis herpetiformis May see osteoporosis May have infertility or increased risk of miscarriage May see hypertransaminasemia

(continued)

IMPLICATIONS

Monitor current research for changes in endocrine function resulting from these chemotherapy agents.

EVALUATION

Monitor growth velocity.

Monitor puberty.

IgA tissue transglutaminase (tTG) antibodies have high sensitivity and specificity; if IgA deficient, need IgG tissue transglutaminase antibodies

Refer to gastroenterologist if positive for further workup (small bowel biopsy to confirm diagnosis).

↓ Stool fat, ↓ serum folate, ↓ serum ferritin, ↓ IGF-1, ↓ IGFBP-3

TYPE	EFFECT
(Celiac Disease)	Treatment (gluten withdrawal): • Will see rapid catch-up growth • ↓ Symptoms • IGF-1 and IGFBP-3 normalize • Should achieve normal final height Neurologic disorders seen: • Peripheral neuropathy • Cerebellar ataxia • Epilepsy • Multiple sclerosis • Migraine Increased risk for certain types of cancers: • Non-Hodgkin's lymphomas • Enteropathy-associated T-cell lymphoma • Small intestine adenocarcinoma • Esophageal and oropharyngeal carcinomas
Crohn's Disease	A third to two thirds of patients will have impaired growth at diagnosis, probably due to malnutrition from malabsorption and anorexia, chronic inflammation, inadequacy of trace minerals in diet, and use of glucocorticoids. Treatment consists of enteral and parenteral nutrition, steroids, and sometimes surgery.
Chronic Liver Disease	Impaired growth caused by ↓ food intake, fat and fat-soluble vitamin malabsorption, trace element deficiencies, and abnormalities of GH-IGF system Linear growth often poor even after transplant due to exogenous glucocorticoids and immunosuppressive agents

May have magnesium and zinc deficiency

↓ IGF-1 levels

↑ Sedimentation rate

Diagnosis requires gastroenterologist referral for endoscopy and biopsy.

30% may have final height deficits.

↓IGF-1, ↓IGF-2, ↓IGFBP-3, ↑GH secretion (acquired GH resistance syndrome)

GH normal

Free IGF may be ↓ as IGFBP-3 is ↑

Long-term growth improvement with use of alternate-day glucocorticoids

GH therapy for 18 months enhances growth rates and increases height.[5]

TYPE	EFFECT

RENAL DISEASE

Chronic Renal Insufficiency (CRI)	Conditions that impair renal function impair growth.
	Uremia and renal tubular acidosis can cause growth failure before other clinical manifestations become evident.
	Poor growth from inadequate formation of 1,25-dihydroxycholecaliferol with resultant osteopenia, ↓ caloric intake, loss of electrolytes, metabolic acidosis, protein wasting, insulin resistance, chronic anemia, compromised cardiac function, impairment of GH and IGF production and action
	Chronic glucocorticoid therapy can exacerbate growth retardation by ↓ GH release and blunting IGF-1 action at growth plates.
Nephropathic Cystinosis	Acquired hypothyroidism contributes to inadequate growth.
Nephrotic Syndrome	Poor growth
Renal Transplant	Growth may be slowed.
	Height at time of transplant and use of alternate-day glucocorticoid therapy correlate with final height.
	Cumulative dose of prednisone has negative impact on height.
	Sex, age at transplant, diagnosis, and number of transplants do not affect final height.

May see normal or ↑ GH levels, depending on degree of renal failure

End-stage renal disease has ↑ GH production.

↓ Hepatic IGF production due to ↓ hepatic GH receptor gene expression; IGF-1 and IGF-2 levels usually normal

↑ Serum IGFBPs (especially IGFBP-1) may inhibit IGF action.

Those with low vitamin D levels can benefit from replacement therapy

Growth hormone therapy is approved for CRI patients at a weekly dosage of up to 0.35 mg/kg of body weight, divided into daily subcutaneous injections. Growth hormone therapy may be continued up to the time of renal transplantation. To optimize therapy for patients who require dialysis, the following injection schedule guidelines are recommended:

- Patients on hemodialysis should receive their own injection at night just before going to sleep, or at least 3-4 hours after their hemodialysis to prevent hematoma formation from heparin.
- Patients with chronic cycling peritoneal dialysis (CCPD) should receive their injection in the morning after they have completed dialysis.
- Patients with chronic ambulatory periotneal dialysis (CAPD) should receive their injection in the evening at the time of the overnight exchange.

Monitor thyroid function.

↓ IGF-1 and ↓ IGFBP-3 due to urinary loss of IGF-1/IGFBP complexes

Watch for ↓ GH secretion, normal IGF-1 and IGFBP-1, ↑ IGFBP-3.

GH important to improve growth velocity and absolute height prior to transplant and may be useful after transplant

EFFECTS OF CANCER THERAPY AND CHRONIC ILLNESS

⑩

TYPE	EFFECT
CHRONIC ANEMIA	
Sickle Cell Disease	Growth failure, delayed adolescent growth spurt, and delayed menarche observed
	Probably due to impaired oxygen delivery to tissues, ↑ work of cardiovascular system, and impaired nutrition
Thalassemia	Chronic anemia, chronic transfusions and accompanying hemosiderosis, and iron overload may contribute to endocrine deficiencies, such as impaired glucose metabolism.
	Growth failure common, especially in adolescents
PULMONARY DISEASE	
Asthma	↓ Growth, even without glucocorticoid therapy
	Mean height and growth velocity and degree of growth failure are related to severity of asthma.
	Delayed puberty associated with growth deceleration in early teen years
	Impaired nutrition, ↑ energy requirements along with chronic stress (especially with nocturnal asthma and enhanced endogenous glucocorticoid production) lead to poor linear growth.
	Glucocorticoid therapy further impairs growth.

EVALUATION

Adolescent growth and final adult height may be normal.

Monitor growth carefully.

GH-IGF system probably does not have important role in growth impairment.

May have impaired IGF-1 synthesis, hypothyroidism, gonadal failure, and hypogonadotropic hypogonadism

GH resistance is suggested by adequate GH production with ↓ IGF-1 levels.

GH treatment increases growth at least initially.

Oral glucose tolerance test (OGTT) if iron overload present

Synthetic glucocorticoids have greater suppression of growth than equivalent doses of alternate-day or aerosolized therapy.

Adrenal gland function may be impaired due to glucocorticoid therapy.

Impaired growth not associated with abnormalities of GH-IGF axis

Normal adult height usually achieved

TYPE	EFFECT
Bronchopulmonary Dysplasia	Use of dexamethasone in neonatal period can cause transient cessation of growth.
	Long-term hypoxemia, poor nutrition, chronic pulmonary infections, and reactive airway disease are responsible for poor growth.
	May see short-term adrenal suppression from dexamethasone, normal after 1 month off therapy
Cystic Fibrosis	Decreased growth and delayed sexual maturation due to chronic pulmonary infection with bronchiectasis, pancreatic insufficiency with exocrine and endocrine inadequacy, malabsorption and malnutrition
	Increased risk of diabetes mellitus (see pp. 76-96 for specialized treatment)
	Alteration of vitamin D metabolism; potentially affects skeletal mineralization but does not diminish growth
Chronic Infection	Cytokines from inflammatory response to infection affect endocrine system.
	Impaired mineral and nutrient metabolism
	Impaired growth
	Remodeling of bone

EVALUATION

Monitor growth closely.

Growth is poor throughout early childhood but accelerates by 8 years of age.

Corticosteroid replacement for VLBW infants on dexamethasone until 1 month off therapy—can perform CRH stimulation test for verification

Degree of growth retardation related closely to severity and variability of pulmonary disease

Improved nutrition useful

Adult heights of surviving patients approach normal range.

GH may be beneficial by ↑ growth velocity, ↑ nitrogen retention, ↑ protein, and ↓ fat stores.

TYPE	EFFECT

IMMUNOLOGIC DISEASE

Acquired Immunodeficiency Syndrome

Treatment Options

Antiretroviral therapy may improve weight gain.

Appetite stimulants (megesterol acetate), anticytokine-directed supplements (dietary N-3 fatty acids), anabolic steroids, growth hormone, and metabolic inhibitors (hydrazine sulfate) may reverse weight loss and wasting syndrome.

HIV-associated lipodystrophy is a syndrome that occurs in individuals who have HIV and are receiving antiretroviral therapy (particularly protease inhibitors). On average, it develops 18 months after initiation of therapy and is a progressive disease. The severity is directly proportional to the patient's age, duration of disease, and length of protease inhibitor therapy.

Growth

Growth failure common, especially in those with more infections and ↓ CD4 counts

Height is more likely to be affected than weight.

Adrenal

Involvement by opportunistic infections (cytomegalovirus [CMV], mycobacteria, cryptococci, toxoplasma, and pneumocystis)

Neoplasms (lymphoma and Kaposi's sarcoma) affect adrenals.

Adrenal medulla is primary site.

May see areas of focal and generalized hemorrhage affecting both medulla and cortex

Ketoconazole (common drug in HIV therapy) is known to inhibit adrenal function.

Hypoadrenalism from drugs (ketoconazole or rifampin)

Hyponatremia from drugs (pentamidine and vidarabine)

Hypocalcemic tetany secondary to Mg^{2+} loss from drugs (amphotericin B and aminoglycosides)

Hyperkalemia from Na^+ channel inhibitory effect of drug (trimethoprim)

Thyroid

Affected by opportunistic infections (CMV, Kaposi's sarcoma, cryptococcal infections, pneumocystis carinii)

Antibiotic therapy for infections listed above may ↓ size of goiter, and thyroid function tests may normalize.

Hypothyroidism may be result of drugs (ketoconazole, rifampin, and interferon).

(continued)

May see normal GH and IGF-1 levels

May see $\downarrow Na^+$, hypotension, $\downarrow K^+$ or $\uparrow K^+$, vomiting, diarrhea, and fever

Usually not seen to have definite adrenal insufficiency

Hyponatremia may be due to renal and/or gastrointestinal losses or SIADH.

Usually see normal cortisol levels

Most have normal cortisol response to ACTH, with intact HPA axis and normal adrenal mineralocorticoid pathway.

May have abnormal thyroid function tests but no clinical evidence of hypothyroidism

Possibility of central hypothyroidism

(continued)

TYPE	EFFECT
(Acquired Immunodeficiency Syndrome)	**Gonads** Delayed puberty Testes may be affected by infection or neoplasm. May see changes in testicular function, spermatogenesis, and Leydig cell atrophy Decreased libido and impotence May see hypogonadism and gynecomastia from drug (ketoconazole) **Pancreas** Lesions seen due to CMV toxoplasmosis, Kaposi's sarcoma, lymphoma, and pancreatitis Hypoglycemia from drugs (pentamidine and trimethoprim-sulfamethoxazole) **Parathyroid** Lesions reported on autopsy; no clinical dysfunction reported
Growth hormone (0.1 mg/kg/day for 7 days) Serostim (a growth hormone) is FDA approved for those with HIV wasting syndrome and has been shown to increase weight, increase lean body mass, and improve physical endurance. Patients must be on antiretroviral therapy (ARV) to qualify. GhRH has recently been shown to be effective in increasing GH levels in HIV patients with muscle wasting.	**Hypothalamus and Pituitary** Panhypopituitarism due to toxoplasmosis Posterior pituitary lesions seen with disseminated CMV • ↑ Body weight, nitrogen retention • ↑ Energy expenditure, lipid oxidation, and glucose flux • ↓ Protein oxidation, resulting in ↑ total-body cell mass

EVALUATION

May see delayed bone age

Monitor testicular volume for atrophy.

Monitor for hypogonadism.

↓ Testosterone and ↓ baseline serum gonadotropin levels

Normal glucose levels usually seen

Watch for ↑ amylase and lipase due to acute pancreatitis.

↑ Ca^{2+}

↓ Parathyroid hormones

↓ Calcitriol

TYPE	EFFECT
Chronic Parasite Infestation	May see growth failure and poor weight gain

CARDIAC DISEASE

Congenital Heart Disease With Cyanosis or Chronic Congestive Failure	Growth failure (27% below 3rd percentile for height and weight, 70% below 50th percentile)

Chronic congestive heart failure associated with malabsorption that includes protein-losing enteropathy, intestinal lymphangiectasia, and steatorrhea

Degree of cyanosis and hypoxia correlates with degree of growth impairment.

Corrective surgery may restore normal growth, frequently after phase of catch-up growth. |

RESOURCES

American Brain Tumor Association
2720 River Rd.
Des Plaines, IL 60018
1-847-827-9910
FAX 1-847-827-9918
PATIENT LINE 1-800-886-2282
www.abta.org

American Cancer Society—The Cancer in Children Resource Center
National Home Office
1599 Clifton Rd. NE
Atlanta, GA 30329
1-800-ACS-2345
www.cancer.org

Association of Pediatric Hematology/ Oncology Nurses (APHON)
4700 W. Lake Ave
Glenview, IL 60025-1485
1-847-375-4724
FAX 1-847-375-6478
www.aphon.org

Childhood Cancer Guides
www.childhoodcancerguides.org

Leukemia and Lymphoma Society
1311 Mamaroneck Ave., Suite 310
White Plains, NY 10605
1-914-949-5213
1-800-955-4572
FAX 1-914-949-6691
www.leukemia.org

EVALUATION

Monitor growth.

Inadequate caloric intake; may see anorexia and vomiting

↑ Cardiac and respiratory work causes ↑ basal metabolic rate; therefore food intake that should be adequate for weight is inadequate for normal growth.

Adequate caloric support, ↓ hypoxia and heart failure necessary for growth prior to surgery

May need to have calorie-dense feedings to restrict fluids

Calcium supplementation may be needed due to use of diuretics.

Iron replacement necessary to maintain enhanced rate of erythropoiesis

CureSearch for Children's Cancer
4600 East-West Highway, Suite 600
Bethesda, MD 20814
1-800-458-6223
www.curesearch.org

National Brain Tumor Society
22 Battery Street, Suite 612
San Francisco, CA 94111-5520
1-415-834-9970
1-800-770-8287
FAX 1-415-834-9980
www.braintumor.org

National Cancer Institute
Public Inquiries Office
6116 Executive Boulevard, Suite 300
Bethesda, MD 20892-8322
1-800-422-6237
www.cancernet.nci.nih.gov

Pituitary Network Association
16350 Ventura Blvd., Suite 231
Encino, CA 91436
1-805-499-2262
1-800-462-9211
FAX 1-805-499-1523
www.pituitary.org

Children's Oncology Group
Family handbook on treatment,
support, and follow-up care
*www.childrensoncologygroup.
org/index.php/family-handbook*

⑪ SYNDROMES

OVERVIEW

A *syndrome* is defined as a group of physical features and symptoms that occur together and are believed to stem from the same cause. Individuals with a particular syndrome share many, but usually not all, of the features and symptoms described. In addition to dysmorphic features, children with genetic disorders can have short or tall stature, obesity, and failure to thrive, and be referred to an endocrinologist for further evaluation. The diagnosis of a specific syndrome assists in the treatment, anticipatory guidance, and genetic counseling for children and their families.

HISTORY

Complete endocrine history with careful attention to the following:

HPI/ROS Birth history with time of onset of symptoms, growth patterns

Medical history Obesity; hypogonadism; short stature; obesity with short stature; tall stature; precocious puberty; congenital anomalies; prenatal history, including maternal chronic illness and exposure to teratogens; infections or trauma; neonatal course; current medications

Family history Three-generation pedigree; familial height, weight, onset of sexual maturation, ethnicity, consanguinity, advanced maternal age. History of neonatal or childhood deaths, mental retardation, seizures, and developmental delay or genetic disorders in other members of the family are all extremely important in the initial evaluation.

Social Development

PHYSICAL EXAMINATION

Complete endocrine physical examination with careful attention to the following:

Height, weight, head circumference, chest circumference, upper/lower segment ratio, arm span, hand/foot lengths, measurements of proximal and distal segments of the limbs, ear length, nasal philtrum, pupillary distance, phallic size, testicular volume and bone lengths, ± presence of metacarpal shortening

Assessment of unusual features (dysmorphic features)

Minor/major anomalies (documented with photographs)

For proper measurement of inner canthal distance and hand and foot lengths, see Fig. 11.1.

DIAGNOSTIC TESTING

See tables for diagnostic testing for specific syndromes.

This section offers a brief synopsis of some genetic disorders with an endocrine component. Presenting features, specific diagnostic evaluation, treatment, and considerations for the transition into adulthood are discussed. For a more complete description of clinical features and inclusive listing of genetic disorders, refer to *Smith's Recognizable Patterns of Human Malformation*.[1]

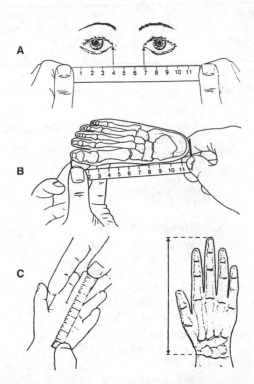

Figure 11.1 **A,** Measurement of inner canthal distance, **B,** length of foot, and **C,** length of hand. (From Hall JG, Allanson JE, Gripp KW, et al. Handbook of Normal Physical Measurement, 2nd ed. Oxford: Oxford University Press, 2007. Reprinted by permission of Oxford University Press.)

DIAGNOSIS	CLINICAL FINDINGS	DIAGNOSTIC FINDINGS

Bartter's Syndrome

A disorder caused by some structural or functional disturbance of the luminal sodium, potassium, chloride co-transporter located in the ascending loop of Henle

Mutations in the renal Na-K-2Cl co-transporter gene have already been demonstrated.

Mostly sporadic occurrence; also autosomal recessive inheritance

Pertinent History

Family history of consanguinity; severe form associated with polyhydramnios, premature delivery

In infancy:
- Failure to thrive
- Poor feeding
- Vomiting
- Constipation
- Weakness
- Dehydration

In childhood:
- Muscle weakness, cramps
- Urinary frequency
- Intellectual impairment

Chronic diuretic use

May have mental retardation

Physical Findings

Normal height and weight at birth; deceleration of growth velocity in infancy and childhood, with growth failure in 75% of patients with early onset

Final height in the low-normal to below-normal percentiles

Normal blood pressure (BP)

Delayed sexual maturation

May have sensorineural deafness

Laboratory Tests

Blood
↑ Renin, aldosterone, parathormone
↓ K^+, Na^+, ionized Ca^+

Urine
↓ Prostaglandin E2 excretion, Ca^+, Cl^-, K^+

Amniocentesis
↑ Aldosterone in amniotic fluid can help identify diagnosis prenatally.

Ultrasound
Early-onset nephrocalcinosis, nephrolithiasis

Radiologic Studies

Bone density: osteopenia

Bone age: delayed

MANAGEMENT/EDUCATION	EVALUATION
Correction of metabolic alkalosis and electrolyte imbalances	Follow-up height, weight, and hydration status each visit
Potassium chloride supplements up to 10 years of age	
Prostaglandin synthetase inhibitors: indomethacin or salicylates	Monitor electrolytes closely to maintain balance.
If unresponsive to indomethacin, oral KCl and spironolactone or triamterene useful in treatment of hypokalemia	
Referral to early intervention program	

11

SYNDROMES

DiGeorge Sequence

Patients with DiGeorge sequence have hypocalcemia arising from parathyroid hypoplasia, thymic hypoplasia, and cardiac defects, mostly of the outflow tract. Hypoplasia of the parathyroid predisposes infants to hypoparathyroidism and subsequent hypocalcemia in the neonatal period. Patients present with tetany and seizures (Fig. 11-2).

DIAGNOSIS	CLINICAL FINDINGS	DIAGNOSTIC FINDINGS
DiGeorge Sequence Heterogenous cause Majority of cases caused by microdeletion of 22q11.2 Also can be associated with prenatal exposure to alcohol, Accutane, chromosomal abnormalities Overall birth prevalence: 1 in 4,000	**Pertinent History** Prenatal exposure to alcohol, retinoic acid, maternal diabetes mellitus Neonatal hypocalcemia, which may present as tetany or seizures Infants may present with congenital cardiac defects: • Aortic arch anomalies • Ventricular septal defect • Patent ductus arteriosus • Tetralogy of Fallot Varying degrees of developmental delay with moderate to severe delay in up to half of cases *(continued)*	**Laboratory Tests** Molecular or fluorescence in situ hybridization (FISH) analysis: microdeletion in chromosome 22q11 (most cases); also found in chromosome 10p13 ↓ Ca+ ↓ Mg+ ↑ Phosphate ↓ or undetectable intact parathyroid hormone, 1,25 hydroxy-vitamin D, B cell, and T cell counts Immunoglobulin levels may be ↓. Audiologic testing ECG

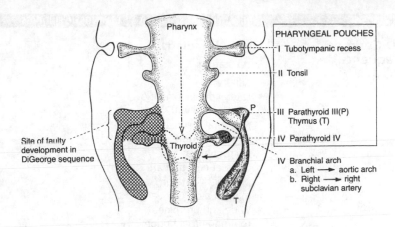

Figure 11.2 DiGeorge sequence. (From Jones KL, ed. Smith's Recognizable Patterns of Human Malformation, 6th ed. Philadelphia: Elsevier Saunders, 2006.)

MANAGEMENT/EDUCATION	EVALUATION
Management of hypocalcemia to prevent hypoxic episodes and prevent development deficits (see pp. 56-57)	Follow-up for hypocalcemia (see pp. 56-57)
Seizure management in early infancy	Consider evaluation for features of velocardiofacial syndrome since there is a microdeletion in same chromosomal region.[1]
Referral to pediatric cardiologist and necessary surgical correction if needed	
If blood transfusion is needed, use irradiated blood.	
May have deficiency in cellular immunity, placing at high risk for severe infectious disease	
May have impaired IgG responses to immunization with bacterial polysaccharides	
Referral as needed for speech therapy and early intervention	

Education

Reinforce medication compliance with family.

DIAGNOSIS	CLINICAL FINDINGS	DIAGNOSTIC FINDINGS
(DiGeorge Sequence)	**Physical Findings** Short stature Facial: • Lateral displacement of inner canthi with short palpebral fissures • Short philtrum, micrognathia • Low-set ears that are posteriorly rotated, making a circular ear • Wide and prominent root and nasal bridge • Prominent U-shaped lips Thymus: hypoplasia to aplasia Parathyroids: hypoplasia to absent	
Down Syndrome Trisomy 21 Incidence: 1 in 660 newborns In advanced maternal age, the risk of occurrence is 1%. In translocation cases with a parent who is a carrier, the risk of recurrence is higher. Mosaicism usually leads to less severe phenotype.	**Pertinent History** Advanced maternal age ↑ Frequency of common illnesses: • Rhinitis • Conjunctivitis • Ear infections Varying degrees of mental retardation *(continued)*	**Laboratory Tests** Karyotype: complete trisomy 21 (94% of cases) Thyroid function tests (TFTs) (congenital hypothyroidism can occur, as well as acquired) At 4 months of age or older, may do TRH stimulation test to rule out subclinical hypothyroidism and for those with elevated TSH and normal T4, free T4 *(continued)*

MANAGEMENT/EDUCATION	EVALUATION

Medications

1-Thyroxine replacement in hypothyroidism

Vitamin supplement therapy is available, but controversial on exact benefits.

GHT has been used in patients with deficiency, although somewhat controversial due to the increased risk of leukemia in this patient population.

Referral to pediatric cardiologist and ophthalmologist for initial evaluation; follow-up based on diagnostic findings

Referral to pediatric surgeon for correction of abnormalities

(continued)

Follow-up for hypothyroidism (see pp. 218-222)

Each visit check for hip dislocations (can occur up to age 10)

Follow-up every 3 months for patients on GH and/or thyroid hormone replacement.

Complications from heart defects are leading cause of mortality.

(continued)

DIAGNOSIS	CLINICAL FINDINGS	DIAGNOSTIC FINDINGS
(Down Syndrome)	**Physical Findings** Major features in neonate: • Poor Moro reflex • Hyperflexion of joints • Excess skin on back/neck, flat facial profile • Slanted palpebral fissures • Anomalous auricles • Dysplasia of pelvis • Dysplasia of midphalanx of fifth finger • Simian crease Growth: short stature Linear growth velocity ↓ between 6 and 24 months, then again during adolescence Final height achieved by 15 years of age • Weight later in life Facies: • Brachycephaly with flat occiput • Late closure of fontanels • Small nose with low nasal bridge with inner epicanthal folds Skin: • Cutis marmorata • Dry skin Eyes: speckling of iris (Brushfield spots) *(continued)*	Complete blood count (CBC), LFTs, plasma amino acids, vitamin A **Radiologic Studies** Radiographs of atlanto-occipital junction by 3 years of age Baseline ECG (congenital heart defects include atrioventricular canal, ventricular septal defect, tetralogy of Fallot, atrial septal defect, and patent ductus arteriosus) Audiologic evaluation (50%-70% have hearing loss) Ophthalmologic evaluation (due to ↑ incidence of ocular defects) Consider GH evaluation in children with abnormal growth velocity who cross down channels on growth curve.

MANAGEMENT/EDUCATION	EVALUATION

Referral to pediatric dentist by the age of 2 with close follow-up; follow recommendations for antibiotic prophylaxis for dental procedures if coronary heart disease present.

Referral to early intervention programs from birth

Referral to genetics for genetic counseling

For children with atlantoaxial instability or those who have not been evaluated, contact sports and somersaults should be restricted.

Education

Promote good dental hygiene with frequent brushing and flossing; close supervision in younger child.

Inform parents about eligibility of special programs available through Public Law 99-457 and 94-142; public laws can assist with school planning and mainstreaming.

In young adulthood, assist families with decisions regarding independent living and placement in group homes.

Cardiology follow-up as an adult for mitral valve prolapse and aortic regurgitation

Baseline amino acids, ammonia, and vitamin A levels prior to start of vitamin therapy

SYNDROMES

DIAGNOSIS	CLINICAL FINDINGS	DIAGNOSTIC FINDINGS
(Down Syndrome)	Ears: • Small, sometimes prominent • Fluid accumulation in middle ear Hands: • Short metacarpals, phalanges • Fifth finger clinodactyly • Distal position of palmar axial triradius (84%) • Ulnar loop dermal ridge pattern of all digits Feet: wide gap between first and second toes Genitalia: • Males: relatively small penis • Decreased testicular volume May have incomplete sexual development	
Kallmann's Syndrome Gonadotropin deficiency causing sexual infantilism associated with anosmia or hyposmia and defective formation of the olfactory bulb	**Pertinent History** Delayed adrenarche History: • Diabetes • Cleft lip and palate • Renal agenesis • Neurosensory deafness • Osteopenia Family history of anosmia and/or sexual infantilism	**Laboratory Tests** Prepubertal FSH, LH ↓ Testosterone + Response to GnRH stimulation **Radiologic Studies** Imaging studies of urinary system
(continued)	*(continued)*	*(continued)*

MANAGEMENT/EDUCATION	EVALUATION
Testosterone replacement therapy for males	Follow-up every 1-3 months based on endocrine therapies
Estrogen/progesterone therapy for females (see pp. 386-387)	Monitor height, weight, progression of sexual development for those on replacement therapy.
Follutein or human menopausal gonadotropin used with luteinizing LH or HCG has stimulated fertility in male and female patients.	Monitor height, weight, progression of sexual development for those on replacement therapy.
GnRH given via infusion may be used to induce ovulation. Long-term treatment in males increases chances to conceive children	Monitor for side effects of replacement therapy.

(continued)

DIAGNOSIS	CLINICAL FINDINGS	DIAGNOSTIC FINDINGS
(Kallmann's Syndrome) The region where the olfactory bulb forms and GnRH cells originate before migration to the hypothalamus is the same. Incidence: • Males, 1 in 10,000 • Females, 1 in 50,000 Autosomal dominant, autosomal recessive, and X-linked recessive genes have been documented. In the X-linked form, the gene has been mapped to the distal part of the short arm of X chromosome (Xp22.3).	**Physical Findings** Normal or tall stature Eye—ocular abnormalities: • Coloboma • Optic disc dysplasia • Myopia • Strabismus Genitalia: • Micropenis • Cryptorchidism	MRI of brain to evaluate olfactory groove; will have absent olfactory bulbs (unilateral or bilateral) Bone age: delayed by 2 to 6 years due to absence of sex steroids Sensorineural hearing evaluation
Klinefelter Syndrome Most common single cause of hypogonadism and infertility With mosaicism, better prognosis for testicular function Incidence: 1 in 500-1,000 male births	**Pertinent History** Development: • Delayed speech, problems with expressive language • Delayed auditory processing, auditory memory leading to decreased ability to read and spell *(continued)*	**Laboratory Tests** Karyotype: 47XXY Other chromosomal variants include XXXY, XXY/XY (mosaicism) and XXYY (may be found on amniocentesis prenatally). ↑ LH ↑ FSH ↓ Testosterone Azospermia *(continued)*

MANAGEMENT/EDUCATION	EVALUATION

Education

Instruct patients receiving testosterone therapy of side effects such as gynecomastia, which is usually transient.

Provide psychologic counseling and emotional support.

Medications

At 11-12 years of age, initiate testosterone replacement therapy: enanthate or cipionate injections biweekly or monthly.

Surgical intervention for gynecomastia may be indicated (10% of individuals).

Education

Males with gynecomastia have the same risk of breast cancer as women. Teach technique for breast self-examination.

Follow-up for testosterone therapy every month

Height, weight, sexual development

Recheck testosterone level to achieve normal levels.

Scoliosis screening each visit

(continued)

(continued)

DIAGNOSIS	CLINICAL FINDINGS	DIAGNOSTIC FINDINGS
(Klinefelter Syndrome)	Behavior problems are common, as well as difficulty with psycho-social adjustment. In adult males, ↓ libido **Physical Findings** Growth: • Long limbs with low upper/lower segment ratio • Tall, slim stature Genitalia: • Relatively small penis and testes from childhood • Testes remain small through adulthood (<2.5 ml), and penis is usually normal in size. • Other than small testicles, normal development of secondary sexual characteristics May have a lack of facial and body hair and gynecomastia Hand tremors More skeletal problems and dysmorphic features are associated with karyotypes that include ≥2 X chromosomes.	**Radiologic Studies** Chest X-ray for increased incidence of mediastinal tumor

MANAGEMENT/EDUCATION	EVALUATION
Anticipatory guidance for parents of early-diagnosed patients that there are varying degrees of psychologic problems	In adulthood, individuals have an increased incidence of developing non–insulin-dependent diabetes mellitus (NIDDM), lupus erythematosus, thyroiditis, and germ cell tumors of the mediastinum.
As an adult, counseling regarding infertility and the option of adoption	

SYNDROMES ⑪

DIAGNOSIS	CLINICAL FINDINGS	DIAGNOSTIC FINDINGS

Marfan Syndrome

A connective tissue, autosomal dominant disorder causing mutations in a fibrillin gene located on chromosome 15q21.1 FBN1

Fibrillin is a glycoprotein that is a major component of the suspended ligament of the eye as well as elastin in the aorta.

Pertinent History

Neonatal presentation most severe, progressive

Expression and severity of clinical features vary from family to family.

Obstructive sleep apnea

Physical Findings

Ocular:
- Lens subluxation, usually upward
- Myopia
- Retinal detachment

Cardiovascular:
- Dilatation with or without dissecting aneurysm of ascending aorta
- Mitral valve prolapse

Skeletal:
- Tall stature
- Long, thin extremities
- Arachnodactyly
- Hyperextensibility of the joints
- Bony overgrowth
- Scoliosis
- Pectus deformity

Confirmation of diagnosis based on major and minor clinical criteria affecting skeletal, ocular, CV systems; family history

Four major diagnostic criteria:
- Dilatation of aorta
- Ectopia lentis
- Dural ectasia
- Four of eight skeletal features[3]

Molecular testing: FBN1 mutation

Radiologic Studies

ECG shows aortic dilatation.

X-ray for scoliosis screen

Ophthalmology exam

Comprehensive management with a team approach:
- Cardiologist
- Geneticist
- Ophthalmologist
- Orthopedist
- Cardiothoracic surgeon

Diagnosis and prevention of scoliosis

Surgical correction of scoliosis or pectus deformation may be necessary.

Orthotics and arch support for treatment of pes planus

Beta-adrenergic blocking agents are started on diagnosis to reduce the rate of aortic dilatation.

Surgical repair of aorta when maximal measurement is 5 cm in adults or older children,[3] or rate ↑ each year, or aortic regurgitation occurs

Prophylaxis for subacute bacterial endocarditis prior to dental work

Ophthalmology evaluation and follow-up

Correction of refractive error prevents further complications.

Education

Restrict:
- Contact sports
- Competitive sports
- Weight lifting
- Isometric exercises
- Activities that cause joint injury or pain

Avoid agents that stimulate the CV system:
- Decongestants
- Caffeine

Avoid LASIK correction of refractive errors.

Prenatal testing for pregnancies at ↑ risk is possible if family mutation is known.

Severity of case is the best indicator of survival.

Early diagnosis and management improve life expectancy.

Cardiovascular complications are leading cause of death.

ECG annually; more frequently when indicated

Young adulthood: intermittent surveillance of aorta by CT or MRI

Annual ophthalmology exam

SYNDROMES

⓫

DIAGNOSIS	CLINICAL FINDINGS	DIAGNOSTIC FINDINGS

McCune-Albright Syndrome (MAS)

Sporadic occurrence resulting from a GNAS genetic mutation encoding the alpha subunit of the G protein. G proteins affect production of cyclic adenosine monophosphate (cAMP). In MAS, it is constantly turned on, leading to overstimulation of growth and function of gonads, adrenal cortex, and specific pituitary cells.

Severity of clinical expression depends on number of cells and areas of body that are involved.

Frequency in females to males is 3:2.

Pertinent History

Early presentation of precocious puberty, with menstruation occurring prior to the development of breasts or pubic hair; 85% of cases develop menstrual bleeding as the first symptom before 2 years of age.

Hyperthyroidism, hyperparathyroidism, pituitary adenomas, Cushing's syndrome, hyperprolactinemia

Family history: bone dysplasia

Physical Findings

Bone: Multiple areas of fibrous dysplasias (most common in long bones and pelvis) may progress during childhood, resulting in fractures, asymmetry, and/or deformity.

Skin:
- Café au lait spots—irregular brown pigmentation, most commonly on sacrum, buttocks, upper spine, shoulders; unilateral (50%)

Laboratory Tests

May have ↑ T3, ↓ TSH

May have ↑ cortisol, ↓ ACTH

Adrenal function not suppressed by dexamethasone

↑ Estradiol, ↓ FSH, ↓ LH

Luteinizing hormone–releasing hormone (LHRH) stimulation test: no response indicating gonadotropin-releasing hormone (GnRH) independent of hypothalamic-pituitary axis

↑ GH levels

↑ Prolactin

Radiologic Studies

MRI of the brain and pituitary gland to rule out possibility of adenoma of pituitary

Skeletal survey:
- Widespread cystic bony changes
- Fractures and deformities of long bones
- Bony lesions in base of skull

Advanced bone age

Pelvic ultrasound may reveal ovarian cysts and/or nodular adrenal hyperplasia.

(continued)

Medications

Precocious puberty
- Tamoxifen
- Ketoconazole

GnRH analogs used alone are not effective.

Other investigational oral medications include aromatase inhibitors, which block estrogen synthesis: letrozole[4]

Hyperthyroidism
- Propylthiouracil (PTU)
- Methimazole

Acromegaly
Surgery if pituitary adenoma secreting GH

Medical management includes:
- Dopamine agonists
- Somatostatin analogs
- Growth hormone receptor antagonist

Bone dysplasias
No medical treatment at this time, although investigational treatment with bisphosphonates has shown improvement.[5]

Surgical procedures such as grafting, pinning, and casting may be used for fractures.

Education

Provide information regarding side effects of thyroid therapy and other medications used to block estrogen synthesis.

In some individuals, regular puberty occurs in adolescence.

These patients should be managed with extreme caution during procedures due to increased bone fragility.

Follow-up based on level of endocrine involvement (see pp. 40-41, pp. 198-201, and pp. 224-227)

Transition to adulthood depends on severity of bone and endocrine involvement.

Many women are fertile and can bear children normally.

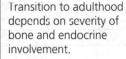

DIAGNOSIS	CLINICAL FINDINGS	DIAGNOSTIC FINDINGS
(McCune-Albright Syndrome)	Coarse facial features, enlargement of the hands and feet, arthritis as a result of excessive GH secretion Thyroid: may have presence of multinodular goiters	
Noonan Syndrome Incidence: 1 in 1,000-2,500 Gene-mapped chromosome 12q24.1 Autosomal dominant inheritance also has been documented. Has been called *male Turner Syndrome* Can affect males and females	**Pertinent History** Congenital heart defects Feeding difficulties in neonatal period May have mild mental retardation. Learning disabilities Lack of sexual development **Physical Findings** Growth: normal size at birth, with subsequent growth retardation Affects height, weight, bone development Adult height: • Males, 162.5 cm • Females, 152.7 cm Short stature (80%)	**Genetic Mutations** PTPN11 (50% of cases) Diagnosis mostly made based on presence of clinical features at this time. Chromosome testing: linkage analysis using chromosome 12 markers is promising for future diagnosis. Chromosome analysis in female to differentiate from Turner Syndrome May have ↓ GH levels (<10 ng/ml in response to stimulation testing) Sex hormone profile may indicate hypogonadism. Thrombocytopenia may be present, indicating an associated coagulopathy found in some individuals.

(continued)

MANAGEMENT/EDUCATION	EVALUATION

GH therapy shows significant improvement in near final height. Earlier age of initiation of treatment and longer prepubertal duration of treatment allow improved height SDS at pubertal onset and near adult height.[6]

Sex hormone replacement therapy to improve secondary sexual characteristics in hypogonadism

Surgical intervention may be indicated for cardiac, skeletal, or genitourinary problems.

Hematologic evaluation prior to any surgical procedure to rule out possibility of bleeding disorder

Precautions for malignant hyperthermia: Anesthesiologists must be informed that child has Noonan Syndrome so anesthetic triggering agents will be avoided.

Encourage family and patient participation in Noonan support group.

Follow-up for patients on GH therapy every 3 months (see pp. 158-166)

Due to incidence of cardiomyopathy and its variable course in each individual, cautious use of GH is essential, as well as cardiology follow-up.

Follow-up every month for patients on sex hormone replacement therapy; evaluation based on clinical exam, sex hormone levels in pubertal range

Fertility may be impaired but is normal in females and in males with descended testes.

DIAGNOSIS	CLINICAL FINDINGS	DIAGNOSTIC FINDINGS
(Noonan Syndrome)	Facies: • Epicanthal folds • Ptosis of eyelids • Hypertelorism • Low nasal bridge • Down-slanting palpebral fissures • Low-set and/or abnormal ears • Anterior dental malocclusion • ↑ Width of mouth • Prominent, protruding retrognathia Neck: • Low posterior hairline • Short or webbed neck Thorax: • Shield chest • Pectus excavatum or pectus carinatum • Cubitus valgus Cardiovascular: Pulmonary valve stenosis is most common defect. Hypertrophic cardiomyopathy Hepatosplenomegaly in first year of life Genitalia: • Small penis • Cryptorchidism • Delayed puberty	

MANAGEMENT/EDUCATION	EVALUATION

DIAGNOSIS	CLINICAL FINDINGS	DIAGNOSTIC FINDINGS

Prader-Willi Syndrome (PWS)

Results from the lack of expression of genes located on the paternally derived "PWS region" of chromosome 15q11-q13 by deletion, uniparental disomy (both maternal 15 and no paternal copy, and imprinting defects)

Prevalence: 1 in 8,000 to 1 in 20,000 live births

PWS is considered today the most common genetic cause of life-threatening obesity.

Most common characteristics:
- Short stature
- Obesity
- Hypogonadism
- Mental deficiency

Pertinent History
Prenatal Period

Decreased fetal activity

Breech presentation

Nonterm delivery

1st stage (neonatal and early infancy):
- Neonatal hypotonia
- Weak cry
- Developmental delay
- Poor suck reflex
- Feeding difficulties, which may require lavage or G-tube feeds

Failure to thrive, poor weight gain

Hypotonia may improve by 8 to 11 months

Temperature instability

Developmental delays: language most delayed

Sit alone: 11-12 months

Crawl: 15-16 months

Walk: 24-27 months

Talk: 10 words, 38-39 months

2nd stage (starts at 2 years of age):
- Onset of hyperphagia leading to obesity
- Continued developmental/psychological motor delay

(continued)

Laboratory Tests

See Butler et al[3] for criteria to prompt diagnostic testing for PWS.

DNA methylation molecular analysis of the Prader-Willi critical region is the most conclusive test (98%) to identify the deletion, uniparental disomy, imprinting defects.

Fluorescence in situ (FISH) analysis shows deletion of hybridization on the long arm of chromosome 15 @ q11-q13.

See Butler et al[7] for more detail on genetic lab testing for PWS.

Initial screening:
- Thyroid panel
- Lipid panel
- IGFBP-3, IGF-1

If obese, fasting glucose, HgbA1c, OGTT, if indicated

In adolescence:
- FSH, LH ↓ to normal
- Estrogens, testosterone ↓ to normal

↓ IGF-1

(continued)

MANAGEMENT/EDUCATION	EVALUATION

Early infancy: Hypotonia may lead to respiratory and feeding problems requiring gavage tube feeding.

Physical Therapy

Essential in treatment of PWS

Respiratory infections may occur due to hypotonia, which leads to poor ventilator capacity. Use antibiotics when infection is present to prevent further respiratory decompensation.[7]

Short Stature/Growth Failure

Growth hormone treatment is indicated in patients with short stature and/or growth failure. Effects on growth, body composition, bone mineral density, and physical function have been reported.[4]

Dietary evaluation and counseling

In older infants and children:
- Control progressive obesity
- Decrease caloric intake to 7-8 cal/cm height for weight loss; 10-14 cal/cm height for weight maintenance.

Family counseling and cooperation; need to make food physically inaccessible

Skin care: Assess regularly for cutaneous infections.

DuoDERM patches, topical antibiotics, and antifungals for skin lesions

Culture and sensitivity for persistent infections

Hypogonadism: sex hormone replacement therapy

Males: testosterone therapy

Infancy: early short-term use for enlargement of micropenis

Adolescence: replacement at biologically appropriate time to improve muscle mass and prevent osteoporosis

(continued)

Early diagnosis leads to appropriate management and referrals for support services, genetic counseling.

Weight Management

Follow-up dependent on level of endocrine component

Height, weight, scoliosis screen each visit

Screening for glucose intolerance if patient is obese.

Regular exams for cutaneous infections; assess pressure points, scalp, perianal area, groin, axillae.

Monitor growth and development in early childhood and every 3 months.

DXA screening in childhood/early adolescence; repeat based on risk factors

Monitor patients on sex hormone replacement.

Clinical and behavior status, bone mineral density

(continued)

⓫

SYNDROMES

DIAGNOSIS	CLINICAL FINDINGS	DIAGNOSTIC FINDINGS
(Prader-Willi Syndrome)	Other features noted: • Speech articulation problems • Foraging for food • Rumination • Unmotivated • Sleepiness • Physical inactivity • ↓ Pain sensitivity • Skin picking or self-injurious behavior • Prolonged periods of hypothermia Obstructive sleep apnea Infants and toddlers usually easygoing, affectionate 3-5 years: • Personality problems • Temper tantrums • Depression • Stubbornness • Obsessive compulsivity • Sudden acts of violence that may or may not be initiated by withholding of food Behavioral/learning problems may be more prominent in teenage years. Decreased incidence of vomiting; vomiting may signal life-threatening illness[6] Amenorrhea (60% of females) *(continued)*	↓ GH levels (<10 ng/mL) on stimulation testing and physiologic secretion (stimulation testing not necessary for approval of GH treatment) Sleep studies for patients with risk factors (See Prader-Willi Syndrome Association (USA) Clinical Advisory Board Consensus Statement 2003[8] for evaluation of breathing abnormalities associated with sleep.) **Radiologic Studies** X-ray of spine may reveal scoliosis. Bone age delayed Body composition analysis Bone mineral density in adolescence/adulthood: osteopenia

MANAGEMENT/EDUCATION	EVALUATION

Females:

Estrogen/progestin therapy for females may be considered especially in presence of amenorrhea or oligomenorrhea and/or osteoporosis.

Cryptorchidism: human chorionic gonadotropin (HCG) treatment biweekly for 4-6 weeks; surgical intervention needed if no response or partial response

Referral to orthopedic surgeon if scoliosis is present.

Preventive treatment of low bone mineral density includes nutrition therapy with prn vitamin D and calcium supplementation, ongoing to prevent osteopenia, osteoporosis.

Instruct family that eating behaviors are part of the syndrome and food must be physically inaccessible. Close supervision of food is necessary for avoiding obesity. Family/caregivers need to make food inaccessible (e.g., locking refrigerators, cabinets containing food, garbage can).

The presence of vomiting may signal a life-threatening illness.[9]

Caretakers should be aware of the decreased pain sensation; signs of infection, fracture, and injury may not be signaled by pain.

Acute or unexpected changes in behavior, mobility, or unusual gait

Reinforce to family that behavior problems are also part of syndrome. Referral to psychiatrist may be necessary.

Educate school nurse and child's teachers about syndrome and level of cognitive deficiency.

Encourage and facilitate family participation in Prader-Willi support groups.

Continue follow-up in adolescence and adulthood to reduce complications of obesity:

- Non–insulin-dependent diabetes mellitus (NIDDM)
- Hyperinsulinism

Individuals vary in their ability to live independently. Assist family in placement of young adult in group home if appropriate.

Educational Evaluation

Monitor school performance.

Psychological and/or educational testing

Transition to Adulthood

GH therapy may be needed to aid in ↑ lean body mass and ↓ fat mass.[10]

SYNDROMES

⑪

DIAGNOSIS	CLINICAL FINDINGS
(Prader-Willi Syndrome)	Excessive daytime sleepiness Level of mental deficiency varies; average IQ is 65 with a range from 20 to 100. **Physical Findings** *Based on age, clinical features vary in extent and severity.* Growth: short stature with decreased growth rate during childhood and adolescence Mean adult height: • Males, 155 cm • Females, 147 cm Craniofacial: • Almond-shaped palpebral fissures • Narrow bifrontal diameter • Thin upper lip • Fish-shaped mouth • Sticky saliva Oral: • Enamel hypoplasia • Dental caries • Malocclusion Eyes/Skin: • Blond to light brown hair with blue eyes and fair skin • Strabismus • Hypopigmentation compared with family members • Sores from excessive skin picking Respiratory abnormalities: sleep-related central and obstructive apnea Hands and feet: • Arrow hands with straight ulnar border • Small for size Genitalia: • Small penis • Cryptorchidism • Hypoplastic labia minora and clitoris Hypotonia: floppy Scoliosis

DIAGNOSTIC FINDINGS	MANAGEMENT/EDUCATION	EVALUATION

DIAGNOSIS	CLINICAL FINDINGS	DIAGNOSTIC FINDINGS

Russell-Silver Syndrome (RSS)

Described by Silver in 1953[11] and Russell in 1954[12]

Large variation in phenotype

Referred to as *primordial dwarfism,* because there is no specific cause for short stature and no identified skeletal dysplasia.

Incidence: 1 in 50,000 to 1 in 100,000 births (milder forms may be more frequent but harder to diagnose)[13]

Uniparental maternal 7 disomy (matUPD7) has been recently described in 10% of individuals[14]; may have milder phenotype[14]

11p15 ICR1 epimutation: can also result in RSS[13]

Pertinent History

Intrauterine growth retardation (IUGR)

Hypoglycemia in infancy and early childhood (2-3 years)

Slow growth with decreased weight for height

Developmental delays

Wilms tumor

Physical Findings

Low birth weight, short length

Large head size for body

Body asymmetry is most distinct feature.

Average height:
- Males, 152 cm
- Females, 144.7 cm

Dysmorphology:
- Clinodactyly of the fifth finger
- Frontal bossing
- Small, triangular face
- Protuberant, low-set and/or posteriorly rotated ears
- Thin upper lip and downturned corners of the mouth
- Small, narrow, pointed chin/jaw

Laboratory Tests

Evaluation of short stature, including GH testing for those with growth retardation (for list of tests, see p. 146)

IGF-1 level low to normal

Radiologic Studies

Bone age

Renal ultrasound in individuals with body asymmetry

(continued)

MANAGEMENT/EDUCATION	EVALUATION

Dietary counseling to increase caloric intake and improve growth

Feeding tube may be necessary to increase caloric intake.

GH therapy (GHT) indicated for small for gestational age children who fail to demonstrate catch-up growth by age 2 years

GHT in documented patients with deficiency

Unknown whether final height is improved favorably with GHT

Speech, occupational, physical, and special education therapies based on individual's needs

Refer to orthopedist for shoe lifts if asymmetry present.

Limb-lengthening surgery may be utilized in leg asymmetry.

Education

Instruct family that most difficult years are the early years of life.

Reinforce that feeding difficulties improve through childhood and are insignificant in adulthood.

Presenting dysmorphology also becomes less prominent as child grows.

Counsel patient and family in dealing with short stature, which poses biggest challenge.

In early infancy and childhood, follow-up every 1-3 months to evaluate adequate weight gain and caloric intake.

Follow-up every 3 months for patients on GHT

SYNDROMES

DIAGNOSIS	CLINICAL FINDINGS	DIAGNOSTIC FINDINGS
(Russell-Silver Syndrome)	Skin: may have café au lait spots Genitalia: • Hypospadias • Cryptorchidism	

Turner Syndrome

Gonadal dysgenesis caused by the absence of 46, XY/X a second X chromosome; also by structural defects resulting in a loss of portions of an X chromosome

Sporadic occurrence with an incidence of 1 in 2,500 live female births

Most consistent features are short stature and gonadal dysgenesis, with or without dysmorphology.

Pertinent History

Primary or secondary amenorrhea 45, X (most common)

History of recurrent otitis media

Development:
• Delays in motor skills (clumsiness)
• Difficulties in math and nonverbal problem solving

Psychosocial: Deficits in social cognition may lead to low self-esteem and depression.

Physical Findings

Growth:
• Gowth retardation in utero
• 2.8 cm less than the mean at birth

Postnatal growth failure from birth and slow growth through childhood and teens; prolonged late-teen growth
(continued)

Laboratory Tests

Diagnosis:
• Karyotype (minimum of 30 cells: mosaicism—46, XX/X)
• ↑ FSH
• ↑ LH
• ↓ Estradiol

Thyroid function tests may indicate hypothyroidism.

Thyroid antibodies: autoimmune thyroiditis

Cardiovascular Screening

Aortic defects common:
• ECG for younger patients
• Cardiac MRI and ECG for older girls and adults
• Discordant BP in extremities

Baseline renal ultrasound to rule out kidney anomalies (most common is horseshoe kidney)

(continued)

MANAGEMENT/EDUCATION	EVALUATION

Medications

GHT for treatment of short stature (early initiation may improve final height)[15]

Low-dose anabolic steroids (oxandrolone) can be considered.[16]

Supplement calcium (1200-1500 mg/day), vitamin D replacement

Ovarian Hormone Replacement

- Age 10-11 years: Monitor spontaneous puberty and FSH level.
- Age 12-13 years: If no spontaneous development and ↑ FSH, start low-dose estrogen and gradually ↑ estrogen dose over 2 years.
- Age 14-16 years: Begin cyclic progesterone after 2 years of estrogen or when breakthrough bleeding occurs.
- Age 14-30 years: Continue full dose at least until age 30.[15]

In patients with a Y chromosome in some cell lines, removal of the streak gonads is necessary due to incidence of gonadoblastomas.

Nursing Considerations

GHT: Early treatment is most effective in maximizing final height and facilitating early catch-up growth.

Anabolic steroids: Consider initiation at bone age of 9-10 years (most effective if used with GH therapy).

(continued)

Follow-up every 3 months with patients on endocrine therapies

Discontinue GH if BA ≥14 or growth velocity <2 cm/yr

Annual lab evaluation:
- Thyroid function testing
- Antithyroid microsomal and thryoglobulin antibodies
- Liver function tests
- Glucose
- Fasting lipid

Celiac screening:
- Tissue transglutaminase IgA every 2-5 years
- Antibodies annually after 8 years

Screen for scoliosis each visit with referral to orthopedic surgeon if necessary.

BP each visit

Cardiologist referral at diagnosis

(continued)

DIAGNOSIS	CLINICAL FINDINGS	DIAGNOSTIC FINDINGS
(Turner Syndrome)	Average height = 143 cm Tendency to become obese Craniofacial: • Narrow maxilla • Small mandible • Inner canthal folds • Prominent, anomalous ears Neck: • Low posterior hairline • Appearance of short neck • Webbed posterior neck • Infants may have excessive skinfolds. Thorax: • Broad chest with widely spaced nipples • Mild pectus excavatum 30%-40% of patients have congenital lymphedema, which may also occur with initiation of growth hormone (GH) or estrogen therapy Musculoskeletal: • Scoliosis • Extremities—elbow, cubitus valgus; short fourth metacarpal Puberty: delayed or incomplete	Audiology: sensorineural hearing testing for hearing loss Baseline bone mineral density: DXA scan; may indicate osteopenia or osteoporosis Psychometric testing may reveal learning disabilities

MANAGEMENT/EDUCATION	EVALUATION

Instruct patients on importance of skeletal loading exercise for bone mineralization.

Refer for psychosocial support and encourage activity in support groups.

Education

Developmental intervention includes:
- Developmental screening at diagnosis and annually or biannually
- Early intervention (OT, PT, ST)
- Educational testing
- Development and implementation of individualized education plan (IEP)
- Vocational counseling
- ADD/ADHD evaluation: 24% prevalence

Instruct patient/family that if patient develops chest pain, he or she must be evaluated immediately.

Inform all providers that patient has Turner syndrome.

Counsel against tobacco and alcohol use.

Early genetic counseling for parents and in early adulthood for patient

---

Echocardiogram for younger patients; MRI, echocardiogram for older girls, adults

BP in all extremities

Cardiologist:
- Check heart
- Aortic valve, arch
- Pulmonary veins

Cardiac follow-up depending on degree of involvement

If normal cardiovascular system and BP, repeat ECG every 5 years, MRI every 5-10 years

ENT and audiology every 1-5 years

Screen for ADHD first to fifth grade

Educational and social progress annually

In adolescents, ↑ risk for metabolic abnormalities, insulin resistance

Monitor lipid profile, glucose, insulin, liver function tests

Rare cases of fertility in women of childbearing years

Ovum donation, in vitro fertilization, and embryo transplantation may be options, as well as adoption.

SYNDROMES ⑪

RESOURCES/SUPPORT GROUPS

Human Growth Foundation
Information on growth and Russell-Silver syndrome, Turner syndrome
Human Growth Foundation
997 Glen Cove Avenue, Suite 5
Glen Head, NY 11545
1-800-451-6434
FAX 1-516-671-4055
www.hgfound.org

Klinefelter Syndrome and Associates
11 Keats Court
Coto de Caza, CA 92679
1-888-999-9428
www.genetic.org/

Magic Foundation
*Information on many endocrine conditions, including
Russell-Silver syndrome and McCune-Albright syndrome*
6645 W. North Avenue
Oak Park, IL 60302
708-383-0808 OR 1-800-3-MAGIC-3
www.magicfoundation.org

National Marfan Foundation (U.S.)
382 Main Street
Port Washington, NY 11050
1-516-883-8712 OR 1-800-8-MARFAN
FAX 1-516-883-8040
www.marfan.org

The Noonan Syndrome Support Group (TNSSG)
P.O. Box 145
Upperco, MD 21155
1-888-686-2224
www.noonansyndrome.org

The Prader-Willi Syndrome Association (U.S.)
8588 Potter Park Drive, Suite 500
Sarasota, FL 34238
1-800-926-4797 OR 941-312-0400
E-MAIL *national@pwsausa.org*
www.pwsausa.org

Turner Syndrome Society of the United States
11250 West Road G
Houston, TX 77065
1-800-365-9944
www.turnersyndrome.org

⑫ STIMULATION TESTING

Please note: Most practitioners develop their own preference for diagnostic agents, testing routine, and protocol format. This section does not address all types of testing or protocols, but does provide a comprehensive overview of stimulation tests commonly used in practice. References provide variation in stimulation testing, including the protocol title, timing of samples, and dosage of the stimulating agent. This chapter is intended to serve only as a reference guide for health care professionals practicing in endocrinology. A pediatric endocrinologist should be readily available on site during stimulation testing and be able to respond immediately to emergent situations before, during, and after the stimulation testing procedure.

ADRENAL DISORDERS

STANDARD ACTH TEST

Indication Screening test for adrenal insufficiency. A very-low-dose test may be useful in assessing adrenal recovery from glucocorticoid suppression.[1]

Preparation Explain the procedure to the patient/family. The patient should be off medication that interferes with ACTH secretion, especially steroids.

Procedure
1. Obtain the baseline cortisol level. Inject Cortrosyn 0.25 mg (Cortrosyn 25 IU, one vial) IV push over approximately 1-2 minutes.[2,3] If using low-dose protocol, use 0.001 mg (1µg) for any age.[1]
2. Subsequent cortisol levels should be obtained at 30 minutes and 60 minutes after administration of Cortrosyn. Protocols vary by dose of Cortrosyn and subsequent timing of cortisol levels.

Nursing considerations Drugs that may falsely increase cortisol levels include corticosteroids, estrogens, and spironolactone.

Interpretation A significant rise of at least 10 µg/dL above baseline in cortisol levels 30 minutes after Cortrosyn and a cortisol level greater than 18-20 µg/dL 60 minutes after Cortrosyn demonstrates normal adrenal secretion of cortisol.[2,3]

RAPID ACTH TEST[1,2,4]

Indication Screening test for adrenal insufficiency. A very-low-dose test may be useful in assessing adrenal recovery from glucocorticoid suppression.

Preparation None

Procedure

1. Cosyntropin (Cortrosyn), a synthetic ACTH derivative, is given IM or IV.
   DOSING   0.10 mg, <1 year of age
             0.15 mg, 1 to 5 years of age
             0.25 mg, older than 5 years
             0.001 mg (1 μg) if using low-dose protocol for any age
2. Blood samples for serum cortisol are drawn at baseline (time 0), and at 30 and 60 minutes after cosyntropin administration.

Nursing considerations Drugs that may cause falsely increased cortisol levels include corticosteroids, estrogens, and spironolactone.

Interpretation Normally, a rise in serum cortisol to >20 μg/dL occurs within 60 minutes of Cortrosyn administration. If the peak serum cortisol is <20 μg/dL, the patient has primary adrenal failure (adrenal glands inadequately stimulated by pituitary ACTH) or chronically suppressed adrenal glands.

ACTH TEST FOR ADRENAL ANDROGEN DISORDERS[2,3]

Indication To assist in the diagnosis of congenital adrenal hyperplasia (CAH) or an adrenal or ovarian tumor

Preparation Explain procedure to patient/family. The patient should be off medication that interferes with ACTH secretion, especially steroids.

Procedure

1. Obtain baseline steroid levels, including those of androstenedione, cortisol, DHEA, DHEA-S, 11-deoxycortisol (Compound S), 17-hydroxyprogesterone (17-OHP), 17-hydroxypregnenolone (17-OH-Preg), deoxycorticosterone (DOC), and testosterone. When ruling out one of the types associated with HTN, a renin is sometimes useful.
2. Cortrosyn 0.25 mg (Cortrosyn 25 IU, one vial) is injected IV push over approximately 1-2 minutes.[2,3]
3. Blood samples are then drawn at 60 minutes after Cortrosyn injection for levels as ordered, possibly androstenedione, cortisol, DHEA, 11-deoxycortisol (Compound S), 17-hydroxyprogesterone (17-OHP), 17-hydroxypregnenolone (17-OH-Preg), and deoxycorticosterone (DOC).

Interpretation The results are determined by considering the difference between the baseline and stimulated sample of steroid levels. One may plot results on the appropriate nomograms or graphs. See specific instructions on graphs for interpretation (Figures 2.3 and 2.4, pp. 26-27).

OVERNIGHT DEXAMETHASONE SUPPRESSION TEST

Indication Useful in screening for glucocorticoid or adrenal androgen overproduction

Preparation Explain procedure to patient/family. Obtain patient's baseline weight.

Procedure Dexamethasone 1 mg (for children <25 kg a dose of 0.5 mg) should be given by mouth at 11:00 PM.[2,5] A fasting cortisol level is drawn at 8:00 AM.

Nursing considerations Evaluate patient for signs of gastric irritation and steroid-induced side effects by monitoring weight, glucose levels, and potassium levels.[5]

Interpretation The test is interpreted by assessing the serum cortisol. Cortisol levels are suppressed in normal individuals to <5 μg/dL. False negatives are extremely rare; patients with cortisol levels between 5-10 μg/dL should have the test repeated. Patients whose cortisol levels fail to suppress to <10 μg/dL should be tested further to evaluate for Cushing's syndrome and its cause.[2,5]

STANDARD DEXAMETHASONE SUPPRESSION TEST

Indication Useful in the diagnosis and differentiation of Cushing's syndrome following inadequate suppression of cortisol on the overnight suppression test

Preparation Explain procedure to patient/family. Obtain patient's baseline weight.

Procedure

1. A standard dexamethasone suppression test requires baseline 24-hour urine collections on days 1-2 for 17-hydroxycorticosteroids (17-OHCS), urinary free cortisol, and creatinine.
2. Part 1: Most often this test is performed as a continuation of the previously described standard dexamethasone suppression test, beginning on day 3. Give the patient a low dose of dexamethasone on days 3-4 (20 μg/kg/day PO to a maximum of 0.5 mg per dose) every 6 hours for 2 days. Adults and older children may be given 0.5 mg every 6 hours for 8 doses.[2] Continue daily 24-hour urine collections and morning serum cortisol levels.
3. Part 2: Give high-dose dexamethasone 2 mg per dose every 6 hours on days 5-6, continuing the 24-hour urine collections as on previous days.[2]
4. Blood for cortisol and DHEA-S should be drawn at 8:00 AM each morning of the test.

Nursing considerations Evaluate patient for signs of gastric irritation and steroid-induced side effects by monitoring weight, glucose levels, and potassium levels.[6]

Interpretation Patients with Cushing's syndrome will rarely suppress, and will maintain elevated urinary free cortisol and urinary 17-OHCS levels. However, by the end of the high-dose part of the test, even the patients with Cushing's syndrome due to excessive pituitary ACTH production (Cushing's disease) should suppress their urinary free cortisol and 17-OHCS levels to <50% of baseline values.[2]

OVERNIGHT METYRAPONE TEST[2,7]

Indication Used to document secondary adrenal insufficiency

Preparation None

Procedure

1. A single dose of metyrapone is given orally between 11 PM and 12 AM with a snack to minimize gastrointestinal discomfort. The dose is 30 mg/kg to a maximum of 1 g.
2. Blood for 11-deoxycortisol, cortisol, and ACTH is drawn at 8 AM.

Nursing considerations Metyrapone should not be used in sick patients or if primary insufficiency (Addison's disease) is suspected. Stay alert for signs of adrenal insufficiency caused by metyrapone. Give metyrapone with food to prevent adverse effects such as nausea.

Interpretation ACTH levels should be elevated. Cortisol should be <8 μg/dL. Serum 11-deoxycortisol should increase to >10 μg/dL.

PUBERTY

GnRH (LHRH) STIMULATION TEST[1]

Indication To determine whether the LH and FSH response suggest a central or peripheral cause for the precocious puberty, and to diagnose delayed puberty or gonadal deficiency. It can also be utilized for assessing dosage appropriateness for GnRH analog.

Due to the unavailability of Factrel, leuprolide acetate is used as an alternative for LHRH stimulation testing.[3,6]

Procedure

GnRH stimulation Obtain baseline estradiol (for females) or testosterone (for males) and FSH and LH. Synthetic GnRH (Factrel) to a maximum dose of 100 μg[3] is given IV push in approximately 30-60 seconds. Blood samples are collected and sent for FSH, LH. Blood samples are recommended at the following times: baseline, 15, 30, 45, 60 and 90 minutes.

Alternatively, synthetic GnRH agonist (leuprolide acetate) 20 μg/kg/dose to a maximum of 500 μg[3] is given by subcutaneous injection. Protocols vary, but Lifshitz[2] recommends that blood samples for LH and FSH then be obtained 3 hours after GnRH. Other protocols indicate sample times at 60, 120, and 180 minutes. A 24-hour postinjection level of estradiol in girls and testosterone in boys is recommended.[3]

Nursing considerations Allergic reactions are exceptionally rare. Inform the patient/family that girls may develop temporary vaginal bleeding within 1 week of the test.

Interpretation Children with true central precocious puberty will show elevated LH levels after stimulation, whereas those with simple precocious thelarche or adrenarche generally maintain LH levels in the prepubertal range after stimulation. Estradiol and testosterone levels 24 hours after injection will be elevated also in children with central precocious puberty. Normal pubertal children should have baseline LH levels 10-40 times higher than prepubertal children and will generally rise to >10 mIU/ml after stimulation.[3]

SINGLE-SAMPLE LH AFTER INJECTION OF DEPOT LEUPROLIDE[3]

Indication Can be used to monitor suppression once initial suppression is verified

Procedure

1. Inject depot formulation at the appropriate time interval.
2. Measure LH 30-60 minutes after the injection of depot leuprolide.

Nursing considerations NPO not necessary

Interpretation The proposed cutoff of LH for treatment efficacy is <3.0 mIU/mL.

THYROID

THYROTROPIN-RELEASING HORMONE (TRH) STIMULATION TEST[3]

Indication The test is used to assess pituitary TSH reserve and prolactin reserve and secretion; to establish TSH suppression by thyroid hormone; to confirm endogenous hyperthyroidism; or to test TSH, GH, LH, or FSH responses in patients with secretory pituitary tumors.

Procedure Thyrotropin-releasing hormone (TRH) 7 μg/kg in children (maximum 400 μg) IVP over a 90-second period

Blood sampling Blood for TSH (for assessment of pituitary reserve) at baseline (0),15, 30, 45, and 60 minutes. The 30-minute sample is most critical. Baseline T3 and T4 should also be obtained. For prolactin, measure at baseline (0), 15, 30, 45, and 60 minutes. For sample of TRH suppression, a single 30-minute sample is enough.

Nursing considerations Transient nausea, sensation of warmth, flushing, mild headache, metallic taste, and/or urge to urinate may occur, lasting <1 minute in some patients. Transient hypertension or hypotension may also occur. Contraindicated in patients with hypertension or cardiac disease. In testing for abnormal prolactin secretion, patients should be off all thyroid medication and chronic aspirin therapy 1 week prior to test.

Interpretation Normally serum TSH concentration rises 5-10 times higher than the basal level following TRH administration. A peak value between 0.1 and 7 mIU/L is a blunted response. Prolactin levels increase 3-5 times the baseline. High baseline prolactin levels without an increase during the test are suggestive, but not diagnostic, of prolactinoma.

PANCREAS

ORAL GLUCOSE TOLERANCE TEST (OGTT)[8]

Indication The test is used to assess glucose tolerance and insulin sensitivity. It is indicated for patients at risk for diabetes mellitus, and for patients with medical conditions associated with impaired glucose tolerance, insulin resistance, or insulin hypersensitivity.

Preparation A dietitian may need to give patient/family dietary instructions. The patient may need to be on a high-carbohydrate diet (generally a minimum of 150 g carbohydrate per day) for 3 days before the test. The patient should be NPO 8-15 hours before the test.

Review current medications and consider discontinuing hyperglycemic and hypoglycemic agents (thiazides, oral contraceptives containing estrogen, salicylates, etc.).

Procedure

1. Insert IV catheter for blood draws.
2. Obtain baseline sample (fasting blood glucose), then Hep-Lock catheter.
3. Give 1.75 g/kg (maximum 100 g) of glucose PO, allowing up to 5 minutes for ingestion. (This can be achieved using a commercially prepared solution, such as glucola, or by mixing glucose with water and lemon juice as a 20% dilution.)
4. Obtain additional blood glucose levels at 30, 60, 120, 180, and 240 minutes after ingestion.

Nursing considerations Standards for the glucose response to OGTT are based on a presumption of adequate dietary carbohydrate intake for the preceding 3 days. The quantitative criteria that have been established for adults may not be appropriate for children. However, it is important to ensure that the test is not performed after a period of reduced intake, such as a fast or illness.

Blood glucose specimens should go to the lab immediately after collection (or be stored on ice) if in red-top tubes, or be collected in gray-top tubes for accurate results.

Interpretation A 2-hour post–oral glucose administration value of <140 mg/dL is normal. A value of 140-199 mg/dL suggests impaired glucose tolerance; ≥200 mg/dL is diagnostic of diabetes mellitus. Elevated values may also indicate Cushing's disease, hemochromatosis, pheochromocytoma, or a CNS lesion. Lower than expected values could indicate the presence of insulinoma, malabsorption syndrome, adrenocortical insufficiency, or hypothyroidism/hypopituitarism. If carbohydrate intake was low during the 3 days prior to the test, insulin response could be impaired, resulting in an exaggeratedly elevated blood glucose value 2 hours after oral glucose administration.

PITUITARY

GROWTH HORMONE TESTING

Interpretation of growth hormone (GH) response to pharmacologic stimuli has changed over the past few years and may vary depending on the practice. A peak GH response of less than 10 ng/mL has historically been considered evidence of GH deficiency. However, one should keep in mind that this standard was selected arbitrarily.[6] Since the response of GH to these stimulants can vary greatly, two different tests are usually performed. The tests may be performed on two separate days or combined in one day.

Different agents cause GH levels to peak at different times; thus giving the medications together can allow shorter testing times. Check with your institution for individual protocols to be used.

ARGININE STIMULATION TEST[9]

Indication Suspected growth hormone deficiency (GHD); useful in diagnosis of adult growth hormone deficiency (AGHD)

Preparation NPO, minimal activity

Medication Arginine HCL 0.5 g/kg (maximum dose 30 g) IV over 30 minutes following an overnight fast. May be used in conjunction with exercise for 10-15 minutes prior to administration to potentiate the response.

Blood sampling Blood for GH at baseline (0), 30, 60, 90, and 120 minutes

Nursing considerations Works by inducing insulin secretion and by blocking somatostatin secretion; should be used with caution in patients with liver and renal disease; may cause hypoglycemia; monitor blood glucose every 30 minutes with vital signs; peak response usually is at the 90-minute sampling.

Interpretation Normal response is a peak GH level 10 ng/mL in children and >5 ng/mL in adults.

CLONIDINE STIMULATION TEST[3]

Indication Suspected GHD

Preparation NPO, minimal activity

Medication Clonidine 0.1 mg/m^2 (maximum dose 250 μg) PO following an overnight fast

Blood sampling Blood for GH at baseline (0), 30, 60, 90, and 120 minutes

Nursing considerations Clonidine is an alpha-adrenergic agonist acting to stimulate hypothalamic growth hormone–releasing hormone (GHRH) secretion. Side effects include hypotension, dizziness, and drowsiness. Blood pressure should be monitored with each blood sample. Because of the long half-life, patients should be instructed to restrict physical activity for at least 6 hours following clonidine administration.

Interpretation Peak GH levels usually occur at the 60-minute sample, with a 30% decrease by 90 minutes. Normal response is at least 1 GH value >10 ng/mL.

INSULIN TOLERANCE TEST[3]

Indication To test GH responsiveness and hypothalamic-pituitary-adrenal axis; test for adult GHD

Preparation NPO, minimal activity

Medication Regular insulin 0.05-0.15 U/kg IV following an overnight fast

Blood sampling Blood is drawn for glucose and GH at 0, 15, 30, 45, 60, 90, and 120 minutes; for cortisol at 0 and 60 minutes (ACTH can also be drawn at 0 and 60 minutes); and at the glucose nadir. A glucometer should be used to check blood glucose levels with each sample.

Nursing considerations Do not leave patient unattended at any time during the study, as severe hypoglycemia requiring medical management may develop. The physician should be readily available. Some institutions recommend that insulin be administered by a physician.

An effective test demonstrates a blood glucose <40 mg/dL or a decrease of 40%-50% below the fasting level. Glucose (D25% 2-4 mL/kg or 50% glucose) should be available immediately for treatment of severe symptoms. If signs of severe hypoglycemia occur (blood glucose <40 mg/dL), patient is symptomatic (rapid pulse, sweating, hot, lethargic), and the signs do not improve by the next scheduled blood sampling, administer glucose (1 mL/kg), but continue to collect serum for GH. At completion of test, administer glucose (0.5-1.0 g/kg) or allow the patient to eat. This test is contraindicated in patients with seizure disorder or cardiac disease.

Interpretation GH levels >10 ng/mL are considered normal in children, >5 ng/mL in adults. Cortisol levels usually exceed 20 μg/dL with hypoglycemia. ACTH should be >50 pg/mL.

L-DOPA STIMULATION TEST[3]

Indication Suspected GHD

NOTE This drug may be made by a compound pharmacist on request.

Preparation NPO, minimal activity

Medication Oral levodopa 125 mg in patients <13.5 kg, 250 mg in patients 13.5-31.5 kg, and 500 mg in patients >31.5 kg; given orally after an overnight fast

Blood sampling Blood for GH at 0, 30, 60, 90, and 120 minutes

Nursing considerations Patients should remain recumbent during test. Side effects include nausea and vomiting, which may occur 1-2 hours after administration. Water may be given during the test.

Interpretation Normal value with at least one GH sample >10 ng/mL occurs at 60 to 90 minutes after administration of L-dopa.

STIMULATION TESTING **12**

GLUCAGON STIMULATION TEST[3]

Indication Suspected GHD; test of choice in infants and young children with suspected GHD. This is a good substitute for insulin-induced hypoglycemia, because the mechanism of inducing GH secretion is by the induction of insulin secretion to compensate for elevated serum glucose levels.

Preparation NPO, minimal activity

Medication Glucagon 0.03-0.1 mg/kg (maximum dose 1 g) administered SQ or IM

Blood sampling Blood for GH at 0, 60, 90, 120, 150, and 180 minutes

Nursing considerations The drug may cause vomiting in some patients; NPO prior to test is recommended. It should not be used in patients who have limited ability to secrete insulin.

Interpretation Normal value with at least one GH sample >10 ng/mL occurs between 2 and 3 hours after glucagon.

GROWTH HORMONE–RELEASING HORMONE STIMULATION TEST[3]

NOTE This agent is currently unavailable commercially but may be reintroduced.

Indication Suspected GHD

Preparation NPO, minimal activity

Medication GHRH 100 μg (1 μg/kg) IVP over a period of 1 minute

Blood sampling Blood for GH at 0, 15, 30, 45, 60, and 90 minutes

Nursing considerations Peak serum GH levels usually occur in the 15- or 30-minute sample. In this case, a 90-minute sample is not necessary.

Flushing, warmth, and local irritation at the IV site are possible.

Interpretation The mean peak GH level in normal children has been reported as 28 ± 2 μg/L. If patient secretes GH in response to GHRH but not to other pharmacologic stimuli that act in the hypothalamus, then a defect in the hypothalamus is suspected.

INSULIN-LIKE GROWTH FACTOR-1 GENERATION TEST[2,10]

Indication To examine GH-receptor function by evaluating its ability to increase serum insulin–like growth factor-1 (IGF-1) levels. It is useful in identifying patients with short stature and degree of GH insensitivity.

STIMULATION TESTING ⑫

Medication Daily doses of GH 0.025-0.05 mg/kg/day for 7 days or 0.1 mg/kg/day for 4 days are given SQ.

Blood sampling When using 0.025-0.05 mg/kg/day, blood sample for serum IGF-1 and IGFBP-3 should be obtained at days 1, 5, and 8. If 0.1 mg/kg/day is used, blood for serum IGF-1 and IGFBP-3 is taken before the first GH injection and 8-16 hours after the fourth injection. Samples on intermediate days may be taken but are not required.

Nursing considerations GH doses should be administered at the same time each day. Children who have GII sensitivity are not good candidates for GII treatment.

Interpretation Normal subjects responded with a mean delta IGF-1 of 230 ng/mL for the low dose of 0.025 mg/kg/day and 322 ng/mL for high dose of 0.05 mg/kg/day. Previous criteria for GH insensitivity include a response of delta over baseline <15 ng/mL for IGF-1.

PHYSIOLOGIC GROWTH HORMONE TESTING

SLEEP[3]

Indication To test physiologic secretion of GH during hours of sleep; can also be done for 12- to 24-hour periods; helpful in diagnosing patients with suspected neurosecretory GHD

Medication No medication is given.

Blood sampling Blood for GH every 20 minutes (sometimes every 30-60 minutes) from onset of sleep for 8 hours. Preferable hours include 11 PM to 7 AM.

Nursing considerations Testing requires admission to the hospital or home testing with a home care service. An IV to Hep-Lock is necessary for frequent sampling. Not more than 5% of total blood volume should be used for laboratory testing in any 2-week period; obtain the absolute minimum whole blood necessary for each sample. To estimate patient blood volume:

- Newborns: 78-86 ml/kg
- 1-12 months of age: 73-78 mL/kg
- 1-3 years of age: 74-82 mL/kg
- 4-6 years of age: 80-86 mL/kg
- 7-18 years of age: 83-90 mL/kg
- Adult: 68-88 mL/kg

Interpretation Results include an evaluation of mean levels, which is the average of the samples collected. A normal response is a mean level >3 ng/mL. Samples can also be evaluated using the Veldhuis and Johnson cluster analysis program. This method looks at the number of episodes of secretion and the half-life of serum GH. There should be 6-10 episodes, with 4 that are >10 ng/mL. Fewer peaks indicate inadequate spontaneous secretion.[5]

EXERCISE[2,5]

Indication To test physiologic GH response to vigorous exercise; may be used as a screening test to evaluate the need for more formal testing for GH secretion

Medication No medication is given. Fasting for 2-4 hours prior to test. Patient exercises on treadmill or bicycle, or climbs stairs for 20 minutes or to maximum tolerance; final heart rate should exceed 120 beats/min

Blood sampling Blood for GH at baseline (0) and immediately after exercise; could also be sampled at end of exercise and 20 and 40 minutes after exercise completion.

Nursing considerations Water can be given freely during test. The child may eat and drink after the first sample obtained at end of exercise.

GLUCOSE SUPPRESSION TEST FOR ACROMEGALY[9]

Indication Suspected autonomous GH hypersecretion

Medication Glucose 1.75 g/kg (maximum 75 g) orally after overnight fasting

Blood sampling Blood for glucose and GH at 0, 30, 60, 90, and 120 minutes

Nursing considerations Water and ambulation are allowed throughout the test. An adequate diet is recommended for 3 days prior to testing. Conditions such as severe liver disease, chronic renal disease, uncontrolled diabetes mellitus, malnutrition, Laron syndrome, and thyrotoxicosis may be associated with inadequate GH suppression.

Interpretation GH levels in patients normally suppress <5 ng/mL, and as low as 2 ng/mL. Failure to suppress in the presence of normally increased blood glucose suggests a pituitary adenoma. Failure to suppress is observed in patients with acromegaly.

WATER DEPRIVATION TEST[9]

Indication To differentiate among the causes of polyuria (not associated with hyperglycemia)

Sampling After an overnight fast, obtain urine and plasma for osmolality, followed by discontinuance of fluid intake. Obtain hourly weights, urine volumes, and hourly urine and plasma for osmolality. To differentiate nephrogenic diabetes insipidus (DI) from central DI, desmopressin acetate (DDAVP) 1 μg IV or 10 μg intranasally is subsequently given.

Miller and Hong McAtee[11] recommend a dose of DDAVP: 0.025 μg/kg up to 1 μg SQ, or 0.25 μg/kg up to 10 μg intranasally.

Nursing considerations Fluid restriction in patients with DI may cause severe extracellular fluid volume depletion. Careful supervision should be maintained, and the test should be aborted if the patient loses more than 3% of body weight. If urine volume has previously exceeded 6 L per day, overnight fasting is contraindicated, and the test should be initiated during the daytime.

Interpretation DI is diagnosed if the urine osmolality is not greater than 300 mOsm/kg before plasma osmolality is greater than 295 mOsm/kg, or if the serum sodium is greater than 143 mmol/L. Alternatively, urine osmolality is measured hourly. Once it has risen by more than 30 mOsm/kg above the preceding hour, the plasma osmolality and serum sodium are measured. After subsequent administration of DDAVP, a rise in urine osmolality >9% indicates a normal renal response.

STIMULATION TESTING

12

⓭ LABORATORY TESTING

The reference values listed herein are meant to be used as a guide only. Values and ranges vary considerably among laboratories that employ a variety of assays for the tests listed. Check with the laboratory that your institution uses.

TEST/RANGE/COLLECTION	PHYSIOLOGIC BASIS
Acetoacetate, serum or urine 0 mg/dL Urine sample should be fresh. *Tube type* _____ *Amount* _____	Acetoacetate, acetone, and β-hydroxybutyrate contribute to ketoacidosis when oxidative hepatic metabolism of fatty acids is impaired. Proportions in serum vary, but are generally 20% acetoacetate, 78% β-hydroxybutyrate, and 2% acetone.
Adrenocorticotropic Hormone (ACTH), plasma AM 15-100 pg/mL 10-80 ng/L (SI units) PM <50 pg/mL <50 ng/L (SI units) Heparinized venous blood Chill blood tube to prevent enzymatic action. Fasting sample *Tube type* _____ *Amount* _____	*Test of the anterior pituitary gland function* Evaluate patient for abnormal sleep patterns. With a normal sleep pattern, the ACTH level is highest between 4 and 8 AM and lowest around 9 PM.

INTERPRETATION	CONSIDERATIONS
Present in Diabetic ketoacidosis (DKA) Alcoholic ketoacidosis Prolonged fasting Severe carbohydrate restriction with normal fat intake	Nitroprusside test is semiquantitative; it detects acetoacetate and is sensitive down to 5-10 mg/dL. Trace = 5 mg/dL, small = 15 mg/dL, moderate = 40 mg/dL, large = 80 mg/dL β-hydroxybutyrate is not a ketone and is not detected by the nitroprusside test. Acetone is also not reliably detected by this method. Failure of test to detect β-hydroxybutyrate in ketoacidosis may produce a seemingly paradoxical increase in ketones with clinical improvement as nondetectable β-hydroxybutyrate is replaced by detectable acetoacetate.

Increased in
Addison's disease
Cushing's disease
Ectopic ACTH syndrome
Stress
Adrenogenital syndrome (congenital adrenal hyperplasia)
 	
Decreased in
Secondary adrenal insufficiency
Cushing's syndrome
Hypopituitarism
Adrenal adenoma or carcinoma
Steroid administration
	Stress and pregnancy can increase levels.
	
	Recently administered radioisotope scans can affect levels.
	
	Drugs that ↑ levels:
	  Estrogens Amphetamines
	  Ethanol Insulin
	  Vasopressin Metyrapone
	  Aminoglutethimide Spironolactone
	
	Drugs that ↓ levels:
	  Corticosteroids

TEST/RANGE/COLLECTION	PHYSIOLOGIC BASIS
Alanine Aminotransferase (ALT, SGPT, GPT), serum 0-35 U/L *Tube type* _____ *Amount* _____	ALT is an intracellular enzyme involved in amino acid metabolism. Present in large concentrations in liver and kidney, and in smaller amounts in skeletal muscle and heart. Released into the bloodstream when tissue is damaged, especially in liver injury.

Alkaline Phosphatase, serum or plasma	Enzyme originating mainly in bone, liver, and placenta. Rises in proportion to new bone cell production.
Infant	150-420 U/L	
2-10 years	100-320 U/L	
11-18 years (boy)	100-390 U/L	
11-18 years (girl)	100-320 U/L	
Adult	30-120 U/L	

Tube type _____
Amount _____

Androstenedione, serum

Androstenedione is a precursor of cortisol, aldosterone, testosterone, and estrogen.

	Range (mean) (ng/dL)		
Preterm infants (male/female)			
26-28 wk (at day 4)	92-892 (254)		
31-35 wk (at day 4)	80-446 (207)		
Fullterm infants (male/female)			
1-7 days	20-290 (150)		
1-12 mo	6-68 (23)		
Prepubertal children	8-50 (24)		

	Female	Male	
Tanner 2	42-100 (65)	31-65 (45)	
Tanner 3	80-190 (123)	50-100 (67)	
Tanner 4	77-225 (131)	48-140 (82)	
Tanner 5	80-240 (160)	65-210 (105)	
Adult	85-275 (165)	78-205 (115)	

Tube type _____
Amount _____

INTERPRETATION	CONSIDERATIONS
Increased in Acute viral hepatitis, biliary tract obstruction, cirrhosis, liver abscess or cancer, right heart failure, ischemia or hypoxia, injury to liver or extensive trauma. Concomitant use of drugs that cause cholestasis or hepatotoxicity **Decreased in** Vitamin B_6 deficiency	Monthly evaluation is recommended for patients prior to and during the first year after initiation of thiazolidinedione therapy.
Increased in Rickets, hyperpara-thyroidism (accompanied by hyper-calcemia), liver disease, bone disease **Decreased in** Hypophosphatemic rickets, dwarfism, malnutrition, hypothyroidism	Used as tumor marker and index of liver and bone disease when correlated with other clinical findings

Increased in Adrenal tumor, congenital adrenal hyperplasia (CAH) ectopic ACTH-producing tumors, ovarian tumor, Cushing's syndrome, polycystic ovarian syndrome (PCOS; Stein-Leventhal syndrome)
 	
Decreased in Primary and secondary adrenal insufficiency
 	
Exogenous testosterone therapy
	Recent radioactive scan may invalidate test results.
	
	Drugs that may ↑ levels:
	    Corticotropin
	    Clomiphene
	    Metyrapone
	
	Drugs that may ↓ levels:
	    Steroids

⑬

LABORATORY TESTING

TEST/RANGE/COLLECTION	PHYSIOLOGIC BASIS
Anti 21 Hydroxylase Antibody, serum Children and adults <1.0 U/ml Freeze specimen. *Tube type* _____ *Amount* _____	Adrenal autoantibodies react with the steroid 21-hydroxylase. These can be detected by radioimmunoassay even before the development of adrenal insufficiency. This is an effective screen for auto-immune adrenalitis in patients with symptoms of adrenal insufficiency. Predicts Addison's disease in patients with clusters of other autoimmune disorders.
Aspartate Aminotransferase (AST, SGOT, GOT), serum 0-35 IU/L *Tube type* _____ *Amount* _____	AST is an intracellular enzyme involved in amino acid metabolism. Present in large concentrations in liver, skeletal muscle, brain, red blood cells, and heart. Released into the bloodstream when tissue is damaged, especially in liver injury.
Autoantibodies, serum Islet cell antibodies (ICA) IA-2 GAD65 GM2	Autoantibodies directed against pancreatic islet cells; includes GAD, IA-2, insulin, ganglioside (GM2) antibody, IgG/IgM, and other cell proteins

INTERPRETATION	CONSIDERATIONS
Present in Addison's disease Autoimmune polyglandular syndrome types 1 and 2	
Increased in Acute viral hepatitis, biliary tract obstruction, cirrhosis, liver abscess or cancer, right heart failure, ischemia or hypoxia, injury to liver or extensive trauma. Concomitant use of drugs that cause cholestasis or hepatotoxicity. **Decreased in** Vitamin B_6 deficiency	Monthly evaluation is recommended for patients prior to and during the first year after initiation of thiazolidinedione therapy.
These assays are used for diagnosing pancreatic islet beta cell autoimmune disease. ICAs are present in serum during the prediabetic phase and predict development of type 1 disease.	If either insulin antibody or glutamic acid decarboxylase antibody is negative, then IA-2 antibody is ordered.

TEST/RANGE/COLLECTION	PHYSIOLOGIC BASIS
β-Hydroxybutyrate, serum <3 mg/dL *Tube type* _____ *Amount* _____	See Acetoacetate, p. 314.
Bicarbonate (HCO₃), venous or arterial Preterm 18-26 mEq/L Full term 20-25 mEq/L >2 yr 22-26 mEq/L *Tube type* _____ *Amount* _____	HCO_3 is a salt that results from the incomplete neutralization of carbonic acid. It may result from the passing of an excess of carbon dioxide into a solution of a base.
C-peptide, serum 0.8-4.0 ng/mL Fasting sample preferred *Tube type* _____ *Amount* _____	C-peptide is an inactive by-product of the cleavage of pro-insulin to active insulin. Its presence indicates endogenous release of insulin.
Calcitonin, serum Double antibiotic RIA Fasting sample preferred Cord blood 25-150 pg/mL Newborn 70-348 pg/mL Children <25-70 pg/mL Adults <25-150 pg/mL *Tube type* _____ *Amount* _____	Hormone secreted by C cells or parafollicular cells of thyroid gland. Inhibits bone resorption by regulating activity and number of osteoblasts. Secreted in direct response of elevated blood calcium levels. May contribute to excessive loss of calcium.

INTERPRETATION	CONSIDERATIONS
See Acetoacetate, p. 315.	
Increased in Potassium or chloride depletion, vomiting, loss of gastric juice, hypoparathyroidism ***Decreased in*** Neonatal hypocalcemia, DKA, hyperparathyroidism, renal tubular acidosis	
Increased in Renal failure, ingestion of oral hypoglycemic drugs, insulinomas, β-cell transplants	Test is most helpful to assess endogenous insulin production in diabetic patient receiving insulin as well as to detect factitious insulin injection (increased insulin, decreased C-peptide).
Increased in Medullary thyroid cancers; pernicious anemia; chronic renal failure; C cell hyperplasia; lung, breast, and pancreas cancers; pregnancy; newborns	Screening of family members of patients with proven medullary thyroid cancer recommended

TEST/RANGE/COLLECTION	PHYSIOLOGIC BASIS
Calcium (Ca^{2+}), serum, plasma Preterm <1 wk 6-10 mg/dL Full term <1 wk 7-12 mg/dL Child 8-10.5 mg/dL Adult 8.5-10.5 mg/dL *Tube type* _____ *Amount* _____	Measures total calcium in blood. Used as a measure of parathyroid function, calcium metabolism, and evaluation of malignancies.
Calcium, 24-hour urine <4 mg/kg per 24 hours *Amount* _____	Used to determine the function of the parathyroid gland.
Calcium/Creatinine Ratio, Ca/Cr (mg/mg) <7 mo 0.86 7-18 mo 0.6 19 mo-6 yr 0.42 Adults 0.22 Random urine sample *Amount* _____	Used as a screen for hypercalciuria.

INTERPRETATION	CONSIDERATIONS
Increased in Hyperparathyroid, excess intake of vitamin D **Decreased in** Rickets, hypoparathyroidism **Normal with increased BUN in** Hyperparathyroidism **Normal with abnormal PO$_4$ in** Rickets **Normal with decreased albumin in** Hypercalcemia	↑Intake of magnesium and phosphates and excessive use of laxatives may ↓ level. Taking calcium supplement shortly before specimen collection will result in a falsely elevated value.
Increased in Hyperparathyroidism, glucocorticoid excess, Fanconi's syndrome, vitamin D intoxication, sarcoidosis, metastatic malignancies, myeloma with bone metastasis, renal tubular acidosis **Decreased in** Hypoparathyroidism, vitamin D deficiency, malabsorption syndrome	**Falsely elevated levels** Due to ↑Na and Mg intake, very high milk intake **Falsely negative levels** ↑Dietary phosphates, alkaline urine
Increased in Osteoporosis of immobilization, renal tubular acidosis, vitamin D intoxication, excessive calcium intake, hyperparathyroidism, steroid use	

⑬

LABORATORY TESTING

TEST/RANGE/COLLECTION	PHYSIOLOGIC BASIS
Chromosome Analysis, karyotype analysis Female 46XX Male 46XY *Tube type* _____ *Amount* _____	Used in diagnosis of endocrine and genetic disorders. There are a variety of staining techniques and cell culture methods used.
Cortisol, plasma or serum 8 AM 5-20 μg/dL (140-550 nmol/L) *Tube type* _____ *Amount* _____	Release of corticotropin-releasing factor (CRF) from the hypothalamus stimulates release of ACTH from the pituitary, which in turn stimulates release of cortisol from the adrenals. Cortisol provides negative feedback to this system. Test measures both free cortisol and cortisol bound to cortisol-binding globulin (CBG). Morning levels are higher than evening levels.
Cortisol, 24-hour urine Adult 10-100 μg/24 hr 27-276 nmol/day (SI units) Adolescent 5-55 μg/24 hr Child 2-27 μg/24 hr Begin 24-hour collection after patient urinates; discard first specimen. Refrigerate throughout collection. Collect last specimen as close as possible to ending time. 50 mL aliquot of a well-mixed 24-hour urine (store frozen) Boric acid as preservative	Test is to evaluate adrenocortical function, especially hyperfunction. An elevated cortisol level in a properly collected urine specimen supports the diagnosis of Cushing's disease in an unstressed patient.

INTERPRETATION	CONSIDERATIONS
See pp. 270-274 for Down syndrome (trisomy 21); pp. 296-299 for Turner syndrome (45X and other abnormalities); pp. 276-279 for Klinefelter syndrome (47XXY). There are a multitude of chromosomal abnormalities that occur. For more references, see Suggested Readings for this chapter on p. 481.	Requires immediate delivery to the laboratory Fluorescence in situ hybridization (FISH) analysis is a type of DNA study used in identifying chromosome deletions. This test needs to be ordered specifically.
Increased in Cushing's syndrome, acute illness, surgery, trauma, septic shock, depression, anxiety, alcoholism, starvation, chronic renal failure, increased CBG (congenital, pregnancy, estrogen therapy) **Decreased in** Addison's disease, decreased CBG (congenital, liver disease, nephrotic syndrome)	Circadian fluctuations in cortisol levels limit usefulness of single measurements unless obtained under physiologic stress (i.e., hypoglycemia) or in the context of standardized suppression or stimulation testing.

Increased in
Cushing's disease
Adrenal adenoma or carcinoma
Ectopic ACTH-producing tumor
Hyperthyroidism
Obesity
Stress
 	
Decreased in
Addison's disease
Hypopituitarism
Hypothyroidism
	Pregnancy and stress can increase cortisol levels.
	
	Test results can be altered by recent radioisotope scans.
	
	Drugs that ↑ levels:
	   Oral contraceptives
	   Danazol
	   Hydrocortisone
	   Spironolactone
	
	Drugs that ↓ levels:
	   Dexamethasone
	   Ethacrynic acid
	   Ketoconazole
	   Thiazides

⑬

LABORATORY TESTING

TEST/RANGE/COLLECTION	PHYSIOLOGIC BASIS
11-Desoxycortisol (Compound S, Metyrapone Test), serum	Used to assess adrenocortical function

Children and adults
  Baseline   <1 μg/dL
  Post Metyrapone
    Single dose   7-18 μg/dL
    Multiple dose   10-25 μg/dL

Freeze specimen.

Tube type _____

Amount _____

17-Hydroxycorticosteroids (17-OCHS), 24-hour urine	Used to assess adrenocortical function

		Because the excretion of cortisol metabolites follows a diurnal variation, a 24-hour collection is necessary.
<8 yr	<1.5 mg/24 hr	
<12 yr	<4.5 mg/24 hr	
Adult male	4.5-10.0 mg/24 hr	
Adult female	2.5-10.0 mg/24 hr	

Begin 24-hour collection after patient urinates; discard first specimen.

Refrigerate throughout collection.

Collect last specimen as close as possible to ending time.

50 mL aliquot of a well-mixed 24-hour urine

Boric acid as preservative

INTERPRETATION	CONSIDERATIONS

Increased in
Adrenal carcinoma
Congenital adrenal hyperplasia
  (11β-OH deficiency)

Decreased in
Congenital adrenal hyperplasia
  (17α-OH deficiency)

Ordered at each clinic visit to assess adequate suppression of adrenal androgens. Rising levels are consistent with decreasing suppression of adrenal androgens.

Increased in
Cushing's syndrome
Pituitary tumor
Adrenal tumor
Bilateral adrenal hyperplasia
Ectopic ACTH-producing tumor
Acromegaly
Thyrotoxicosis
Severe hypertension
Stress

Decreased in
Addison's disease
Adrenal infarction
Adrenal hemorrhage
Surgical removal of the adrenals
Congenital adrenal hypoplasia
Adrenal suppression from steroid
  therapy
Hypopituitarism
Hypothyroidism
Adrenogenital syndrome

Emotional and physical stress may cause ↑ in adrenal activity.

Drugs that ↑ 17-OHCS:
  Chloral hydrate
  Chlorpromazine
  Etazolamide
  Colchicine
  Erythromycin
  Meprobamate
  Paraldehyde
  Quinidine
  Quinine
  Spironolactone

Drugs that ↓ 17-OHCS:
  Estrogens
  Oral contraceptives
  Phenothiazines
  Reserpine

TEST/RANGE/COLLECTION	PHYSIOLOGIC BASIS

17-Ketosteroids (17-KS), 24-hour urine

Child <12 yr	<5 mg/24 hr
Child 12-15 yr	5-12 mg/24 hr
Adult male	7-25 mg/24 hr
	24-88 μmol/day
	(SI units)
Adult female	4-15 mg/24 hr
	14-52 μmol/day
	(SI units)

Begin 24-hour collection after patient urinates; discard first specimen.

Refrigerate throughout collection.

Collect last specimen as close as possible to ending time.

50 mL aliquot of a well-mixed 24-hour urine

Boric acid as preservative

Test is used to measure adrenocortical function by measuring 17-KS in the urine. 17-KSs are metabolites of the nontestosterone androgenic sex hormones that are secreted from the adrenal cortex and the testes.

Since most of the excreted androgen hormones are derived from the adrenal cortex, this test is very useful in diagnosing adrenocortical dysfunction.

Dehydroepiandrosterone (DHEA), serum

Major steroid product of the adrenal cortex.

	Range (ng/dL)	Mean (ng/dL)
Premature infants (at day 4)		
26-28 wk	236-3,640	941
31-35 wk	80-3,150	811
Full-term infants		
3 days	65-1,250	570
7-30 days	50-760	285
1-6 mo	26-385	113
6-12 mo	20-100	40
Prepubertal children		
1-6 yr	20-130	29
6-8 yr	20-275	93
8-10 yr	31-345	156

Tube type _____

Amount _____

INTERPRETATION	CONSIDERATIONS

Increased in Congenital adrenal hyperplasia; pregnancy; ACTH administration; Cushing's syndrome; testosterone- or estrogen-secreting tumor of the adrenals, ovaries, or testes; severe stress or infection; hyperpituitarism; ovarian neoplasia

Decreased in Addison's disease, hypogonadism, hypopituitarism, myxedema, severe debilitating disease, nephrosis, gout, castration, thyrotoxicosis

Stress may increase adrenal activity.

Drugs that may cause ↑ 17-KS:
Antibiotics
Chlorpromazine
Dexamethasone
Phenothiazines
Quinidine
Secobarbital
Spironolactone

Drugs that may cause ↓ 17-KS:
Estrogen
Oral contraceptives
Probenecid
Promazine
Reserpine
Salicylates
Thiazide diuretics

Increased in Polycystic ovarian syndrome, adrenal carcinomas, Cushing's syndrome, congenital adrenal hyperplasia, premature adrenarche

Decreased in Adrenal adenoma (nonfunctioning)

Tanner Stage	Age (yr)	Range (ng/dL)	Mean (ng/dL)
Puberty: male			
1	<9.8	31-345	156
2	9.8-14.5	110-495	300
3	10.7-15.4	170-585	390
4	11.8-16.2	160-640	395
5	12.8-17.3	250-900	505
Puberty: female			
1	<9.2	31-345	156
2	9.2-13.7	150-570	330
3	10.0-14.4	200-600	385
4	10.7-15.6	200-780	430
5	11.8-18.6	215-850	540

TEST/RANGE/COLLECTION	PHYSIOLOGIC BASIS

DHEA Sulfate (DHEA-S), serum

	Range (μg/dL)	Mean (μg/dL)
Premature infants (at day 4)		
26-28 wk	123-882	392
31-35 wk	122-710	398
Full-term infants		
3 days	88-356	160
7-30 days	5-111	—
1-6 mo	5-48	—
Prepubertal children		
1-6 yr	<5-57	11
6-8 yr	9-72	21
8-10 yr	13-115	50

Tube type _____

Amount _____

Major adrenal 19-carbon steroid

More than 99% of DHEA is sulfated before secretion.

Deoxycorticosterone (DOC), serum

Newborn: Levels are markedly elevated at birth and decrease rapidly during the first week to the range found in older infants.

	Range (ng/dL)	Mean (ng/dL)
Premature infants (at day 4)		
26-28 wk	20-105	47
Full-term infants		
1-12 mo	7-49	23
Prepubertal children	2-34	10.9
Pubertal/adult	2-19	7.1

Tube type _____

Amount _____

Decreased production of cortisol in 11β-hydroxylase deficiency and 17α-hydroxylase deficiency results in the accumulation of DOC, causing hypertension.

INTERPRETATION	CONSIDERATIONS			

Increased in
Adrenal carcinoma
Cushing's syndrome
Congenital adrenal hyperplasia
Premature adrenarche

Decreased in
Adrenal adenoma (nonfunctioning)

Tanner Stage	Age (yr)	Range (µg/dL)	Mean (µg/dL)
Puberty: male			
1	<9.8	13-83	36
2	9.8-14.5	42-109	93
3	10.7-15.4	48-200	122
4	11.8-16.2	102-385	206
5	12.8-17.3	120-370	230
Puberty: female			
1	<9.2	19-144	40
2	9.2-13.7	34-129	72
3	10.0-14.4	32-226	88
4	10.7-15.6	58-260	120
5	11.8-18.6	44-248	148

⑬

LABORATORY TESTING

Increased in
11β-hydroxylase deficiency
Adrenal carcinoma

Degree of elevation corresponds to degree of biosynthetic block.

TEST/RANGE/COLLECTION	PHYSIOLOGIC BASIS
Endomysial Antibodies (EMA), serum Negative in normal individuals; also negative in celiac disease patients adhering to gluten-free diet *Tube type* _____ *Amount* _____	Includes presence and titer of circulating antiendomysial IgA antibodies Useful for the diagnosis of celiac disease and for monitoring adherence to gluten-free diet
Estradiol Prepubertal children 1-10 years <1.0 ng/dL *Tube type* _____ *Amount* _____	Major sex steroid for females Produced by the ovaries Responsible for breast development and ovarian differentiation and development
Fluorescence In Situ Hybridization (FISH), blood Normally, a probe will hybridize in two places, indicating the presence of two homologous chromosomes. If a probe from the chromosome segment being examined hybridizes to only one of the patient's chromosomes, the patient has a deletion. If additional material is found, the probe will hybridize in three places instead of two. *Tube type* _____ *Amount* _____	A technique in which a labeled chromosome-specific DNA segment or probe is hybridized to metaphase, prophase, or interphase chromosomes and then is visualized under a fluorescence microscope. FISH can be used to test for missing or additional chromosomal materials as well as chromosome arrangements.

INTERPRETATION	CONSIDERATIONS
Presence of antibodies associated with a history of gastrointestinal disorders is consistent with celiac disease or dermatitis herpetiformis, which are caused by a sensitivity to gluten.	Strict avoidance of gluten in the diet will control disease activity, and antibodies will disappear with time.

LABORATORY TESTING

Increased in Precocious puberty (girls), McCune-Albright syndrome, gynecomastia

Decreased in Delayed puberty (girls), Turner syndrome

Tanner Stage	Age (yr)	Range (ng/dL)	Mean (ng/dL)
Puberty: male			
1	<9.8	0.5-1.1	0.8
2	9.8-14.5	0.5-1.6	1.1
3	10.7-15.4	0.5-2.5	1.6
4	11.8-16.2	1.0-3.6	2.2
5	12.8-17.3	1.0-3.6	2.1
Puberty: female			
1	<9.2	0.5-2.0	0.8
2	9.2-13.7	1.0-2.4	1.6
3	10.0-14.4	0.7-6.0	2.5
4	10.7-15.6	2.1-8.5	4.7
5	11.8-18.6	3.4-17.0	11.0

DiGeorge, velocardiofacial, CATCH22 syndrome, FISH with DNA probes for DiGeorge chromosome region of chromosome 22 (22q11.2) Prader-Willi/Angelman syndrome FISH with DNA probes for PWS/AS critical region 15q11-q13	This is a separate test from a chromosome analysis. Must order FISH analysis for specific region or disorder Check with laboratory for specimen requirements and procedures.

TEST/RANGE/COLLECTION	PHYSIOLOGIC BASIS

Follicle-Stimulating Hormone (FSH), serum ICMA

	Range (mIU/mL)	Mean (mIU/mL)
Infants (4 wk-1 yr)		
Male	0.16-4.1	1.0
Female	0.24-14.2	7.2
Prepubertal (2-8 yr)		
Male	0.26-3.0	0.98
Female	1.0-4.2	2.1

Tube type _____

Amount _____

PHYSIOLOGIC BASIS

Anterior pituitary hormone that stimulates the growth of graafian follicles and activates sperm-forming cells

FSH is a glycoprotein produced by the anterior pituitary gland and regulated by GnRH and feedback by gonadal steroid hormones. It is useful in the diagnosis of gonadal dysfunction.

Gliadin Antibodies, serum
IgG and IgA antibodies

IgA

<2 years	<50 U/mL (negative)
	50-100 U/mL (weak positive)
	>100 U/mL (positive)
≥2 years	<25 U/mL (negative)
	25-50 U/mL (weak positive)
	>50 U/mL (positive)

IgG

<2 years	<50 U/mL (negative)
	50-100 U/mL (weak positive)
	>100 U/mL (positive)
≥2 years	<25 U/mL (negative)
	25-50 U/mL (weak positive)
	>50 U/mL (positive)

Tube type _____

Amount _____

INTERPRETATION	CONSIDERATIONS			

Increased in
Central precocious puberty
Gonadotropin-secreting pituitary
tumors
Menopause
Germinal cell aplasia
Gonadal dysgenesis

Decreased in
Delayed puberty, peripheral sexual
precocity
Hypothalamic GnRH deficiency
Pituitary insufficiency
Isolated FSH deficiency
Isolated gonadotropin deficiency
Hyperprolactinemia

Tanner Stage	Age (yr)	Range (mIU/mL)	Mean (mIU/mL)
Puberty: male			
1	<9.8	0.26-3.0	0.98
2	9.8-14.5	1.8-3.2	2.5
3	10.7-15.4	1.2-5.8	2.9
4	11.8-16.2	2.0-9.2	4.4
5	12.8-17.3	2.6-11.0	6.1
Puberty: female			
1	<9.2	1.0-4.2	2.1
2	9.2-13.7	1.0-10.8	4.0
3	10.0-14.4	1.5-12.8	5.1
4	10.7-15.6	1.5-11.7	6.4
5	11.8-18.6	1.0-9.2	4.9

Increased in
Celiac disease or other gluten-sensitive
enteropathics

False positives are possible since other gastrointestinal disorders may induce circulating antigliadin antibody, Crohn's disease, food protein intolerance, and postinfection malabsorption.

LABORATORY TESTING 13

TEST/RANGE/COLLECTION	PHYSIOLOGIC BASIS
Glucose, serum 60-115 mg/dL (3.3-6.3 mmol/L) *Tube type* _____ *Amount* _____	Normally, the glucose concentration in extracellular fluid is closely regulated so that a source of energy is readily available to tissues and so that no glucose is excreted in the urine.
Growth Hormone (GH), serum 0-5 ng/mL Genetics: Gene for GH is located on chromosome 17. *Tube type* _____ *Amount* _____	Growth hormone is a single-chain polypeptide of 191 amino acids that induces the generation of insulin-like growth factors, which directly stimulate collagen and protein synthesis. GH levels fluctuate considerably during the day, with maximal GH secretion at night.
Growth Hormone–Binding Protein (GHBP), serum |	**pmol/L** | Infancy	50-280 | Childhood	60-620 | Puberty	70-780 | Adult	65-310 | Store and ship frozen. *Tube type* _____ *Amount* _____	GHBP is derived from the extracellular domain of the growth hormone receptor and from the GH receptor gene. Circulating levels of GHBP reflect GH receptor levels and activity. Levels are low in early life, rise through childhood, and plateau during puberty and adulthood. Low levels are associated with degree of GH resistance.

INTERPRETATION	CONSIDERATIONS
Increased in Diabetes mellitus, Cushing's syndrome, chronic pancreatitis. *Drugs:* corticosteroids, phenytoin, estrogen, thiazides ***Decreased in*** Pancreatic islet cell disease with increased insulin, insulinoma, adrenocortical insufficiency, hypopituitarism, diffuse liver disease, malignancy, infant of a diabetic mother, enzyme deficiency diseases. *Drugs:* insulin, ethanol, propranolol, sulfonylureas, tolbutamide, other oral hypoglycemic agents	See pp. 76-78 for diagnosis of diabetes mellitus. See pp. 66-67 for diagnosis of hypoglycemia.
Increased in Acromegaly, Laron dwarfism (defective GH receptor), starvation. *Drugs:* arginine, levodopa, clonidine ***Decreased in*** Pituitary dwarfism, hypopituitarism, aging, IGF deficiency, obesity	Random GH levels are not useful in the diagnosis of GH deficiency in children. (See GH testing, p. 307.)
Increased in Estrogen treatment, familial short stature with high GHBP, obesity, early pregnancy ***Decreased in*** Laron dwarfism, other inherited abnormalities of the GH receptor, impaired nutrition, diabetes mellitus, hypothyroidism, chronic liver disease	Useful in identifying persons with GH resistance caused by genetic abnormalities of the GH receptor

⑬

LABORATORY TESTING

TEST/RANGE/COLLECTION	PHYSIOLOGIC BASIS

Human Chorionic Gonado-tropin (HCG), beta-subunit, serum
 	
Children
  Newborn-puberty   <5 mIU/ml
Adults
  Males and non-
    pregnant females   <5 mIU/ml
 	
Tube type _____
Amount _____
	Used as a marker in the diagnosis of pregnancy, testicular and trophoblastic tumors

Hemoglobin A1c (glycosylated hemoglobin), whole blood or packed cells Nondiabetic 3.9%-6.9% (method-dependent) *Tube type* _____ *Amount* _____	During the life span of each red blood cell, glucose combines with hemoglobin to produce a stable glycated hemoglobin. The level of glycated hemoglobin is related to the mean plasma glucose level during the prior 1-3 months.
17-Hydroxyprogesterone (17-OH prog), serum	Measures cortisol precursor; used to assess adrenocortical function

		ng/dL
Males	Prepubertal	0-81
	Adult	36-154
Females	Prepubertal	0-92
	Adult (follicular)	15-102
	Adult (luteal)	150-386

Tube type _____
Amount _____

INTERPRETATION	CONSIDERATIONS
Increased in Testicular and ovarian teratomas, pregnancy, multiple pregnancy, hydatidiform mole, choriocarcinoma, and seminoma	Interfering factors: Lipemia, hemolysis

⓮ LABORATORY TESTING

INTERPRETATION	CONSIDERATIONS
Increased in Diabetes mellitus, splenectomy. Falsely high results can occur depending on the method used and may be due to presence of hemoglobin F or uremia. ***Decreased in*** Any condition that shortens red blood cell life span (hemolytic anemias, congenital spherocytosis, acute or chronic blood loss, sickle cell disease, hemoglobin-opathies)	Test is used to monitor long-term control of blood glucose. Development and progression of chronic complications of diabetes are related to the degree of altered glycemia. Measurement of HgbA1c is recommended quarterly. Reference ranges are method-specific. Comparing HgbA1c to blood glucose

4%	60 mg/dL	9%	210 mg/dL
5%	90 mg/dL	10%	240 mg/dL
6%	120 mg/dL	11%	270 mg/dL
7%	150 mg/dL	12%	300 mg/dL
8%	180 mg/dL	13%	330 mg/dL

INTERPRETATION	CONSIDERATIONS
Increased in Congenital adrenal hyperplasia (21-OH and 11β-OH deficiency)	Infant serum contains substances that may cross react with assay and artificially ↑ level unless separated by chromatography.

TEST/RANGE/COLLECTION	PHYSIOLOGIC BASIS

17-Hydroxypregnenolone (17-OH preg), serum

Used to assess adrenocortical function

	Range (ng/dL)	Mean (ng/dL)
Premature infants (at day 4)		
26-28 wk	124-841	471
31-35 wk	26-568	248
Full-term infants		
At 3 days	7-77	36
Female		
1-12 mo	13-106	31
Male		
1-12 mo	Levels increase after first week to peak values ranging from 40-200 ng/dL between 30 and 60 days. Values then decline to prepubertal range before 1 year.	
Prepubertal children	3-90	38

Tube type _____

Amount _____

| INTERPRETATION | CONSIDERATIONS |

Increased in
Forms of congenital adrenal
  hyperplasia (3-β hydroxysteroid
  dehydrogenase deficiency)

Tanner Stage	Age (yr)	Range (ng/dL)	Mean (ng/dL)
Puberty: male			
1	<9.8	30-90	38
2	9.8-14.5	5-115	51
3	10.7-15.4	10-138	57
4	11.8-16.2	29-180	80
5	12.8-17.3	24-175	97
Puberty: female			
1	<9.2	3-82	31
2	9.2-13.7	11-98	49
3	10.0-14.0	11-155	70
4	10.7-15.6	18-230	91
5	11.8-18.6	20-265	108
Adults			
Male		27-199	103
Female			
Follicular		15-70	46
Luteal		35-290	165

13

LABORATORY TESTING

TEST/RANGE/COLLECTION	PHYSIOLOGIC BASIS

Insulin, serum

Following a 4- to 12-hour fast

	Range (μU/mL)	Mean (μU/mL)
Infants and prepubertal children	<2-13	5.9
Pubertal children and adults	<2-17	7.0

Tube type _____

Amount _____

Measures levels of insulin, either endogenous or exogenous

Insulin-like Growth Factor 1 (IGF-1 or somatomedin C)

Age (yr)	Females (ng/mL)	Males (ng/mL)
1-2	45-222	99-254
3-4	36-202	36-202
5-6	32-259	57-260
7-8	65-278	97-352
9-10	52-330	49-461
11-12	80-723	101-580
13-14	142-855	199-658
15-16	176-845	236-808
17-18	152-668	165-526
19-30	126-382	138-410

Check lab for special handling and reference range. (See pp. 398-399.)

Tube type _____

Amount _____

Involved in stimulating growth, regulated by GH and nutritional status. Synthesized in many tissues and acts via insulin receptors. The liver is major source of IGF-1, which circulates bound to binding proteins.

INTERPRETATION	CONSIDERATIONS
Increased in Insulin-resistant states (e.g., obesity, type 2 diabetes mellitus, uremia, glucocorticoids, acromegaly), liver disease, surreptitious use of insulin or oral hypoglycemic agents, insulinoma (pancreatic islet cell tumor) ***Decreased in*** Type 1 diabetes mellitus, hypopituitarism (untreated)	Measurement of serum insulin level has little clinical value except in the diagnosis of fasting hypoglycemia or insulin-resistance syndromes (i.e., type 2 diabetes, polycystic ovarian syndrome). C-peptide should be used as well as serum insulin to distinguish insulinoma from surreptitious insulin use, since C-peptide will be absent with exogenous insulin administration. (See C-peptide, pp. 320-321.)
Increased in Acromegaly Gigantism ***Decreased in*** Isolated GH deficiency Hypopituitarism Laron dwarfism Undernutrition Liver disease	Test is useful in screening for GH deficiency. Serum levels are relatively constant during the day. Serum IGF-1 levels are age-dependent, being lowest in the <5 age group. Glucocorticoids inhibit growth-promoting actions of somatomedins.

13

LABORATORY TESTING

TEST/RANGE/COLLECTION	PHYSIOLOGIC BASIS

Insulin-like Growth Factor– Binding Protein 3 (IGFBP-3), serum

IGFBP-3s bind IGF-1 and IGF-2 with high affinity. Transports approximately 95% circulating IGFs. IGFBP-3 levels are GH dependent.

Age (yr)	mg/L
2	0.8-3.9
3	0.9-4.3
4	1.0-4.7
5	1.1-5.2
6	1.3-5.6
7	1.4-6.1
8	1.6-6.5
9	1.8-7.1
10	2.1-7.7
11	2.4-8.4
12	2.7-8.9
13	3.1-9.5
14	3.3-10.0
15	3.5-10.0
16	3.4-9.5
17	3.2-8.7
18	3.1-7.9
19	2.9-7.3

Check lab for special handling and reference range.

Tube type _____

Amount _____

Karyotype

See Chromosome analysis, pp. 324-325.

INTERPRETATION	CONSIDERATIONS
Increased in Acromegaly ***Decreased in*** Hypopituitarism Isolated GH deficiency Poorly controlled diabetes Caloric and protein restriction (less affected by malnutrition than IGF-1)	Clinically useful in assisting in differentiating between GH-deficient and non–GH-deficient short children.

TEST/RANGE/COLLECTION	PHYSIOLOGIC BASIS
Lactate, plasma 5-20 mg/dL *Tube type* _____ *Amount* _____	Severe tissue anoxia leads to anaerobic glucose metabolism with production of lactic acid.

Luteinizing Hormone (LH) (electrochemiluminescence [ECL] assay)

	Range (mIU/mL)	Mean (mIU/mL)
Infants (2 wk-1 yr)	0.02-7.0	—
Prepubertal (2-8 yr)	0.02-0.3	0.07

Tube type _____
Amount _____

A glycoprotein produced by anterior pituitary gland. Production is regulated by gonadotropin-releasing hormone (GnRH) and feedback by gonadal sex hormones. In females, LH stimulates ovulation and the production of estrogen and progesterone. In males, LH controls Leydig's cell secretion of testosterone.

INTERPRETATION	CONSIDERATIONS

Increased in Lactic acidosis, ethanol ingestion, sepsis, shock, liver disease, diabetes ketoacidosis, muscular exercise, hypoxia, type I glycogen storage disease, fructose 1,6 diphosphatase deficiency, pyruvate dehydrogenase deficiency.
Drugs: phenformin, isoniazid toxicity, metformin toxicity

Lactic acidosis should be suspected when there is a markedly increased anion gap (>18 mEq/L) in the absence of other causes (e.g., renal failure, ketosis, ethanol, methanol, or salicylate). Lactic acidosis is characterized by lactate levels >5 mmol/L in association with metabolic acidosis.

Increased in Central precocious puberty, luteal phase in menstrual cycle, primary hypogonadism, Turner syndrome, gonadotropin-secreting pituitary tumors, menopause

Decreased in Prepubertal children, delayed puberty, hypothalamic hypogonadism, ectopic steroid hormone production, GnRH analog treatment, peripheral sexual precocity, premature thelarche

Tanner Stage	Age (yr)	Range (mIU/mL)	Mean (mIU/mL)
Puberty: male			
1	<9.8	0.02-0.3	0.09
2	9.8-14.5	0.2-4.9	1.8
3	10.7-15.4	0.2-5.0	1.9
4-5	11.8-17.3	0.4-7.0	2.6
Puberty: female			
1	<9.2	0.02-0.18	0.06
2	9.2-13.7	0.02-4.7	0.72
3	10.0-14.4	0.10-12.0	2.3
4-5	10.7-18.6	0.4-11.7	3.3

Adults	Range (mIU/mL)
Menstruating women (based on normal-cycling females)	
Follicular	2-9
Peak	18-49
Luteal	2-11
Post-menopausal women	20-70
Men	1.5-9.0

13

LABORATORY TESTING

TEST/RANGE/COLLECTION	PHYSIOLOGIC BASIS
Magnesium (Mg²⁺), serum 1.3-2.1 mEq/L or 0.65-105 mmol/L *Tube type* _____ *Amount* _____	Important for the absorption of calcium from the intestines and in calcium metabolism
Microalbumin, urine	Protein/creatinine ratio: Determine ratio of protein (mg/dL) and creatinine (mg/dL) concentrations in a randomly collected spot urine during normal ambulation.
Molecular Analysis, Prader-Willi/Angelman Syndrome, blood Interpretive report identifies a normal or abnormal methylation pattern in the Prader-Willi/Angelman syndrome critical region *Tube type* _____ *Amount* _____	Southern blot analysis is utilized to identify parental origin of deletion or uniparental disomy by detecting differences in methylation within Prader-Willi syndrome/Angelman syndrome critical region.

INTERPRETATION	CONSIDERATIONS
Increased in Renal failure, Addison's disease, hyperparathyroidism, hypothyroidism, diabetes ketoacidosis (before treatment), dehydration, use of antacids containing Mg^{2+} **Decreased in** Hypoparathyroidism, possible neonatal hypocalcemia, chronic diarrhea, chronic renal disease, aldosteronism, hyperaldosteronism, malabsorption syndromes	Hemolysis may cause falsely elevated levels. Prolonged salicylate therapy, lithium, and magnesium products (antacids, laxatives) will cause falsely elevated levels, especially when renal damage is present.
Normal urinary protein: Normal urinary creatinine is <0.2 in older children and <0.5 during the first few months of life. All aberrant ratios should be confirmed with a 24-hour urine collection for proteinuria.	Increased activity may result in false-positive results.
	The southern blot analysis does not distinguish between a deletion in the paternally derived chromosome 15 (15q11.2-13), maternal uniparental disomy (mUPD), or the presence of an imprinting mutation. Additional cytogenetic studies or molecular genetic analysis is required to distinguish these possibilities.

TEST/RANGE/COLLECTION	PHYSIOLOGIC BASIS
Osmolality, serum 282-303 mOsm/kg water *Tube type* _____ *Amount* _____	Measure of solute concentration in the blood. Controlled by the hypothalamic-posterior pituitary regulation of vasopressin secretion for modification of renal free water excretion. It is useful in the assessment of fluid and electrolyte balance.
Osmolality, urine 200-1192 mOsm/kg water *Tube type* _____ *Amount* _____	Measure of solute concentration in the urine and reflective of the kidney's concentrating ability. Regulated by vasopressin and the kidneys. It is useful in diagnosis and management of fluid and electrolyte disorders.
Parathyroid Hormone (PTH), serum **Midregion specific radioimmunoassay** <10-65 pg/mL (with normal calcium) Fasting sample *Tube type* _____ *Amount* _____	Polypeptide hormone; factors in the regulation of calcium concentration in extracellular fluid

INTERPRETATION	CONSIDERATIONS
Increased in Diabetes insipidus Dehydration Hyperglycemia Hypernatremia Alcohol poisoning **Decreased in** Syndrome of inappropriate ADH secretion (SIADH) Overhydration Hyponatremia	Obtain urine for osmolality simultaneously.
Increased in SIADH Dehydration Liver disease Heart disease **Decreased in** Diabetes insipidus Overhydration Hypokalemia	Obtain urine for osmolality with simultaneous serum osmolality.
Increased in Pseudohypopara- thyroidism, vitamin D deficiency, rickets, vitamin A and D intoxication, hyperparathyroidism and Graves' disease **Decreased in** Hypoparathyroidism	↑ Lipids interfere with results. Milk ingestion may falsely lower levels.

TEST/RANGE/COLLECTION	PHYSIOLOGIC BASIS

Phosphorus (PO₄), plasma, serum

	mg/dL
Newborn	4.9-9.0
0-15 yr	3.2-6.3
Adult	2.7-4.5

Tube type _____

Amount _____

Phosphate is required for generation of bony tissue and aids in metabolism of lipids and glucose.

Plasma Renin Activity, plasma

Age	ng/mL/hr
0-3 yr	<16.6
3-6 yr	<6.7
6-9 yr	<4.4
9-12 yr	<5.9
12-15 yr	<4.2
15-18 yr	<4.3

Do not leave at room temperature; must chill tube.

Tube type _____

Amount _____

Renin is an enzyme released by the kidney in response to sodium depletion and hypovolemia. It activates the renin-angiotensin system, stimulating aldosterone production from the adrenal cortex.

INTERPRETATION	CONSIDERATIONS
Increased in Renal insufficiency, ↑vitamin D intake, healing fractures, bone tumors, hypocalcemia, Addison's disease, acromegaly, hypoparathyroidism ***Decreased in*** Rickets, hyperinsulinism, hyperparathyroidism	Normally high in children May be falsely ↑ by hemolysis Vitamin D may ↑. Laxatives may ↑. If PO_4 ↑ and Ca^{2+} ↓, be alert for arrhythmias and muscle twitching.
Increased in Essential, malignant, and renovascular hypertension; Addison's disease; Bartter's syndrome; cirrhosis, hypokalemia, hemorrhage ***Decreased in*** Salt-retaining steroid therapy, antidiuretic hormone therapy	Try to perform test with patient in an upright position. Posture affects levels. Renin is ↑ in the upright position and ↓ in the recumbent position. Values are higher early in the day and in patients on low-salt diets. Drugs that may affect test results: 　Antihypertensives 　Diuretics 　Estrogens 　Oral contraceptives 　Vasodilators

⓭

LABORATORY TESTING

TEST/RANGE/COLLECTION	PHYSIOLOGIC BASIS
Potassium, serum <10 days of age 4.0-6.0 mEq/L >10 days of age 3.5-5.0 mEq/L *Tube type* _____ *Amount* _____	Intracellular K concentration is about 150 mEq/L, whereas the serum K is about 4 mEq/L. The ratio is important in maintaining membrane electrical potential in excitable neuromuscular tissue. Serum concentration is so small that minor changes in concentration have significant consequences.

Progesterone, serum		Used to evaluate function of the corpus luteum and confirm ovulation

	ng/dL
Preovulation	20-150
Midcycle	300-2400
Pregnancy	>2400

Tube type _____
Amount _____

INTERPRETATION	CONSIDERATIONS

Increased in ↑Potassium intake, excessive dietary intake, excessive IV intake, ↓potassium loss, acute or chronic renal failure, Addison's disease, hypoaldosteronism, aldosterone-inhibiting diuretics such as spironolactone, triamterene, acidosis, infection, crush injury to tissues
 	
Decreased in ↓Potassium intake, deficient dietary intake, deficient IV intake, excessive potassium loss as in diarrhea, vomiting, diuretic use, hyperaldosteronism, Cushing's syndrome, renal tubular acidosis
	Exercise of the forearm with a tourniquet in place, heelstick or traumatic phlebotomy, may ↑ K levels.
	
	Drugs that may ↑ levels:
	    Aminocaproic acid, antibiotics, antineoplastic drugs, captopril, epinephrine, heparin, histamine, isoniazid (INH), lithium, mannitol, potassium-sparing diuretics, potassium supplements, succinylcholine
	
	Drugs that may ↓ levels:
	    Acetazolamide, aminosalicylic acid, amphotericin B, carbenicillin, cisplatin, potassium-wasting diuretics, glucose infusions, insulin, laxatives, lithium carbonate, penicillin G sodium, phenothiazines, aspirin, sodium polystyrene (Kayexalate)

Increased in Pregnancy Adrenal neoplasm Ovarian neoplasm **Decreased in** Amenorrhea	Recent use of isotopes may affect test results. Drugs that may interfere with test include estrogen and progesterone.

⑬

LABORATORY TESTING

TEST/RANGE/COLLECTION	PHYSIOLOGIC BASIS

Prolactin, serum

	Range (ng/mL)	Mean (ng/mL)
Newborn (1-7 days)	30-495	188
Children and adults		
Male	3-18	8.8
Female	3-24	12.6

Tube type _____

Amount _____

A protein hormone secreted by the anterior pituitary gland and the placenta. May play a role in the number of developing follicles in the follicular phase of menstrual cycle. Associated during and following pregnancy stimulation of breast development and milk production.

Sex Hormone–Binding Globulin (SHBG), serum

	Range (µg/dL)
Infants (1 mo-2 yr)	1.5-6.3
Prepubertal children (2-8 yr)	1.8-5.5
Pubertal males	0.4-2.5
Pubertal females	0.9-3.2
Adult males	0.5-1.5
Adult females	1.0-3.0

Tube type _____

Amount _____

Used in diagnosis of polycystic ovarian syndrome

Sex Hormone–Binding Globulin (SHBG) IRMA, serum

	Range (nmol/L)
Infants (1 mo-2 yr)	60-252
Prepubertal children (2-8 yr)	72-220
Pubertal males	16-100
Pubertal females	36-125
Adult males	20-60
Adult females	40-120

Tube type _____

Amount _____

INTERPRETATION	CONSIDERATIONS
Increased in Hypothalamic pituitary tumor Stress (physical and emotional) Antidepressants Breast-feeding (nipple stimulation) Hypothyroidism ***Decreased by*** Bromocriptine Dopamine and dopamine analogs	Stress from venipuncture can falsely elevate prolactin level. Hyperprolactinemia inhibits gonadotropin secretion and produces hypogonadism in males and females with low or low-normal LH and FSH levels.
Increased in Oral contraceptive users ***Decreased in*** Polycystic ovarian syndrome	

TEST/RANGE/COLLECTION	PHYSIOLOGIC BASIS

Sodium, serum

	mEq/L
Newborn	134-144
Infant	134-150
Child	136-145
Adult	136-145

Tube type _____

Amount _____

Sodium salts are the major determinants of extracellular osmolality. Sodium content of the blood is the result of a balance between dietary intake and renal excretion.

Aldosterone causes conservation of sodium by decreasing renal losses. Natriuretic hormone increases renal losses of sodium. ADH controls reabsorption of water at the distal tubules of the kidney, which affects sodium serum levels.

Testosterone, serum

	Range (ng/dL)	Mean (ng/dL)
Premature infants (at day 4)		
Male		
26-28 wk	59-125	91
31-35 wk	37-198	126
Female		
26-28 wk	5-16	11
31-35 wk	5-22	12
Full-term infants		
Newborn male	75-400	200
Newborn female	20-64	39
Prepubertal children		
1-10 yr	<3-10	4.9

Tube type _____

Amount _____

Major sex steroid for males; produced by the testes

Small amount produced by the ovaries and adrenal glands in females

INTERPRETATION	CONSIDERATIONS

Increased in ↑Sodium intake, excessive dietary intake, excessive sodium in IV fluids, ↓sodium loss, Cushing's syndrome, hyperaldosteronism, excessive free body water loss, excessive sweating, excessive thermal burns, diabetes insipidus, osmotic diuresis

Decreased in ↓Sodium intake, deficient dietary intake, deficient sodium in IV fluids, ↑sodium loss, Addison's disease, diarrhea, vomiting or nasogastric aspiration, diuretic administration, chronic renal insufficiency, ↑free body water, excessive oral water intake, excessive IV water intake, congestive heart failure, SIADH, ascites, peripheral edema, pleural effusion, salt-wasting congenital adrenal hyperplasia

Recent trauma, surgery, or shock may cause increased levels.

Drugs that may ↑ levels:
Anabolic steroids Laxatives
Antibiotics Methyldopa
Clonidine Carbenicillin
Corticosteroids Estrogens
Cough medicines Oral contraceptives

Drugs that may ↓ levels:
Carbamazepine ACE inhibitors
Diuretics Captopril
Sodium-free IV Triamterene
  fluids Nonsteroidal
Sulfonylureas   anti-inflammatory
Haloperidol   drugs (NSAIDs)
Heparin Vasopressin
Tricyclic
  antidepressants

13

LABORATORY TESTING

Increased in
Precocious puberty (male)
Androgen resistance
Testotoxicosis
Congenital adrenal hypoplasia
Polycystic ovarian disease
Ovarian tumors

Decreased in
Delayed puberty (male)
Gonadotropin deficiency
Testicular defects

Tanner Stage	Age (yr)	Range (ng/dL)	Mean (ng/dL)
Puberty: male			
1	<9.8	<3-10	4.9
2	9.8-14.5	18-150	42
3	10.7-15.4	100-320	190
4	11.8-16.2	200-620	372
5	12.8-17.3	350-970	546
Puberty: female			
1	<9.2	<3-10	4.9
2	9.2-13.7	7-28	18
3	10.0-14.4	15-35	25
4	10.7-15.6	13-32	22
5	11.8-18.6	20-38	28

TEST/RANGE/COLLECTION	PHYSIOLOGIC BASIS

Free Thyroxine Index (FTI)

1.25-4.2

Thyroglobulin (Tg), serum

Age	Range (ng/dL)	Mean (ng/dL)
1-12 mo	12-113	42
Prepubertal	5.2-72	29
Pubertal and adults	<3-39	16

Tube type _____

Amount _____

Thyroglobulin is a large protein from which thyroxine is synthesized and cleaved.

Thyroid Antibodies, serum

Antithyroglobulin

Negative	≤1:40
Borderline	1:80
Significant	1:160-1:640
Very significant	>1:640

Antithyroperoxidase (anti-TPO)

Negative	<1:400
Borderline	1:400
Significant	1:1,600-1:6,400
Very significant	>1:6,400

Tube type _____

Amount _____

Autoantibodies formed against the thyroid autoantigens thyroglobulin and thyroidal peroxidase

Presence of one or both of these is a useful indicator of autoimmune thyroid disease.

INTERPRETATION	CONSIDERATIONS
Calculated: T4 radioimmunoassay × T3 resin uptake (T4 RIA × T3 RU)	FTI estimates how much T4 is present compared with thyroid-binding globulin (TBG). It can correct for variations in TBG, and can help determine if abnormal amounts of T4 are present as a result of abnormal amounts of TBG.
Increased in Hyperthyroidism, subacute thyroiditis, untreated thyroid carcinoma (except medullary carcinoma) ***Decreased in*** After total thyroidectomy, presence of thyroglobulin autoantibodies, TSH deficiency. May be normal or decreased in primary hypothyroidism, Hashimoto's thyroiditis, transient neonatal hypothyroidism.	Tg can be used as a reliable tumor marker for thyroid cancer.
Present in Hashimoto's thyroiditis, hyperthyroidism. May be normal or increased in primary hypothyroidism.	

⑬

LABORATORY TESTING

TEST/RANGE/COLLECTION	PHYSIOLOGIC BASIS

Tissue Transglutaminase (tTG)

>2 yr	
Negative	<25U/mL by ELISA
Weak positive	25-50 U/mL
Positive	>50 U/mL

Tube type _____

Amount _____

IgA, IgG antibodies to gliadin (wheat protein)

Thyroid-Stimulating Hormone (TSH), serum

Age	Normal Range (mIU/mL)
Cord	<2.5-17.4
1-3 days	<2.5-13.3
1-4 wk	0.6-10.0
1-12 mo	0.6-6.3
1-15 yr	0.6-6.3
16-50 yr	0.2-7.6

Tube type _____

Amount _____

Thyrotropin (TSH) is secreted by the pituitary gland and regulates the synthesis and release of thyroxine (T4) and triiodothyronine (T3) by the thyroid gland. TSH production is stimulated by thyrotropin-releasing hormone (TRH) from the hypothalamus and inhibited by circulating free T4 and T3.

TSH Receptor Antibody (TSH-binding inhibition index)

Normal	<10
Indeterminate	10-14
Positive	>15

Tube type _____

Amount _____

An autoantibody formed against the TSH receptor autoantigen. May be an inhibitory (TBII) or a stimulating (TSI) antibody.

INTERPRETATION	CONSIDERATIONS
Increased in celiac disease False-positive results possible: likely elevated in Crohn's disease, postinfective malabsorption, food protein intolerance (e.g., cow's milk)	If elevated refer to gastroenterology for assessment. Gold standard is intestinal biopsy to confirm diagnosis. Sensitivity of 95% for active, untreated celiac disease if testing both IgA and IgG antibodies. IgA deficiency can cause false-negative tTG, IgA. IgA monitors dietary compliance better in people who can respond to IgA.
Increased in Primary hypothyroidism Decreased thyroid reserve (subclinical hypothyroidism) TSH-dependent hyperthyroidism Thyroid hormone resistance ***Decreased in*** Graves' disease Autonomous thyroid hormone secretion TSH deficiency (secondary hypothyroidism) Thyrotoxicosis	TSH surge peaks 80-90 mIU/mL in term newborn within 30 minutes after birth. After 1 week, values are within adult range. Low T4 and T3 in the presence of low or normal TSH suggest hypothalamic or pituitary dysfunction.
Increased in Transient neonatal hypothyroidism. May be negative or increased in primary hypothyroidism, Hashimoto's thyroiditis, Graves' disease, neonatal Graves' disease.	

TEST/RANGE/COLLECTION	PHYSIOLOGIC BASIS
Thyroxine, Free (free T4), serum	Measures the unbound form of thyroxine

Free T4 in preterm/term infants

Estimated Gestational Age	Normal Range (ng/dL)
29-30 wk	0.3-1.2
31-32 wk	0.2-1.6
33-34 wk	0.5-1.4
35-36 wk	0.5-1.7
37-38 wk	0.6-1.9

Age	Range (ng/dL)
1-10 days	0.6-2.0
>10 days	0.7-1.7

Tube type _____

Amount _____

TEST/RANGE/COLLECTION	PHYSIOLOGIC BASIS
Thyroxine by Radioimmuno-assay (T4 RIA), serum	Measures total amount of bound and unbound thyroxine in the blood

Age	Range (μg/dL)
Cord	6.6-17.5
1-3 days	11.0-21.5
1-4 wk	8.2-16.6
1-12 mo	7.2-15.6
1-5 yr	7.3-15
6-10 yr	6.4-13.3
11-15 yr	5.6-11.7
16-20 yr	4.2-11.8

Tube type _____

Amount _____

INTERPRETATION	CONSIDERATIONS
Increased in Graves' disease, neonatal Graves' nonthyroidal illness, especially psychiatric, use of drugs such as amiodarone, high-dose beta-blockers	Normal range is assay dependent.
Decreased in Hypothyroidism, TSH deficiency, Hashimoto's thyroiditis, nonthyroidal illness, use of phenytoin. Decreased or normal in sick euthyroid syndrome	
Increased in Hyperthyroidism, neonatal Graves' disease, increased thyroxine-binding globulin (TBG) disease, concomitant use of drugs such as high dose beta-blockers and amiodarone (may cause hyperthyroidism or hypothyroidism)	
Decreased in Primary hypothyroidism, TSH deficiency, low TBG, use of drugs such as phenytoin, lithium, carbamazepine, and androgens. May be normal or decreased in Hashimoto's thyroiditis. Decreased or normal in sick euthyroid syndrome	

13

LABORATORY TESTING

TEST/RANGE/COLLECTION	PHYSIOLOGIC BASIS
Thyroxine-Binding Globulin (TBG), serum	Thyroid hormone transport protein

Age	Normal (mIU/mL)
Cord	0.7-4.7
1-3 days	—
1-4 wk	0.5-4.5
1-12 mo	1.6-3.6
1-5 yr	1.3-2.8
6-20 yr	1.4-2.6
21-50 yr	1.2-2.4

Tube type _____

Amount _____

TEST/RANGE/COLLECTION	PHYSIOLOGIC BASIS
Resin Triiodothyronine Uptake (T3 RU), serum	Measures thyroid hormone binding (not T3)

25%-35%

Tube type _____

Amount _____

TEST/RANGE/COLLECTION	PHYSIOLOGIC BASIS
Reverse Triiodothyronine (rT3), serum	Newborns reach adult levels at about 1 week of age. In adults rT3 is about one third of the total T3 concentration. Can be used to differentiate sick euthyroid syndrome from hypothyroidism.

Age	Range (ng/dL)
Newborns	90-250
Children	10-50
Adults	10-50

Tube type _____

Amount _____

INTERPRETATION	CONSIDERATIONS
Variable in T4 protein-binding abnormalities; otherwise normal **Increased in** TBG excess **Decreased in** TBG deficiency	
Increased in Thyroxine-binding globulin (TBG) deficiency, hyperthyroidism, nonthyroid illness **Decreased in** Hypothyroidism, TBG excess, secondary hypothyroidism	
Increased in Graves' and neonatal Graves' disease. Increased or normal in sick euthyroid syndrome. **Decreased in** Primary hypothyroidism, transient neonatal hypothyroidism, Hashimoto's thyroiditis, TSH deficiency	Newborn values reach the adult range by 1 week.

TEST/RANGE/COLLECTION	PHYSIOLOGIC BASIS
Triiodothyronine by Radioimmunoassay (T3 RIA), serum	The metabolically active thyroid hormone

Age	Range (ng/dL)
Cord	14-86
1-3 days	100-380
1-4 wk	99-310
1-12 mo	102-264
1-5 yr	105-269
6-10 yr	94-241
11-15 yr	83-213
16-20 yr	80-210

Tube type _____

Amount _____

25-OH Vitamin D (calcifediol), serum	Required for normal calcium and phosphorus metabolism

Age	Range (ng/mL)
Newborns	5-42
Children	10-55

Tube type _____

Amount _____

1,25-(OH)₂ Vitamin D (calcitriol), serum	Action is to promote absorption of both phosphorus and calcium from the gut. Enhances bone metabolism by encouraging release of available calcium and phosphorus from the bone as well as reabsorption of calcium and phosphorus into the bone matrix protein that is required for bone growth, modeling, and general skeletal strengthening.

Age	Range (pg/mL)
Newborns	8-72
Infants and children	15-90

Tube type _____

Amount _____

INTERPRETATION	CONSIDERATIONS
Increased in Hyperthyroidism (T3 is often elevated to a greater degree than T4 or free T4), high TBG ***Decreased in*** Hypothyroidism, low TBG; decreased or normal in sick euthyroid syndrome	
Increased in Hypervitaminosis ***Decreased in*** Vitamin D deficiency rickets	
Increased in Possible in vitamin D deficiency rickets ***Decreased in*** Vitamin D deficiency rickets	

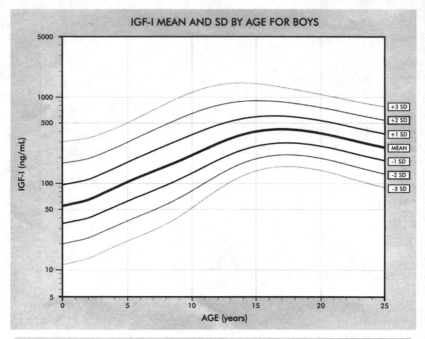

IGF-I MEAN AND SD BY AGE FOR BOYS

FOR BOYS

ACCESSION NUMBER

DATE DRAWN

DATE REPORTED

PATIENT INFORMATION

PATIENT NAME

AGE

DOB

TANNER STAGE

HEIGHT

WEIGHT

REFERRING PHYSICIAN

TEST RESULTS	REFERENCE RANGE
IGF-I (ng/mL)	IGF-I (ng/mL)
IGFBP-3 (ng/mL)	IGFBP-3 (ng/mL)
BONE AGE	Refer to table on back of pad for reference ranges

The composite data presented in this nomogram was log normalized, and the means and standard deviations were plotted using smoothed-spline curve-fit generated by a computerized statistical software program. The nomogram represents the reference table on the back cover; please refer to the table for actual values.

Diagnostic Systems Laboratories, Inc., 445 Medical Center Blvd., Webster, Texas 77598-4217
Tel: +1.281.332.9678 +1.800.231.7970 Fax: +1.281.338.1895 Email: mktg@dslabs.com
GERMANY: Diagnostic Systems Laboratories, Deutschland GmbH, Kleines Feldlein 4, 74889 Sinsheim, Tel: +49.7261.92160, Fax: +49.7261.921699
ITALY: Diagnostic Systems Laboratorium Italia, Via Gracia 25/2, 35020 Padova, Tel: +39.49.760.844, Fax: +39.49.760.855
INDIA: Diagnostic Systems Laboratories India Pvt. Ltd., 44, Udyog Bhavan, Sonawala Road, Goregaon (East), Mumbai - 400063, Tel: +91.22.871.7344, Fax: +91.22.871.7300

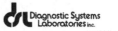

IGF-I FOR GIRLS

ACCESSION NUMBER	
DATE DRAWN	DATE REPORTED

PATIENT INFORMATION

PATIENT NAME		
AGE	DOB	TANNER STAGE
HEIGHT	WEIGHT	
REFERRING PHYSICIAN		

TEST RESULTS	REFERENCE RANGE
IGF-I (ng/mL)	IGF-I (ng/mL)
IGFBP-3 (ng/mL)	IGFBP-3 (ng/mL)
BONE AGE	Refer to table on back of pad for reference ranges

LABORATORY TESTING ⑬

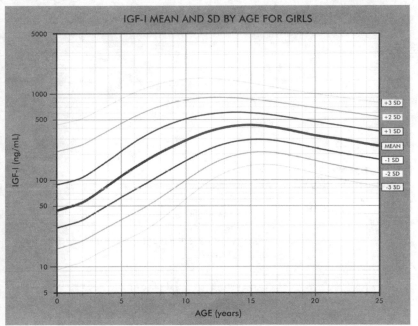

IGF-I MEAN AND SD BY AGE FOR GIRLS

IGF-I (ng/mL) vs AGE (years)

+3 SD
+2 SD
+1 SD
MEAN
-1 SD
-2 SD
-3 3D

The composite data presented in this nomogram was log normalized, and the means and standard deviations were plotted using smoothed-spline curve-fit generated by a computerized statistical software program. The nomogram represents the reference table on the back cover; please refer to the table for actual values.

Diagnostic Systems Laboratories, Inc., 445 Medical Center Blvd., Webster, Texas. 77598-4217
Tel. +1.281.332.9678 +1.800.231.7970 Fax +1.281.338.1895 Email: mktg@dslabs.com
GERMANY. Diagnostic Systems Laboratories, Deutschland GmbH, Kleines Feldlein 4, 74889 Sinsheim , Tel. +49.7261.92160, Fax +49.7261.921699
ITALY. Diagnostic Systems Laboratories Italia, Via Grazia 25/2, 35020 Padova, Tel. +39.49.760.844, Fax +39.49.760.655
INDIA. Diagnostic Systems Laboratories India Pvt. Ltd., A4, Udyog Bhavan, Sonawala Road, Goregaon (East), Mumbai - 400063, Tel. +91.22.871.7344, Fax +91.22.871.7300

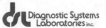

Diagnostic Systems Laboratories inc.

©1997 DSL, Inc.

⑭ PEDIATRIC ENDOCRINE MEDICATIONS

DRUG	HOW SUPPLIED / DOSE AND ROUTE
Alendronate Sodium (Fosamax)	Tabs 5 mg 10 mg 35 mg 40 mg 70 mg
Atorvastatin Calcium (Lipitor) HMG-CoA reductase inhibitor	Tabs 10 mg 20 mg 40 mg 80 mg ─────── *Heterozygous familial and nonfamilial and Mixed dyslipidemia* Starting dose 10 mg qd Dose range 10-80 mg qd There are no pharmacokinetic data on children less than 9 years of age.

SIDE EFFECTS/REMARKS	NURSING CONSIDERATIONS
Headache, blurred vision, abdominal distention, acid regurgitation, gastritis, erythema, photosensitization	Patients should be taught to take first thing in the morning, 30 minutes before eating or drinking. The drug should be taken with water. Patients need to know the importance of remaining upright for 30 minutes to minimize esophageal irritation. Encourage sunscreen use and protective clothing when outside. Contraindicated in pregnancy or lactation.
Nausea, vomiting, dry mouth, anorexia, increased appetite, insomnia, dizziness, muscle achiness, urinary tract infection, peripheral edema, pruritus, dry skin, constipation, flatulence, dyspepsia, and abdominal pain	The patient should be placed on a standard cholesterol-lowering diet before starting this medication and should continue on this diet during treatment. Use of this drug in combination with HMG-CoA reductase inhibitors and fibrates should be avoided. Lipid levels should be checked every 2-4 weeks upon initiation or titration of the dose.

14

PEDIATRIC ENDOCRINE MEDICATIONS

DRUG	HOW SUPPLIED/DOSE AND ROUTE
Bromocriptine Mesylate (Parlodel) Dopamine agonist	Tabs 2.5 mg Caps 5.0 mg *Hyperprolactinemia* Initial: 1.25-2.5 mg PO qd Can be titrated up by an additional 2.5 mg as tolerated every 3-7 days until an optimal therapeutic response is achieved. Safety and efficacy have not been established in children under the age of 15.
Cabergoline (Dostinex) Dopamine agonist	Tabs 0.5 mg *Hyperprolactinemia* Initial: 0.25 mg PO twice a week The drug can then be titrated up to a dosage of 1 mg twice a week. Dosage adjustments should not be made more frequently than every 4 weeks so the physician can assess the patient's response to each dosage level.

SIDE EFFECTS/REMARKS	NURSING CONSIDERATIONS
Nausea, headache, vomiting, orthostatic hypotension, somnolence; less common: nasal stuffiness and constipation	Patients being treated for a macroadenoma should report any persistent watery nasal discharge to their physician.

Side effects can be minimized by beginning treatment with a very small dose at bedtime, always taking the medication with food, and gradually increasing the dose to the recommended amount.

If a patient is intolerant of one drug, he or she may be able to tolerate another drug. |
| Nausea, headache, dizziness, and constipation | Side effects can be minimized by beginning treatment with a very small dose at bedtime, always taking the medication with food and gradually increasing the dose to the recommended amount. |

⑭

PEDIATRIC ENDOCRINE MEDICATIONS

DRUG	HOW SUPPLIED/DOSE AND ROUTE
Calcitriol (Rocaltrol) Synthetic active form of vitamin D_3 Promotes reabsorption of calcium from GI tract	Caps 0.25 μg 0.5 μg Injection 1 μg/mL 2 μg/mL <hr>*Hypocalcemia* 0.25-2 μg/day PO *Hypoparathyroid >5 years of age* 0.225 μg/day PO, may be ↑ at 2-4 week intervals (usual range 0.5-2.0 μg/day) *Hypoparathyroid <5 years of age* 0.25-0.75 μg/day PO (0.04-0.08 μg/kg/day)
Calcium Salts (Os-Cal, Tums, Caltrate, Citracal, Neo-Calglucon) Replacement of calcium in deficiency states	Tabs 650 mg, 1.25 g, 1.5 g Chewable tabs 750 mg, 1.25 g Caps 1.25 g Oral suspension 1.25 g/5 mL Powder 6.5 g/packet Injection 10% (0.45 mEq/mL) 1.1g/5 mL (4.5 mEq/5 mL) <hr>*Supplementation* 45-65 mg/kg/day PO *Neonatal hypocalcemia* 50-150 mg/kg PO (not to exceed 1 g) *Hypocalcemia emergency* Children IV: 1-7 mEq Infants IV: <1 mEq *Hypocalcemic tetany* Children IV: 0.5-0.7 mEq/kg 3-4 × daily Neonate IV: 2.4 mEq/kg/day in divided doses

SIDE EFFECTS / REMARKS	NURSING CONSIDERATIONS
Weakness, headache, somnolence, photophobia, conjunctivitis, rhinorrhea, hypertension, arrhythmias, nausea, vomiting, dry mouth, constipation, metallic taste, polydipsia, anorexia, weight loss, polyuria, nocturia, ↓ libido, albuminuria, pruritus, hypercalcemia, hyperthermia, muscle pain, bone pain	Patients should be assessed for bone pain and/or weakness at each visit. Any indication of hypervitaminosis should be reported to physician. Dose may be taken PO without regard to meals. If dose is missed, take it as soon as possible. *Do not* double up. Vitamin D–rich foods include breads, cereals, fish, fish liver oils, and fortified milk. Calcium-rich foods include bok choy, broccoli, brussels sprouts, cabbage, cauliflower, cheeses, collards, fish, milk, mustard greens, pork, rice, spinach, turnips, and yogurt.
Bradycardia, arrhythmias, cardiac arrest (IV), tingling, syncope (IV), nausea, vomiting, constipation, hypercalciuria, calculi, phlebitis at IV site Drug-Drug: ↑ Risk of cardiac glycoside toxicity; avoid use with thiazide diuretics Drug-Food: Cereals, spinach or rhubarb may ↓ absorption	Take with or 1 hour after meals and at bedtime. Chewable tablets need to be well chewed before swallowing. A full glass of water should be taken. IV may cause burning sensation, peripheral vasodilation, and a ↓ in blood pressure. Use small-bore needle in large vein. Warm IV solution before infusion. Premature dissolution of enteric-coated tablets will occur if they are taken within 1 hour of calcium.

14

PEDIATRIC ENDOCRINE MEDICATIONS

DRUG	HOW SUPPLIED/DOSE AND ROUTE
Carnitine (Carnitor, Levocarnitine, Vitacarn) Amino acid	Tabs 330 mg Caps 250 mg Solution 100 mg/mL (118 mL) Injection 200 mg/mL (5 mL) (preservative free) *For plasma membrane carnitine transporter defect* Children 100 mg/kg/24 hr PO ÷ q6-8h
Chlorothiazide (Diuril, Diurigen) Thiazide diuretic	Tabs 250 mg, 500 mg Suspension 250 mg/5 mL (237 mL) Injection 500 mg (5 mEq Na/1 g) 20-40 mg/kg/24 hr ÷ q12h PO/IV ≥6 mo 20 mg/kg 24 ÷ q12h PO/IV Adults 250-1000 mg/dose qd-qid PO/IV Max. dose 2 g/24 hr

Chorionic Gonado-tropin (HCG)
 	
 Polypeptide hormone
	Injection 10 ml lyophilized multi-dose vials
	               (5000 units or 10,000 units when
	               reconstituted)
	
	 Prepubertal cryptorchidism not due to anatomic obstruction
	 <1 yr 250 IU biw × 5 wk
	 1-5 yr 500 IU biw × 5 wk
	 >5 yr 1000 IU biw × 5 wk
	
	 Regimens vary from 100-4000 IU per injection biw or tiw × 5 wk
	
	 Hypogonadotropic hypogonadism
	 500-1000 units tiw × 3 wk, then biw × 3 wk
	 4000 units tiw × 6-9 mo, then ↑ dose to 2000 units
	    tiw × 3 mo

SIDE EFFECTS/REMARKS	NURSING CONSIDERATIONS
Nausea, vomiting, diarrhea, and fishy body odor	
May increase serum calcium, bilirubin, glucose, uric acid May cause alkalosis, pancreatitis, dizziness, hypokalemia, and hypo-magnesemia	*Use with caution* in liver and severe renal disease. *Avoid IM or SQ administration.*
May cause headache, irritability, restlessness, depression, fatigue, edema, precocious puberty, gyneco-mastia, pain at the injection site, local and systemic hypersensitivity reactions Contraindicated in precocious puberty, prostatic carcinoma, prior allergic reaction to HCG, pregnancy	With cryptorchidism, monitor every 2 weeks for progress of treatment. Surgical repair necessary if testicle(s) fail to descend into scrotal sac Discontinue if signs of precocious puberty occur. Use with caution in cardiac or renal disease, epilepsy, migraines, or asthma. Requires refrigeration after reconstitution.

14

PEDIATRIC ENDOCRINE MEDICATIONS

DRUG	HOW SUPPLIED/DOSE AND ROUTE
Clomiphene Citrate (Clomid, Serophene) Ovulatory stimulant	Tabs 50 mg *Gynecomastia* 100 mg PO qd × 6 mo NOTE Use and dosage outside of product labeling *Ovulation* 50 mg PO qd × 5 days
Desmopressin Acetate (DDAVP, Stimate) Vasopressin analog, synthetic; hemostatic agent	Tabs 0.1, 0.2 mg Nasal solution DDAVP, 100 μg/mL (2.5 mL); Stimate, 1500 μg/mL (2.5 mL); both preparations contain 9 mg/NaCl/mL Injection 4 μg/mL (1, 10 mL); 15 μg/mL (1, 2 mL) Nasal spray 100 μg/mL, 10 μg/spray (50 sprays, 5 mL); contains 7.5 mg NaCl/mL CONVERSION 100 μg = 400 IU arginine vasopressin *Diabetes insipidus* Oral Children Start with 0.05 mg bid; titrate to effect Adult Start with 0.05 mg bid; titrate dose to effect; usual dose range: 0.1-0.2 mg/24 hr ÷ bid-tid Intranasal 3 mo-12 yr 5-30 μg/24 hr ÷ qd-bid Adults 10-40 μg/24 hr ÷ qd-tid; titrate dose to achieve control of excessive thirst and urination; max. intranasal dose: 40 μg/24 hr IV/SQ 2-4 μg/24 hr ÷ bid *(continued)*

SIDE EFFECTS/REMARKS	NURSING CONSIDERATIONS
May cause hot flashes, nausea, stomach discomfort, or visual disturbances.	Not indicated for individuals with liver disease Therapy should begin 5 days after onset of menses. If menses absent, therapy can be started anytime.
May cause headache, nausea, hyponatremia, nasal congestion, abdominal cramps, and hypertension	*Use with caution* in hypertension and coronary artery disease. SQ or IV injection may be substituted at approximately 10% of intranasal dose. Adjust fluid intake to decrease risk of water intoxication. Peak effects: 1-5 hr with intranasal route; 1.5-3 hr with IV route; and 2-7 hr with PO route For hemophilia A and von Willebrand's disease, administer dose intranasally 2 hours before procedure; administer IV dose 30 minutes before procedure.

⑭

PEDIATRIC ENDOCRINE MEDICATIONS

DRUG	HOW SUPPLIED / DOSE AND ROUTE
(Desmopressin Acetate)	*Hemophilia A and von Willebrand's disease*
	Intranasal 2-4 μg/kg/dose
	IV 0.2-0.4 μg/kg/dose over 15-30 min
	Nocturnal enuresis (>6 yr)
	Oral 0.2 mg at bedtime, titrated to 0.6 mg to achieve desired effect
	Intranasal 20 μg at bedtime, range 10-40 μg; divide dose by 2 and administer each one-half dose per nostril
Dexamethasone (Decadron and others) Corticosteroid See steroid equivalency table, p. 424.	Tabs 0.25, 0.5, 0.75, 1, 1.5, 2, 4, 6 mg
	Elixir 0.5 mg/5 mL (some preparations contain 5% alcohol)
	Oral solution 0.1, 1 mg/mL (some solutions contain 30% alcohol)
	Injection 4, 10, 20, 24 mg/mL (sodium phosphate; some preparations contain benzyl alcohol)
	Injection 8, 16 mg/mL (acetate)
	Physiologic replacement
	PO/IM/IV 0.5-0.75 mg/m^2/24 hr ÷ q6-12h
	Stress dosing
	PO/IM 2-4 times the physiologic replacement dose. Give preoperatively and post-operatively with gradual decrease to maintenance.
	Anti-inflammatory
	Children 0.08-0.3 mg/kg/24 hr PO, IV, IM ÷ q6-12h
	Adults 0.75-9 mg/24 hr PO, IV, IM ÷ q6-12h

SIDE EFFECTS / REMARKS	NURSING CONSIDERATIONS

Mood changes Nausea Seizures Abdominal distention Hyperglycemia GI bleeding Diarrhea *With prolonged use:* Cushingoid effects Hypothalamic-pituitary-adrenal axis suppression Cataracts Glaucoma ↓ Bone mineral density ↓*Effects with:* Barbiturates Ephedrine Phenytoin Rifampin Sudden withdrawal may precipitate an adrenal crisis.	Consider for patients on glucocorticoid therapy >1 month. Must be used in conjunction with mineralocorticoid (Florinef) where applicable Contraindicated in patients with systemic fungal infections Growth and development of children on corticosteroids should be closely monitored. May mask signs of infection Patients should be monitored regularly for BP and serum electrolytes.

DRUG	HOW SUPPLIED/DOSE AND ROUTE
Diazoxide (Hyperstat, Proglycem) Antihypoglycemic agent	Injection 15 mg/ml Caps 50 mg Suspension 50 mg/mL (30 mL); contains 7.25% alcohol *Hyperinsulinemic hypoglycemia* (due to insulin-producing tumors) Newborns and infants 8-15 mg/kg/24 hr divided q8-12h PO Children and adults 3-8 mg/kg/24 hr divided q8-12h PO
Dihydrotachysterol (DHT) Vitamin D analog Promotes absorption of calcium and phosphorus	Oral solution 0.2 mg/mL Tablets 0.125, 0.2, 0.4 mg Capsules 0.125 mg *Hypoparathyroid* 1-5 mg/day initially for 4 days, then 0.5-1.5 mg/day

SIDE EFFECTS/REMARKS	NURSING CONSIDERATIONS
Fluid and sodium retention Hypertrichosis GI disturbances Rash Hypotension Hyperuricemia	If given IV route, must be given over 15 minutes to avoid hypotension If given PO route, hyperglycemic effect occurs within 1 hour with a duration of 8 hours
No side effects if taken within range of daily requirements *Drug-drug interactions:* Cholestyramine, colestipol or mineral oil ↓ absorption. Use with thiazide diuretics may result in hypercalcemia. Glucocorticoids ↓ effectiveness. Use with cardiac glycosides ↑ risk of arrhythmias. Requirements ↑ with phenytoin, hydantoin anticonvulsant, sucralfate, barbiturates, and primidone.	Observe for hypocalcemia. May be taken PO without regard to meals. Liquid should be measured accurately with provided calibrated dropper. Vitamin D–rich foods include breads, cereals, fish, fish liver oils, and fortified milk. Calcium-rich foods include bok choy, broccoli, brussels sprouts, cabbage, cauliflower, cheeses, collards, fish, milk, mustard greens, pork, rice, spinach, turnips, and yogurt.

14

PEDIATRIC ENDOCRINE MEDICATIONS

DRUG	HOW SUPPLIED/DOSE AND ROUTE
Ergocalciferol (Calciferol) Vitamin D$_2$ Promotes absorption of calcium and phosphorus	Liquid 8000 units/mL Caps 50,000 units Tabs 50,000 units Injection 50,000 units/mL *Vitamin D deficiency* Initial 1000-4000 units/day Maintenance 400 units/day *Hypoparathyroid* 50,000-200,000 units/day
Estrogen, Conjugated (Premarin) Major sex hormone for females	Tabs 0.3, 0.625, 0.9, 1.25, 2.5 mg Vivelle dot (patch) 0.025, 0.0375, 0.05, 0.075, 0.10 mg *Female hypogonadism* 0.3-0.625 mg PO qd, administered cyclically (e.g., 3 weeks on and 1 week off) Start 0.025 mg patch twice weekly. Patches can be cut to achieve desired smaller doses. In clinical studies of delayed puberty due to female hypogonadism, breast development was induced by doses as low as 0.15 mg. The dose can be gradually titrated upward at 6-12 month intervals as needed to achieve appropriate bone age advancement and eventual epiphyseal closure.

SIDE EFFECTS / REMARKS	NURSING CONSIDERATIONS
No side effects if taken within range of daily requirements *Drug-drug interactions:* Cholestyramine, colestipol, or mineral oil decreases absorption. Use with thiazide diuretics may result in hypercalcemia. Glucocorticoids ↓ effectiveness. Use with cardiac glycosides ↑ risk of arrhythmias. Requirements ↑ with phenytoin, hydantoin anticonvulsant, sucralfate, barbiturates, and primidone.	May be taken orally without regard to meals. Liquid should be measured accurately with provided calibrated dropper. May be mixed with juice, cereal, or food. Injection is oil-based; avoid IV administration. Vitamin D–rich foods include breads, cereals, fish, fish liver oils, and fortified milk. Calcium-rich foods include bok choy, broccoli, brussels sprouts, cabbage, cauliflower, cheeses, collards, fish, milk, mustard greens, pork, rice, spinach, turnips, and yogurt.
Headaches, nausea, breast tenderness Anticonvulsants, rifampin, and tetracyclines will cause estrogen to be less effective.	Should not be used during pregnancy Thyroid replacement therapy may need to be increased when an estrogen product is added to therapeutic regimen. Place patch on clean, dry area of abdomen. Rotate sites.

⑭

PEDIATRIC ENDOCRINE MEDICATIONS

DRUG	HOW SUPPLIED / DOSE AND ROUTE
Ethinyl Estradiol (Desogen, Ortho-Cept; Ortho-Novum 777; Ortho Tri-Cyclen) Contraceptive agent/ hormone replacement	Tabs 0.15 mg desogestrel and 30 μg ethinyl estradiol 0.5/0.75/1.0 mg norethindrone and 35 μg ethinyl estradiol 0.18/0.215/0.250 mg norgestimate and 35 μg ethinyl estradiol *Estrogen replacement* 0.02 mg PO qd for 6-12 months, then need to cycle The estrogenic potency of the current synthetic low-dose oral contraceptive pill is 5 to 6 times more potent than 0.625 mg Premarin.
Fludrocortisone Acetate (Florinef) Corticosteroid	Tab 0.1 mg *Addison's disease* 0.1 mg/daily PO Dose may vary from 0.1 mg 3 times/wk to 0.2 mg/daily. *Salt-losing congenital adrenal hyperplasia* 0.1-0.2 mg/daily PO
Furosemide (Furomide, Lasix, and others) Loop diuretic	Tabs 20, 40, 80 mg Injection 10 mg/mL Oral liquid 10 mg/mL (60, 120 mL), 40 mg/5 mL *IM, IV, PO* Neonates 0.5-1 mg/kg/dose q8-24h; max. PO dose: 6 mg/kg/dose, max. IV dose: 2 mg/kg/dose Infants and children 0.5-2 mg/kg/dose q6-12h; max. dose: 6 mg/kg/dose Adults 20-80 mg/24 hr ÷ q6-12h; max. dose: 600 mg/24 hr *Continuous IV infusion* Children and adults 0.05 mg/kg/hr, titrate to effect

SIDE EFFECTS/REMARKS	NURSING CONSIDERATIONS
Headaches, nausea, vomiting Anticonvulsants, rifampin, and tetracyclines will cause estrogen to be less effective.	Thyroid medication dose may need to be increased when an estrogen product is added.
Hypertension, edema, cardiac enlargement, congestive heart failure, potassium loss, hypokalemic alkalosis Drug interactions may occur with digitalis, oral anticoagulants, anti-diabetic drugs, aspirin, barbiturates, phenytoin, rifampin, anabolic steroids, and estrogen.	Contraindicated in patients with systemic fungal infections Growth and development of children on corticosteroids should be closely monitored. May mask signs of infection Patients should be monitored regularly for BP and serum electrolytes.
Ototoxicity may occur in presence of renal disease, especially when used with aminoglycosides. May cause hypokalemia, alkalosis, dehydration, hyperuricemia, bone loss/decreased bone mineral density, and increased calcium excretion.	Use with caution in hepatic disease. Prolonged use in infants may result in nephrocalcinosis. Max. rate of intermittent IV dose 0.5 mg/kg/min.

14

PEDIATRIC ENDOCRINE MEDICATIONS

DRUG	HOW SUPPLIED/DOSE AND ROUTE
Glucagon HCl Antihypoglycemic agent	Injection 1, 10 mg/vial Also available in preassembled emergency kit: 1 mg *Hypoglycemia* Neonates/infants 0.2-0.3 mg/kg/dose IM, IV, SQ Children <20 kg 0.5 mg Children >20 kg, adults 1.0 mg IV, IM, SQ
Histrelin Acetate (Supprelin) GnRH agonist	Injection 30-day kit of single-use vials 3 strengths available: 200 μg/mL, 500 μg/mL, 1000 μg/mL Implant 50 mg Insert 1 per year. *Central precocious puberty* 10 μg/kg/day, can titrate up to 20 μg/kg/day SQ. One implant per year. Use LH and estradiol or testosterone to evaluate adequacy of dose. Levels should be suppressed.
Hydrocortisone (Solu-Cortef, Hydrocortone, Cortef) Corticosteroid	Hydrocortisone base (tabs) 5, 10, 20 mg Injection Na phosphate 50 mg/mL Na succinate (Solu-Cortef) 100, 250, 500, 1,000 mg/vial Acetate (Hydrocortone) 25, 50 mg/mL *Physiologic replacement* PO 0.5-0.75 mg/kg/day or 20-25 mg/m^2/day $\div$ q8h IM 0.25-0.35 mg/kg/dose or 12-15 mg/m^2/day qd Stress dosing: Generally 2-3 times the physiologic replacement dose, depending on the severity of the illness or stress

SIDE EFFECTS / REMARKS	NURSING CONSIDERATIONS
Nausea, vomiting may occur.	Rebound hypoglycemia may occur.
Do not delay starting glucose infusion/treatment while awaiting effect of glucagon.	
Skin reactions may occur at the site of injection.	Recommend giving injection at the same time each day.
There is an increased risk of diabetes, cardiovascular disease, and osteoporosis in adults.	Girls may experience vaginal bleeding during first month of treatment.
Hypertension, euphoria, insomnia, acne, hyperglycemia, growth suppression, immunosuppression	Monitor BP and weight.
	Give with meals to decrease GI upset.
Adrenal suppression	
There may be bruising, pain, soreness, erythema, and swelling after implant insertion.	

14

PEDIATRIC ENDOCRINE MEDICATIONS

DRUG	HOW SUPPLIED/DOSE AND ROUTE
Indomethacin (Indocin) Nonsteroidal anti-inflammatory agent	Caps 25, 50 mg Sustained-release caps 75 mg Injection 1 mg Suppositories 50 mg Suspension 25 mg/5 mL *Anti-inflammatory* >14 years of age 1-3 mg/kg/24 hr PO ÷ tid-qid; max. dose: 200 mg/24 hr Adults 50-150 mg/24 hr PO ÷ bid-qid; max. dose: 200 mg/24 hr
Leuprolide Acetate for Depot Suspension (Lupron Depot-PED) GnRH agonist	Injection 7.5, 11.25, 15 mg Comes in two types of kit packaging: 1. A prefilled, dual-chamber syringe 2. A vial and ampule *Central precocious puberty* IM 0.3 mg/kg every 4 weeks (minimum dose of 7.5) Starting dose is dictated by child's weight: <25 kg 7.5 mg 25-37.5 kg 11.25 mg >37.5 kg 15 mg If downregulation is not achieved, the dose should be titrated upward in increments of 3.75 mg.
Leuprolide Acetate for Injection GnRH agonist	Injection 2.8 mL multiple-dose vial, 5 mg/mL *Leuprolide acetate stimulation test* 20 μg/kg SQ

SIDE EFFECTS / REMARKS	NURSING CONSIDERATIONS
Contraindicated in active bleeding, coagulation defects, necrotizing enterocolitis, and renal insufficiency May cause decreased urine output, platelet dysfunction, and GI blood flow	Monitor renal and hepatic function before and during use. Fatal hepatitis reported in treatment of juvenile rheumatoid arthritis Pregnancy category changes to D if used for >48 hours or after 34 weeks' gestation or close to delivery.
Injection site reaction, including erythema, inflammation, pain, or sterile abscess Use of ELA-Max or Numby Stuff prior to injection may help to reduce pain. The long-term effect on fertility after treatment with GnRH analogs is unknown. During the first 2 months of therapy, a female may experience menses or spotting.	Inform family that observation of clinical signs/symptoms and, sometimes, repeat GnRH stimulation testing are used to assess biochemical suppression. Requires IM administration, since the drug would be rapidly destroyed within the GI tract if given orally
Mild erythema at injection site is possible. Patients with known sensitivity to benzyl alcohol can have erythema and induration at injection site.	Leuprolide is inactivated if ingested orally. Inspect solution in vial for discoloration or particles.

⑭

PEDIATRIC ENDOCRINE MEDICATIONS

DRUG	HOW SUPPLIED/DOSE AND ROUTE
Levothyroxine Sodium (Synthroid, Levoxyl, Levothroid, and others) Thyroid hormone	Tabs 25, 50, 75, 88, 100, 112, 125, 137, 150, 175, 200, 300 μg IV, IM 50%-75% of oral dosage Injection 0.2 mg/vial, 0.5 mg/vial Starting dose 10-15 μg/kg/day for congenital hypothyroidism *Recommended Doses of Levothyroxine Based on Body Weight*

Age	Dose
0-1 mo	12-18 μg/kg
0-6 mo	10-12 μg/kg
6-12 mo	8-10 μg/kg
1-5 yr	6-8 μg/kg
5-10 yr	2-4 μg/kg
10-14 yr	2-4 μg/kg
>15 yr	2-3 μg/kg
Adult	1.6 μg/kg

SIDE EFFECTS/REMARKS	NURSING CONSIDERATIONS
Uncorrected adrenal insufficiency Symptoms of hyperthyroidism, rash, growth disturbances, hypertension, diarrhea, weight loss, arrhythmias	Adjust dose every 2-4 weeks to achieve therapeutic effect. Need to rule out adrenal insufficiency before starting thyroxine replacement. If adrenal insufficiency present, need to correct this before starting thyroxine replacement. Medication administration for infant: Crush pill and mix with water, formula, breast milk, or small amount of food. *Do not* mix with soy formula. Administer shortly after preparation. Give daily dose in AM if restlessness occurs after administration.

Conditions that alter levothyroxine requirements ↑ requirements for T4:
- Pregnancy
- GI disease, including celiac disease, inflammatory bowel disease, and jejunoileal bypass small bowel resection

Drugs that impair T4 absorption:
- Aluminum hydroxide
- Calcium carbonate
- Cholestyramine
- Ferrous sulfate
- Omeprazole
- Soya oil
- Soy-containing milk

Drugs that increase T4 clearance:
- Carbamazepine
- Phenobarbitol
- Phenytoin
- Rifampin
- Sertraline

(continued)

PEDIATRIC ENDOCRINE MEDICATIONS 14

DRUG	HOW SUPPLIED/DOSE AND ROUTE
(Levothyroxine Sodium)	

Lidocaine 2.5%, Prilocaine 2.5% (Emla Cream)	Disk	1 g in occlusive dressing
	Tube	5 g with dressing, 30 g tube size
Topical anesthetic	Children	
	<37 wk gestational age	Not recommended
	0-3 mo (<5 kg)	Max. 1 g per 10 cm² applied up to 1 hour
	3-12 mo (>5 kg)	Max. 2 g per 20 cm² applied up to 4 hours
	1-6 yr (>10 kg)	Max. 10 g per 100 cm² applied up to 4 hours
	7-12 yr (≥20 kg)	Max. 20 g per 200 cm² applied up to 4 hours
	Adults	
	Minor dermal procedures	Apply 1 disk, or 2.5 g cream in thick layer with occlusion dressing over 20-25 cm² for at least 1 hour.
	Major dermal procedures	Apply 2 g per 10 cm² in thick layer with occlusive dressing for at least 2 hours.

SIDE EFFECTS / REMARKS	NURSING CONSIDERATIONS
	Drugs that increase thyroxine: • Estrogen • Oral contraceptives Drugs that impair T4 to T3 conversion: • Amiodarone • Beta blockers • Glucocorticoids
Local side effects: Paleness, erythema, changes in temperature sensation, edema, itching Contraindicated in methemoglobinemia If child is under 12 months of age, do not use with methemoglobinemia-inducing drugs (e.g., acetaminophen, sulfonamides, nitrates, phenytoin, phenobarbital). Toxicity may be potentiated by Class I antiarrhythmics (tocainamide, mexiletine).	Clean and disinfect area prior to administration. Avoid mucous membranes, eyes, and tympanic membrane. Do not ingest, apply to large areas, or apply for period longer than recommended.

14

PEDIATRIC ENDOCRINE MEDICATIONS

DRUG	HOW SUPPLIED/DOSE AND ROUTE
Lidocaine Topical 4% (ELA-Max)	Topical anesthetic cream available in 5 g and 30 g tube size
	Indicated for the temporary relief of minor skin pain. For topical use only.
	A thick layer of cream is applied to intact skin. Do not leave on for more than 2 hours.
	A single application of cream in a child weighing less than 10 kg should not be applied over an area larger than 100 cm^2.
	A single application of cream in a child weighing between 10 kg and 20 kg should not be applied over an area larger that 200 cm^2.
Mecasermin (Increlex [rDNA origin])	Injection 10 mg/mL (4 ml vial); multiple-dose vial
	Severe primary IGFD
	Starting dose: 0.04-0.08 mg/kg (40 to 80 μg/kg) BID SQ.
	If well tolerated for 1 week, dose should be increased by 0.04 mg/kg per dose to the maximum dose of 0.12 mg/kg BID.

SIDE EFFECTS/REMARKS	NURSING CONSIDERATIONS
Local reactions (erythema or edema) at application site	When applied to young children, supervision is required to avoid accidental ingestion of cream.
Allergic and anaphylactic reactions	Consult doctor for use in children under 2 years of age.
Systemic reactions (rare), including CNS and cardiovascular manifestations	
Contraindicated in persons with known sensitivity or allergy to lidocaine or other topical anesthetics	
For external use only	
Avoid mucous membranes.	
Hypoglycemia, tonsillar hypertrophy, intracranial hypertension, mild elevations in AST, ALT, and LDH, lipohypertrophy, bruising at injection site, otitis media, headache, dizziness, vomiting, arthralgia, thickening of soft tissues of face, scoliosis, slipped capital femoral epiphysis	Give shortly before or after (± 20 minutes) a meal or snack
Has not been studied in children under 2 years of age	If the patient is unable to eat for any reason, that dose should be withheld.
Contraindications: Should not be used for growth promotion in presence of closed epiphysis.	Subsequent doses should never be increased to make up for one or more omitted doses.
In the presence of active or suspected neoplasia; d/c if neoplasia develops	If hypoglycemia occurs with recommended doses, despite adequate food intake, the dose should be reduced.
IV administration	Injection sites should be rotated to a different site each injection.
In patients with allergy to mecasermin or any of the inactive ingredients (benzyl alcohol)	Patients should avoid high-risk activities within 2-3 hours after dosing, especially at initiation of treatment, until well-tolerated dose is established.
	Store unopened vials in refrigerator. Once opened, keep refrigerated and use within 30 days.
	Do not freeze.
	Keep out of direct heat and bright light.

PEDIATRIC ENDOCRINE MEDICATIONS

DRUG	HOW SUPPLIED/DOSE AND ROUTE
Medroxyproges-terone Acetate (Provera) Progestin	Tabs 2.5, 5, 10 mg *Secondary amenorrhea* 5-10 mg/day PO for 5-10 days In conjunction with estrogen therapy to induce endometrium shedding, estrogens are given on days 1-21 of the cycle, adding a progestin 5-10 mg PO on days 15-21 of each month. Withdrawal bleeding usually occurs within 3-7 days after discontinuing progestin.
Metformin (Glucophage) Antihyperglycemic agent	Tabs 500, 850,1000 mg *Type 2 diabetes mellitus* Children The usual starting dose of Metformin is 500 mg twice a day, given with meals. Dosage increases should be made in increments of 500 mg weekly, up to a maximum of 2000 mg per day, given in divided doses. The maximum daily dose is 2000 mg in pediatric patients (10 to 16 years of age). Adults The usual starting dose of Metformin is 500 mg twice a day or 850 mg once a day, given with meals. *(continued)*

SIDE EFFECTS / REMARKS	NURSING CONSIDERATIONS
Breast tenderness; galactorrhea; skin reactions including urticaria, pruritus, edema, generalized rash; thrombophlebitis; pulmonary embolism; breakthrough bleeding, spotting, change in menstrual flow; change in weight; cholestatic jaundice; mental depression; nausea; changes in libido; changes in appetite	Patients on progestin therapy and combination estrogen-progestin drugs should be monitored closely for thrombophlebitis, pulmonary embolism, and cerebral thrombosis/embolism.
Contraindicated in patients with thrombophlebitis, thromboembolic disorders, cerebral apoplexy, liver dysfunction, known or suspected malignancy of breast or genital organs, undiagnosed vaginal bleeding, as a diagnostic test for pregnancy, pregnancy	Instruct patients to report any early manifestations of chest or calf pain, dyspnea, numbness in extremity, dizziness, or visual disturbance.
	May reduce the effectiveness of hypoglycemic agents by decreasing glucose tolerance
	Minimize GI upset by taking with food.
Tansient GI symptoms (diarrhea, nausea, vomiting, abdominal bloating, flatulence, and anorexia) can be minimized by gradual dose escalation and taking the drug with meals.	Instruct patient to take with meals.
Contraindicated in patients with impaired renal function or any condition associated with hypoxemia, dehydration, or sepsis from an increased risk of lactic acidosis—a rare but serious complication of metformin therapy	Instruct patient to seek medical attention if experiencing any of the following symptoms that may be associated with lactic acidosis: malaise, myalgia, difficulty breathing, sleepiness, and nonspecific abdominal discomfort or pain.
	Ensure that patient knows the location of the nearest emergency room.

PEDIATRIC ENDOCRINE MEDICATIONS ⑭

DRUG	HOW SUPPLIED / DOSE AND ROUTE
(Metformin)	Dosage increases should be made in increments of 500 mg weekly or 850 mg every 2 weeks, up to a total of 2000 mg per day, given in divided doses.
	Patients can also be titrated from 500 mg twice a day to 850 mg twice a day after 2 weeks.
	For patients requiring additional glycemic control, Metformin may be given to a maximum daily dose of 2550 mg per day.
	Doses above 2000 mg may be better tolerated given 3 times a day with meals.
	The maximum daily dose is 2550 mg per day in adults.
Metformin Extended Release (Fortamet, Glucophage XR)	XR 500, 750, 1000 mg
	The usual starting dose of Metformin Extended Release tablets is 500 mg once daily with the evening meal.
	Dosage increases should be made in increments of 500 mg weekly, up to a maximum of 2000 mg once daily with the evening meal.
	Maximum recommended daily dose is 2000 mg in adults.
	Safety and effectiveness of Metformin Extended Release in pediatric patients have not been established.

SIDE EFFECTS/REMARKS	NURSING CONSIDERATIONS

DRUG	HOW SUPPLIED / DOSE AND ROUTE
Metformin Liquid (Riomet)	Solution 100 mg/mL The maximum recommended daily dose of Metformin Liquid is: 2000 mg (20 mL) in pediatric patients (10 to 16 years of age). 2550 mg (25.5 mL) in adults

Methimazole (MMI) (Tapazole)
 	
Antithyroid agent
	Tabs 5, 10 mg
	———
	Initial
	  Children 0.5-1 mg/kg/day PO ÷ q8h
	  Adults 15-60 mg/day PO ÷ tid
	Maintenance
	  Children ⅓-½ of initial dose PO ÷ q8h
	  Adults 5-15 mg/day PO ÷ q8h
	Methimazole is usually ¹⁄₁₀ the PTU dose.

SIDE EFFECTS/REMARKS	NURSING CONSIDERATIONS
Nausea, vomiting, dyspepsia, agranulocytosis, fever, liver disease, central nervous system reactions (headache, drowsiness, vertigo), dermatitis, urticaria, malaise, arthralgias, hypothyroidism	Administer doses with food. Ensure that the family understands that they must report symptoms of fever, sore throat, joint pain, and rash so a complete blood count can be drawn to evaluate for the possibility of agranulocytosis, a side effect of therapy.
Drug interactions may occur with lithium, potassium iodide, and iodinated glycerol.	
Does not block the release of preformed, stored thyroid hormones; therefore it takes 4-8 weeks to achieve euthyroid state.	
MMI is more potent (tenfold) than PTU and has a longer half-life (12-16 hr vs 2-4 hr) than PTU.	

14

PEDIATRIC ENDOCRINE MEDICATIONS

DRUG	HOW SUPPLIED/DOSE AND ROUTE

Methylpredniso-lone (Depo-Medrol, Solu-Medrol)
 	
Corticosteroid
	Injection Depo-Medrol: 40 mg/mL and 80 mg/mL
	              Solu-Medrol: 40, 125, 500, and 1000 mg
	              with diluent
	Tabs 2, 4, 16, 24, 32 mg
	
	Children (anti-inflammatory or immunosuppressive)
	  Oral, IM, IV 0.117-1.66 mg/kg/d q6-12h in
	                    divided doses
	
	Adults
	  Oral 2-60 mg in 1-4 divided doses
	  IM (methylpred- 10-80 mg once daily
	     nisolone acetate)

Nafarelin Acetate (Synarel) GnRH analog	Nasal spray 0.5 oz bottle (10 mL) concentration: 2 mg/mL Each spray delivers 200 μg. The spray bottle is intended to deliver 60 sprays. *Central precocious puberty* Starting dose: 1600 μg/day. This dose is achieved by two sprays (400 μg) into each nostril in the morning and 2 sprays into each nostril in the evening, a total of 8 sprays per day. The dose can be titrated up to 1800 μg/day. This dose can be achieved by 3 sprays (600 μg into alternating nostrils three times a day, a total of 9 sprays per day).

SIDE EFFECTS / REMARKS	NURSING CONSIDERATIONS
Cardiovascular: Edema, hypertension *Central nervous system:* Headache, vertigo, seizures *Dermatologic:* Acne, skin atrophy *Endocrinologic:* Cushing's syndrome, pituitary-adrenal axis suppression, glucose intolerance, hypokalemia, alkalosis *Gastrointestinal:* Nausea, vomiting, peptic ulcer *Neuromuscular:* Muscle weakness, osteoporosis; may retard bone growth *Ocular:* Cataracts, glaucoma	Monitor electrolytes, blood glucose, and BP. Take after meals or with food or milk. If given IV, give slow IV push. If on stress doses of steroids, do not administer live virus vaccines.
Acne, breast enlargement, vaginal bleeding, emotional lability, body odor, and seborrhea (usually transient)	The patient's head should be tilted back slightly, and 30 seconds should elapse between sprays. If the use of a nasal decongestant for rhinitis is necessary, the decongestant should not be used until at least 2 hours after dosing.

⑭

PEDIATRIC ENDOCRINE MEDICATIONS

DRUG	HOW SUPPLIED/DOSE AND ROUTE
Octreotide Acetate (Sandostatin) Somatostatin analog	Injection Ampule: 0.05, 0.1, 0.5 mg/ml (1 mL) Multi-dose vials: 0.2, 1 mg/mL (5 mL) LAR Depot: 5 ml vial of 10 mg, 20 mg, 30 mg kit *Hyperinsulinism* 2-5 μg/kg/day and increase to 20 μg/kg/day SQ, divided q6-8h *Continuous IV infusion* 10 μg/kg/24 hr
Oxandrolone (Oxandrin) Anabolic steroid	Tabs 2.5 mg *Adjunctive therapy for growth in Turner syndrome* 0.06mg/kg/day Tablets can be halved.
Pamidronate Bisphosphonate (Aredia)	IV In clinical trials for children: 0.5 = 1 mg/kg/day for 3 consecutive days every 4-6 months

SIDE EFFECTS/REMARKS	NURSING CONSIDERATIONS
Cholelithiasis, nausea, transient diarrhea, abdominal discomfort, hyperglycemia, headache, transient growth impairment Pain at injection site may occur, so use smallest possible volume to deliver desired dose.	For prolonged storage, Sandostatin LAR Depot should be stored at refrigerated temperatures of 2° C-8° C (36° F-46° F) and protected from light until the time of use. Should remain at room temperature for 30-60 minutes prior to preparation of the drug suspension. After preparation, the drug must be administered immediately.
Virilization, liver toxicity, insulin resistance, bone maturation	Observe for signs of clitoromegaly, hirsutism, acne. Monitor liver functions quarterly. Monitor bone age every 6 months. Discontinue if any of the above are at issue.
Nausea, hypocalcemia, hypokalemia, hypomagnesemia, leucopenia, phlebitis at insertion site, muscle stiffness, fever	Patients should be taught signs and symptoms of hypocalcemia. Diet should contain adequate amounts of vitamin D and calcium (see Calcitriol, pp. 376-377). Dental surgery should be avoided during therapy, because recovery may be prolonged. Patients need encouragement to keep follow-up appointments even after therapy is stopped.

14

PEDIATRIC ENDOCRINE MEDICATIONS

DRUG	HOW SUPPLIED/DOSE AND ROUTE	
Paricalcitol (Zemplar) Vitamin D compound	Caps	1, 2, 4 μg
	Injection vials	5 μg/mL in 1 mL and 2 mL
	PO	1-2 μg/day
	IV	0.04-0.1 μg/kg every other day
	Children 5-19 yr	
	IV	0.04-0.08 μg/kg three times a week
Phentermine Hydrochloride (Adipex, Dapex, Fastin, Obe-Nix, Ona-Mast, Phentercot Phentride, T-Diet, Tora-30, Zantryl) Anorexiant	Tabs 30 mg	
	Exogenous obesity	
	One capsule approximately 2 hours after breakfast for appetite control	
	Not recommended for patients <16 years of age	
Phosphorus Supplements (NeutraPhos, K-PHOS Neutral, NeutraPhos-K)	Caps, powder	NeutraPhos: 250 mg P, 7 mEq Na, 7 mEq K NeutraPhos-K: 250 mg P, 14.25 mEq K
	Tabs	K-PHOS Neutral: 250 mg P, 10.9 mEq Na, 1.27 mEq K
	Injection	Na Phosphate: 94 mg P, 4 mEq Na/mL K Phosphate: 94 mg P, 4.4 mEq K/mL
	Oral	Reconstitute in 75 mL water per capsule or packet.
	Children	
	IV	15-45 mg/kg over 24 hours
	PO	30-90 mg/kg/24 hr ÷ tid-qid

SIDE EFFECTS/REMARKS	NURSING CONSIDERATIONS
Edema, palpitations, headaches, somnolence, pruritus, chills, fever, nausea, anorexia, constipation	Pregnancy category C

Encourage foods high in vitamin D and calcium.

Patients should avoid antacids containing magnesium.

Toxicity may manifest as hypercalcemia (see Calcitriol, p. 377, for vitamin D and calcium-rich foods). |
| Primary pulmonary hypertension; palpitations; dry mouth; ↑BP, restlessness, dizziness, tremor, headache, diarrhea, constipation, urticaria, impotence, and changes in libido | Safety and effectiveness in children have not been established.

Medication should only be used for a few weeks. Long-term usage has not been adequately studied.

May be habit forming

Do not drink alcohol while taking this medication. |
| May cause tetany, hyperphosphatemia, hyperkalemia, hypocalcemia

PO administration may cause nausea, vomiting, abdominal pain, diarrhea.

IV administration may cause hypotension, renal failure, arrhythmias, heart block, cardiac arrest with potassium salt. | *Use with caution* in patients with renal impairment. |

⑭

PEDIATRIC ENDOCRINE MEDICATIONS

DRUG	HOW SUPPLIED / DOSE AND ROUTE
Potassium Iodide (SSKI, Iosat, Thyro Block) Antithyroid agent	Tabs 65, 130 mg SSKI (saturated solution) 1 g/mL (30, 240 mL bottles) 10 drops = 500 mg Lugol's solution Potassium iodide 100 mg/mL with iodine 50 mg/mL (15, 473 mL bottles) *Neonatal Graves' disease* 1 drop (Lugol's solution) PO q8h *Thyrotoxicosis in children* 50-250 mg PO tid (about 1-5 drops of SSKI PO tid) *Thyrotoxicosis in adults* 50-500 mg PO tid (1-10 drops if SSKI PO tid)
Prednisone (many brand names) Corticosteroid See steroid equivalency table, p. 424.	Tabs 1, 2.5, 5, 10, 20, 50 mg *Anti-inflammatory/immunosuppressive* 0.5-2 mg/kg/24 hr PO ÷ qd-qid *Acute asthma* 2 mg/kg/24 hr PO ÷ qd-bid Max. dose: 80 mg/24 hr *Nephrotic syndrome* Starting dose: 2 mg/kg/24 hr PO Max. dose: 80 mg/24 hr Further treatment plans individualized; consult nephrologist. *Physiologic replacement (adrenal insufficiency)* 4-6 mg/m^2/24 hr (mean 5) ÷ q12h *Stress dosing* PO 2-4 × the physiologic replacement dose Give preoperatively and postoperatively with gradual decrease to maintenance.

SIDE EFFECTS/REMARKS	NURSING CONSIDERATIONS
Rash, metallic taste, GI upset, headache, rhinitis	Administer with food or milk. Dilute with large quantity of water, juice, or milk. Ideally, should be administered after meals. Contraindicated in pregnancy
Mood changes Seizures Hyperglycemia Diarrhea Nausea Abdominal distention GI bleeding *With prolonged use:* Cushingoid effects Cataract Hypothalamic-pituitary-adrenal axis suppression ↓ Bone mineral density ↓ *Effects with:* Barbiturates Carbamazepine Phenytoin Rifampin Isoniazid ↑ *Effects with:* Estrogen Sudden withdrawal may precipitate an adrenal crisis.	Consider stress dosing for patients on glucocorticoid therapy >1 month.

DRUG	HOW SUPPLIED / DOSE AND ROUTE
Propranolol (Inderal and others) Beta-adrenergic blocker	Tabs 10, 20, 40, 60, 80, 90 mg Solution 20, 40 mg/5 mL Concentrated solution 80 mg/mL Extended release caps 60, 80, 120, 160 mg Injection 1 mg/mL *Thyrotoxicosis* Neonates 2 mg/kg/day ÷ q6-12h Adolescents PO: 10-40 mg/dose q6h and adults IV: 1-3 mg/dose slow (10 min) IV push. May repeat in 4-6 hours.
Salmon Calcitonin (Miacalcin) Hormone	Nasal spray 200 units/spray; 2 mL bottle (14 doses) Injection 200 units/mL SQ or IM; 2 mL vials Not recommended for children *Osteoporosis* Adults 200 units IN daily, alternate nostrils OR 100 units SQ or IM daily

SIDE EFFECTS/REMARKS	NURSING CONSIDERATIONS
Hypoglycemia, hypotension, bronchospasm, heart block, nausea, vomiting, depression, weakness	Bioavailability may be increased in Down syndrome.
Use with caution in asthma, Raynaud's syndrome, heart block, congestive heart failure.	Treatment should never be discontinued suddenly. A gradually decreasing dose titration is necessary.
Use with caution in presence of diabetes mellitus, renal or hepatic disease.	
Nasal spray: Rhinitis and other upper respiratory/nasal symptoms, back pain, GI upset	Encourage diet high in calcium and vitamin D.
Injection: GI upset, flushing, rash, antibody formation, local inflammation	

DRUG	HOW SUPPLIED/DOSE AND ROUTE
Somatropin (HGH) (Genotropin, Humatrope, Norditropin, Nutropin, Nutropin AQ, Omnitrope, Saizen)	Injection

Growth hormone deficiency

Infants with hypoglycemia secondary to GHD	Give an immediate dose of 0.1 mg/kg daily SQ. At 2-4 months of age, dose is reduced to 0.3-0.35 mg/kg/week SQ/IM.
Children	0.16-0.3 mg/kg/week or 0.05 mg/kg/day divided into 7 doses/week SQ
Adolescents/pubertal dosing	Up to 0.7 mg/kg/week divided into 7 doses/week SQ
Adult GHD	0.04-0.08 mg/kg/wk or 0.15 to 0.30 mg/day
Alternate dosing:
Start 0.2 mg/day with a range of 0.15 to 0.3 mg/day, without consideration of weight.

Pediatric idiopathic short stature

0.37 mg/kg/week recommended

Turner syndrome

0.33 – 0.375 mg/kg/week divided into 7 doses/week
Up to 0.067 mg/kg/day or 0.47 mg/kg/week

SHOX deficiency

0.35 mg/kg/week

Pediatric PWS patients

0.24 mg/kg/week recommended

Noonan syndrome

0.066 mg/kg/day

Somatropin (HGH) (Genotropin, Humatrope, Norditropin, Nutropin, Nutropin AQ, Omnitrope, Saizen)

SIDE EFFECTS / REMARKS

Possible side effects include transient or persistent low thyroxine (T4) levels leading to HGH antibody formation, which in rare cases may impede growth; hypothyroidism, slipped capital femoral epiphysis, edema and sodium retention, pseudotumor cerebri (increased intracranial pressure), hyperinsulinism, glucose intolerance, increased risk of leukemia, and acromegaloid features (large hands and feet, coarse facial features).

NURSING CONSIDERATIONS

Adult GHD: Increase dose every 1 to 2 months by increments of 0.1 to 0.2 mg/day based on IGF-1 levels and patient clinical response.

PEDIATRIC ENDOCRINE MEDICATIONS

DRUG	HOW SUPPLIED/DOSE AND ROUTE
Spironolactone (Aldactone) Aldosterone antagonist/ antiandrogenic agent	Tabs 25, 50, 100 mg Suspension 1, 2, 5 mg/mL *Hirsutism* 50-200 mg PO qd, in single or divided doses OR 200-400 mg PO qd, in single or divided doses *Primary aldosteronism* Children 125-375 mg/m²/day PO ÷ bid-qid
Tamoxifen Citrate (Nolvadex) Antiestrogenic agent	Tabs 10, 20 mg *Pubertal gynecomastia* 10 mg PO bid × 3 mo NOTE Use and dosage outside of product labeling
Testolactone (Teslac) Steroid aromatase inhibitor	Tabs 50 mg *Pubertal gynecomastia* 450 mg PO qd for up to 3 mo NOTE Use and dosage outside of product labeling *McCune-Albright syndrome* 40 mg/kg/day ÷ qid

SIDE EFFECTS / REMARKS	NURSING CONSIDERATIONS
Contraindicated in acute renal failure	
Hot flashes, rash, loss of libido, impotence, change in liver enzymes	
Macular/papular erythema, elevation of blood pressure, anorexia, nausea, and vomiting When given in conjunction with oral anticoagulants, anticoagulant effect may be increased. Diarrhea and cramping may be minimized by starting at a low dose and titrating the dose upward at weekly intervals.	

DRUG	HOW SUPPLIED/DOSE AND ROUTE

Testosterone
(Delatestryl,
Depo-Testosterone,
Androderm)

Androgen

Injection	Cypionate: 1, 10 mL (100 mg/mL)
	1, 10 mL (200 mg/mL)
	Enanthate: 1, 5 mL (200 mg/mL)
Androderm patch	2.5, 5.0 mg
AndroGel 1%	2.5 g packet (equivalent to 25 mg testosterone)
	5 g packet (equivalent to 50 mg testosterone)
Metered-dose gel	2.5 g, 5 g (each actuation delivers 1.25 g)

Male pubertal delay

Initial: 50-100 mg IM per month for 4-6 months

Male hypogonadism

Initial: 50-100 mg IM per month for 6-12 months

Titrate upward based on clinical findings and biochemical measurements.

Transdermal patch

Therapy for nonvirilized patients may be initiated with 1 patch (2.5 mg) nightly. Adult starting dose is 2 (2.5 mg) patches.

No data available on patch use in individuals <15 years of age

AndroGel 1%

Apply once daily (AM). Measure serum testosterone 14 days after starting prescription. If serum testosterone is below the normal range, dose should be increased from 5 g to 7.5 g. Can be increased to 10 g maximum. Has not been clinically evaluated in males <18 years of age.

SIDE EFFECTS / REMARKS	NURSING CONSIDERATIONS

Acne, headache, and possible aggressive behavior

Injection: Local inflammation at injection site

Patch: Local site reactions of pruritus, blisters, and erythema

Testosterone such as methandrosteno-lone may decrease the dose require-ment of patients receiving anticoagu-lants. Careful monitoring when starting or stopping testosterone therapy is necessary.

In patients with diabetes, androgens may decrease the blood glucose.

AndroGel 1% and Testoderm patch: Too frequent or persistent penile erections. Nausea, vomiting, changes in skin color, ankle swelling

AndroGel 1%: Breathing disturbances, including those associated with sleep

Androderm patch: Patch should be applied at night to mimic the normal circadian pattern of males. Should not be applied to the scrotal area, nor to areas that have bony prominences.

Rotation of patch sites is important; wait 7 days between use of the same site.

AndroGel 1%: Instruct patient to wash hands with soap and water immedi-ately after application and to cover the application site with clothing after AndroGel has dried. If skin where AndroGel has been applied comes in contact with another person, imme-diate washing of that person's skin with soap and water is necessary. Should not be aplied to the genital area.

AndroGel pump: Pump needs priming before first use by depressing pump three times and discarding any dispensed gel.

Changes in body hair distribution, significant increase in acne, or other signs of virilization of the female partner should be brought to the physician's attention.

14

PEDIATRIC ENDOCRINE MEDICATIONS

Table 14.1   Time Action for Insulin Preparations

Insulin Type	Preparations (generic)*	Onset	Peak	Effective Duration
Rapid-acting	Humalog (lispro) Novalog (aspart) Apidra (glulisine)	5-15 min	30-90 min	<5 hr 5 hr
Short-acting	Regular, human	30-60 min	2-3 hr	5-8 hr
Intermediate-acting	NPH, human	2-4 hr	4-10 hr	10-16 hr
Long-acting	Lantus (glargine) Levemir (detemir)	2-4 hr 3-8 hr	No peak No peak	20-24 hr 5.7-23.2 hr
Fixed combination	70/30 (NPH/regular ratio)	30-60 min	Dual	10-16 hr
	50/50 (NPH/regular ratio)	5-15 min	Dual	10-16 hr
	75/25 (NPH/regular ratio)	5-15 min	Dual	10-16 hr
	70/30 (NPA/aspart ratio)	5-15 min	Dual	10-16 hr

Adapted from Wickersham RM, Novak KK, eds. Facts and Comparisons. St Louis: Wolters Kluwer Health, 2005.
*Most branded products are available in pen delivery systems.

Table 14.2 Insulin Storage Guidelines

Insulin Type		Refrigerated (36° F to 46° F)		Room Temperature (59° F to 86° F)	
		Opened	Unopened	Opened	Unopened
Vials	Humulin R	28 days	Until expiration date	28 days	28 days
	Humalog	28 days	Until expiration date	28 days	28 days
	NovoLog	28 days	Until expiration date	28 days	28 days
	Apidra Novo-Log R (10 mL)	28 days	Until expiration date	28 days	28 days
	Lantus	28 days	Until expiration date	28 days	28 days
	Levemir	28 days	Until expiration date	28 days	28 days
Cartridges	Humalog	28 days	Until expiration date	28 days	28 days
	Lantus	28 days	Until expiration date	28 days	28 days
	Apidra NovoLog, R, N, 70/30	28 days	Until expiration date	28 days	28 days

		Refrigerated Pens Not in Use	Opened Pens in Use
Cartridge pens	NovoLog 70/30 FlexPen delivers 1-60 U/dose in 1 U increments; 3 mL pen fill cartridge; designed for use with NovaPen 3	Until expiration date	28 days
	Humalog (lispro)		
	NovoLog (aspart)		
	Apidra (glulisine)		
Pens	Humalog	Until expiration date	28 days
	NovoLog	Until expiration date	28 days
	Humulin N	Until expiration date	14 days
	NovoLog mix 70/30	Until expiration date	14 days
	Humalog mix 75/25	Until expiration date	10 days

Pens in use (opened) should not be stored in refrigerator.

⑭

PEDIATRIC ENDOCRINE MEDICATIONS

Table 14.3 Potency of Various Oral Steroid Preparations as Related to Cortisol and Florinef

Generic Name	Trade Name	Glucocorticoid Effect Equivalent to 100 mg Cortisol PO	Na+ Retention Effect Equivalent to 0.1 mg Florinef
Hydrocortisone	Cortef	100	20
Prednisolone	Orapred, Pediapred, Millipred, Veripred, Flo-Pred	20	50
Prednisone	Prednisone, Pred-nisone Intensol	25	50
Dexamethasone	Dexamethasone, Dexamethasone Intensol, Baycadron, DexPak	4	No effect
Fludricortisone	Florinef	6.5	0.1

Values estimated by respective pharmaceutical companies. All values in mg.

⑮ CONVERSIONS/FORMULAS/TABLES

WEIGHT

2.2 lb/kg
Weight (pounds) ÷ 2.2 = weight (kilograms)
Weight (kilograms) × 2.2 = weight (pounds)

HEIGHT

2.54 cm/inch
Height (cm) ÷ 2.54 = height (inch)
Height (inches) × 2.54 = height (cm)

BODY MASS INDEX (BMI)

$$\frac{(\text{Weight in kg})}{(\text{Height in cm} \div 100)^2}$$

OR

$$\frac{(\text{Weight in kg})}{(\text{Height in meters})^2}$$

Table 15.1 Percentiles for Body Mass Index in U.S. Boys 5 to 17 Years of Age

Age (yr)	Percentile	Asian	Black	Hispanic	White	U.S. Weighted Mean (A)	NHANES (B)	% Difference*
5	5	13.2	13.7	13.8	13.7	13.7	—	—
	15	14.0	14.4	14.6	14.4	14.4	—	—
	50	15.0	15.5	15.9	15.5	15.6	—	—
	75	15.3	16.2	17.2	16.4	16.5	—	—
	85	15.5	16.8	18.0	17.1	17.2	—	—
	95	17.1	18.1	19.4	18.1	18.3	—	—
6	5	13.3	13.8	13.8	13.8	13.8	12.9	6.7
	15	14.1	14.4	14.7	14.4	14.5	13.4	7.9
	50	15.0	15.5	16.0	15.6	15.6	14.5	7.7
	75	15.5	16.4	17.4	16.6	16.7	—	—
	85	15.7	17.0	18.2	17.3	17.4	16.6	4.5
	95	17.8	18.8	20.2	18.9	19.0	18.0	5.5

Reprinted from Journal of Pediatrics, volume 132, Rosner B, et al, Percentiles for body mass index in US children 5 to 17 years of age, pages 211-222, Copyright 1998, with permission from Elsevier Science.
*(A − B)/B × 100%.

(continued)

Table 15.1   Percentiles for Body Mass Index
in U.S. Boys 5 to 17 Years of Age (*cont'd*)

Age (yr)	Percentile	Asian	Black	Hispanic	White	U.S. Weighted Mean (A)	NHANES (B)	% Difference*
7	5	13.5	14.0	14.0	13.9	13.9	13.2	5.6
	15	14.3	14.6	14.9	14.6	14.7	13.9	5.5
	50	15.2	15.8	16.2	15.8	15.8	15.1	4.9
	75	15.8	16.7	17.7	16.9	17.0	—	—
	85	16.1	17.4	18.6	17.7	17.8	17.4	2.1
	95	18.8	19.9	21.2	19.9	20.0	19.2	4.4
8	5	13.7	14.2	14.2	14.1	14.1	13.6	3.9
	15	14.5	14.8	15.1	14.9	14.9	14.3	4.0
	50	15.6	16.1	16.6	16.2	16.2	15.6	3.7
	75	16.4	17.3	18.3	17.5	17.5	—	—
	85	16.9	18.3	19.5	18.6	18.6	18.1	2.7
	95	20.2	21.3	22.7	21.4	21.5	20.3	5.8
9	5	13.9	14.4	14.4	14.3	14.3	14.0	2.5
	15	14.7	15.1	15.4	15.1	15.1	14.7	2.8
	50	16.0	16.5	17.0	16.6	16.6	16.2	2.7
	75	17.2	18.1	19.1	18.3	18.4	—	—
	85	17.9	19.4	20.7	19.7	19.7	18.9	4.4
	95	21.7	22.9	24.4	23.0	23.1	21.5	7.4
10	5	14.1	14.6	14.7	14.6	14.6	14.4	1.3
	15	15.0	15.4	15.6	15.4	15.4	15.2	1.3
	50	16.6.	17.1	17.6	17.1	17.2	16.7	2.8
	75	18.0	19.0	20.0	19.2	19.2	—	—
	85	19.1	20.6	21.9	20.9	20.9	19.6	6.7
	95	23.2	24.4	25.9	24.5	24.6	22.6	8.8
11	5	14.4	14.9	15.0	14.9	14.9	14.8	0.7
	15	15.4	15.8	16.1	15.8	15.8	15.6	1.3
	50	17.1	17.7	18.1	17.7	17.8	17.3	2.7
	75	18.9	19.9	20.9	20.1	20.1	—	—
	85	20.0	21.6	22.9	21.9	21.9	20.4	7.4
	95	24.3	25.5	27.1	25.6	25.7	23.7	8.6
12	5	14.8	15.3	15.4	15.3	15.3	15.2	0.8
	15	16.0	16.3	16.6	16.3	16.3	16.1	1.5
	50	17.8	18.3	18.8	18.4	18.4	17.9	2.8
	75	19.6	20.6	21.7	20.8	20.9	—	—
	85	20.7	22.3	23.6	22.6	22.6	21.1	7.3
	95	25.1	26.3	27.9	26.4	26.5	24.9	6.5

*(A − B)/B × 100%.

(continued)

Table 15.1 Percentiles for Body Mass Index in U.S. Boys 5 to 17 Years of Age (*cont'd*)

Age (yr)	Percentile	Asian	Black	Hispanic	White	U.S. Weighted Mean (A)	NHANES (B)	% Difference*
13	5	15.4	15.9	15.9	15.9	15.9	15.7	1.0
	15	16.6	17.0	17.3	17.0	17.0	16.6	2.4
	50	18.4	19.0	19.5	19.1	19.1	18.5	3.2
	75	20.2	21.2	22.3	21.5	21.5	—	—
	85	21.2	22.8	24.2	23.2	23.2	21.9	5.9
	95	25.6	26.9	28.5	27.0	27.1	25.9	4.6
14	5	16.0	16.5	16.6	16.5	16.5	16.2	1.9
	15	17.3	17.7	18.0	17.7	17.7	17.2	2.9
	50	19.2	19.7	20.2	19.8	19.8	19.2	3.2
	75	20.8	21.9	23.0	22.1	22.1	—	—
	85	21.8	23.4	24.8	23.7	23.7	22.8	4.1
	95	26.3	27.6	29.2	27.6	27.8	26.9	3.2
15	5	16.7	17.2	17.3	17.2	17.2	16.6	3.7
	15	18.0	18.3	18.6	18.3	18.4	17.8	3.1
	50	19.9	20.5	21.0	20.5	20.6	19.9	3.3
	75	21.5	22.5	23.6	22.8	22.8	—	—
	85	22.5	24.1	25.6	24.5	24.5	23.6	3.9
	95	27.2	28.5	30.1	28.5	28.7	27.8	3.2
16	5	17.3	17.9	18.0	17.9	17.9	17.0	5.1
	15	18.6	18.9	19.2	18.9	19.0	18.3	3.6
	50	20.6	21.2	21.7	21.3	21.3	20.6	3.3
	75	22.2	23.3	24.4	23.6	23.6		
	85	23.4	25.1	26.5	25.4	25.4	24.5	3.9
	95	28.2	29.6	31.2	29.6	29.8	28.5	4.5
17	5	17.8	18.4	18.4	18.3	18.3	17.3	6.0
	15	19.2	19.6	19.9	19.6	19.6	18.7	4.9
	50	21.2	21.7	22.3	21.8	21.8	21.1	3.5
	75	22.9	23.9	25.1	24.2	24.2	—	—
	85	23.8	25.5	27.0	25.9	25.9	25.3	2.3
	95	28.6	29.9	31.6	30.0	30.1	29.3	2.8

*(A − B)/B × 100%.

CONVERSIONS/FORMULAS/TABLES

Table 15.2   Percentiles for Body Mass Index in U.S. Girls 5 to 17 Years of Age

Age (yr)	Percentile	Asian	Black	Hispanic	White	U.S. Weighted Mean (A)	NHANES (B)	% Difference*
5	5	13.0	13.3	13.5	13.0	13.1	—	—
	15	13.6	14.0	14.3	13.7	13.8	—	—
	50	14.5	15.4	15.5	14.9	15.1	—	—
	75	15.2	16.6	17.1	15.8	16.1	—	—
	85	15.7	17.7	18.1	16.5	16.9	—	—
	95	16.6	19.8	19.6	18.1	18.5	—	—
6	5	13.3	13.6	13.8	13.3	13.4	12.8	4.9
	15	13.8	14.2	14.5	14.0	14.1	13.4	4.9
	50	14.6	15.5	15.6	15.0	15.2	14.3	6.0
	75	15.5	17.0	17.5	16.1	16.4	—	—
	85	16.1	18.1	18.5	16.9	17.2	16.2	6.5
	95	17.4	20.7	20.5	18.9	19.3	17.5	10.5
7	5	13.4	13.8	13.9	13.5	13.6	13.2	2.8
	15	14.0	14.4	14.7	14.1	14.3	13.8	3.3
	50	14.9	15.8	15.9	15.3	15.4	15.0	2.8
	75	16.1	17.5	18.0	16.7	17.0	—	—
	85	16.7	18.8	19.2	17.6	17.9	17.2	4.3
	95	18.4	21.8	21.6	20.0	20.4	18.9	8.0
8	5	13.5	13.9	14.0	13.5	13.6	13.5	1.0
	15	14.2	14.6	14.9	14.3	14.4	14.2	1.6
	50	15.3	16.2	16.3	15.7	15.8	15.7	0.7
	75	16.8	18.3	18.8	17.4	17.7	—	—
	85	17.7	19.8	20.2	18.6	18.9	18.2	3.9
	95	19.6	23.1	22.9	21.2	21.7	20.4	6.2
9	5	13.6	14.0	14.1	13.6	13.7	13.9	−1.1
	15	14.4	14.8	15.1	14.5	14.6	14.7	−0.3
	50	15.8	16.7	16.9	16.2	16.4	16.3	0.4
	75	17.7	19.2	19.7	18.3	18.6	—	—
	85	18.8	21.0	21.4	19.7	20.1	19.2	4.6
	95	20.9	24.5	24.3	22.6	23.0	21.8	5.7
10	5	13.9	14.2	14.4	13.9	14.0	14.2	−1.3
	15	14.8	15.2	15.5	14.9	15.0	15.1	−0.4
	50	16.5	17.4	17.6	16.9	17.1	17.0	0.4
	75	18.7	20.2	20.8	19.3	19.6	—	—
	85	20.0	22.3	22.7	21.0	21.4	20.2	5.7
	95	22.4	26.1	25.8	24.1	24.5	23.2	5.8

*(A − B)/B × 100%.

(continued)

Table 15.2   Percentiles for Body Mass Index in U.S. Girls 5 to 17 Years of Age (*cont'd*)

Age (yr)	Percentile	Asian	Black	Hispanic	White	U.S. Weighted Mean (A)	NHANES (B)	% Difference*
11	5	14.3	14.7	14.9	14.4	14.5	14.6	−0.8
	15	15.4	15.8	16.1	15.5	15.6	15.5	0.8
	50	17.3	18.3	18.4	17.7	17.9	17.7	1.1
	75	19.7	21.3	21.9	20.4	20.7	—	—
	85	21.2	23.5	24.0	22.2	22.6	21.2	6.5
	95	23.8	27.6	27.4	25.6	26.1	24.6	6.0
12	5	15.0	15.4	15.5	15.0	15.1	15.0	1.0
	15	16.1	16.6	16.9	16.3	16.4	16.0	2.4
	50	18.2	19.2	19.3	18.6	18.8	18.4	2.1
	75	20.7	22.4	22.9	21.4	21.7	—	—
	85	22.2	24.6	25.1	23.2	23.6	22.2	6.4
	95	25.2	29.1	28.9	27.0	27.5	26.0	5.8
13	5	15.8	16.1	16.3	15.8	15.9	15.4	3.3
	15	16.9	17.4	17.7	17.1	17.2	16.4	5.0
	50	19.0	20.0	20.2	19.4	19.6	19.0	3.2
	75	21.5	23.2	23.8	22.2	22.5	—	—
	85	23.0	25.4	25.9	24.0	24.4	23.1	5.6
	95	26.3	30.3	30.0	28.1	28.6	27.1	5.7
14	5	16.5	16.8	17.0	16.5	16.6	15.7	5.8
	15	17.7	18.1	18.5	17.8	18.0	16.8	6.9
	50	19.6	20.7	20.8	20.1	20.2	19.3	4.9
	75	22.1	23.8	24.3	22.8	23.1	—	—
	85	23.5	25.9	26.4	24.5	24.9	23.9	4.2
	95	26.9	31.0	30.7	28.8	29.3	28.0	4.7
15	5	17.0	17.4	17.5	17.0	17.1	16.0	7.0
	15	18.1	18.6	19.0	18.3	18.4	17.2	7.2
	50	20.0	21.1	21.2	20.5	20.6	19.7	4.8
	75	22.3	24.0	24.6	23.1	23.4	—	—
	85	23.8	26.2	26.7	24.8	25.2	24.3	3.7
	95	27.2	31.3	31.0	29.1	29.6	28.5	3.9
16	5	17.2	17.6	17.8	17.3	17.4	16.4	6.1
	15	18.4	18.9	19.2	18.5	18.7	17.5	6.6
	50	20.2	21.3	21.4	20.7	20.9	20.1	3.8
	75	22.5	24.2	24.8	23.2	23.5	—	—
	85	24.0	26.5	27.0	25.1	25.5	24.7	3.1
	95	27.5	31.6	31.4	29.4	29.9	29.1	2.9

*(A − B)/B × 100%.

(continued)

Table 15.2   Percentiles for Body Mass Index in U.S. Girls 5 to 17 Years of Age (cont'd)

Age (yr)	Percentile	Asian	Black	Hispanic	White	U.S. Weighted Mean (A)	NHANES (B)	% Difference*
17	5	17.5	17.9	18.1	17.6	17.7	16.6	6.6
	15	18.6	19.1	19.5	18.8	18.9	17.8	6.3
	50	20.6	21.6	21.8	21.0	21.2	20.4	4.0
	75	23.0	24.7	25.3	23.7	24.1	—	—
	85	24.5	26.9	27.5	25.5	25.9	25.2	3.0
	95	28.8	33.0	32.8	30.8	31.3	29.7	5.4

Reprinted from Journal of Pediatrics, volume 132, Rosner B, et al, Percentiles for body mass index in US children 5 to 17 years of age, pages 211-222, Copyright 1998, with permission from Elsevier Science.

*(A − B)/B × 100%.

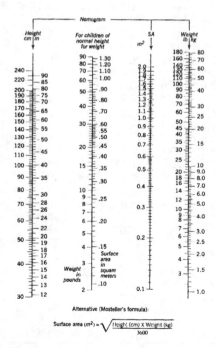

Figure 15.1   Body surface area nomogram. (This figure was published in The Harriet Lane Handbook, Siberry GK, Iannone R, eds, p 295, Copyright Elsevier, 1999.)

BODY SURFACE AREA (BSA)

Body surface area may be approximated if only weight is known by using the following formula:

$$\frac{(\text{Weight in kg} \times 4) + 7}{90 + (\text{Weight in kg})}$$

PREDICTED TARGETED GENETIC ADULT HEIGHT

Genetic potential formula

Boys ([Mother's height + 13 cm] + father's height) ÷ 2
Girls ([Father's height − 13 cm] + mother's height) ÷ 2

GROWTH VELOCITY

$$\frac{\text{Growth in cm}}{\text{Time (weeks)}} \times \frac{\text{Growth in cm}}{\text{Over 1 yr (52 weeks)}} \qquad \text{EXAMPLE} \qquad \frac{2 \text{ cm}}{12 \text{ weeks}} \times \frac{X}{52 \text{ weeks}}$$

TEMPERATURE

Degrees Celsius to degrees Fahrenheit ([9/5] × Temperature) + 32
Degrees Fahrenheit to degrees Celsius (Temperature − 32) × (5/9)

LAB EQUIVALENTS

Serum Osmolality Calculation

Defined as the number of particles per liter, osmolality may be approximated by the following formula:

$$2(Na^+) + \frac{\text{Glucose (mg/dL)}}{18} + \frac{\text{BUN (mg/dL)}}{2.8}$$

Normal range: 285-295 mOsm/L

Anion Gap

Represents anions other than bicarbonate and chloride needed to balance the positive charge of Na:

Anion gap = $Na^+ - (Cl^- + CO_2)$
Normal: 12 mEq/L ± 2 mEq/L

CLITORAL SIZE[3]

See General Endocrine Assessment, p. 8.

PENILE LENGTH[3]

See General Endocrine Assessment, pp. 6-7.

Table 15.3 Blood Pressure Levels for Girls by Age and Height Percentile

Age (yr)	BP Percentile	Systolic BP (mm Hg) Percentile of Height						
		5th	10th	25th	50th	75th	90th	95th
1	50th	83	84	85	86	88	89	90
	90th	97	97	98	100	101	102	103
	95th	100	101	102	104	105	106	107
	99th	108	108	109	111	112	113	114
2	50th	85	85	87	88	89	91	91
	90th	98	99	100	101	103	104	105
	95th	102	103	104	105	107	108	109
	99th	109	110	111	112	114	115	116
3	50th	86	87	88	89	91	92	93
	90th	100	100	102	103	104	106	106
	95th	104	104	105	107	108	109	110
	99th	111	111	113	114	115	116	117
4	50th	88	88	90	91	92	94	94
	90th	101	102	103	104	106	107	108
	95th	105	106	107	108	110	111	112
	99th	112	113	114	115	117	118	119
5	50th	89	90	91	93	94	95	96
	90th	103	103	105	106	107	109	109
	95th	107	107	108	110	111	112	113
	99th	114	114	116	117	118	120	120
6	50th	91	92	93	94	96	97	98
	90th	104	105	106	108	109	110	111
	95th	108	109	110	111	113	114	115
	99th	115	116	117	119	120	121	122
7	50th	93	93	95	96	97	99	99
	90th	106	107	108	109	111	112	113
	95th	110	111	112	113	115	116	116
	99th	117	118	119	120	122	123	124

From National Heart, Lung, and Blood Institute as a part for the National Institutes of Health and the U.S. Department of Health and Human Services. Available at *http://www.nhlbi.nih.gov/guidelines/hypertension/child_tbl.pdf*. Accessed July 22, 2009.
The 90th percentile is 1.28 SD, 95th percentile is 1.645 SD, and the 99th percentile is 2.326 SD over the mean.

Diastolic BP (mm Hg)

Percentile of Height						
5th	10th	25th	50th	75th	90th	95th
38	39	39	40	41	41	42
52	53	53	54	55	55	56
56	57	57	58	59	59	60
64	64	65	65	66	67	67
43	44	44	45	46	46	47
57	58	58	59	60	61	61
61	62	62	63	64	65	65
69	69	70	70	71	72	72
47	48	48	49	50	50	51
61	62	62	63	64	64	65
65	66	66	67	68	68	69
73	73	74	74	75	76	76
50	50	51	52	52	53	54
64	64	65	66	67	67	68
68	68	69	70	71	71	72
76	76	76	77	78	79	79
52	53	53	54	55	55	56
66	67	67	68	69	69	70
70	71	71	72	73	73	74
78	78	79	79	80	81	81
54	54	55	56	56	57	58
68	68	69	70	70	71	72
72	72	73	74	74	75	76
80	80	80	81	82	83	83
55	56	56	57	58	58	59
69	70	70	71	72	72	73
73	74	74	75	76	76	77
81	81	82	82	83	84	84

(continued)

CONVERSIONS/FORMULAS/TABLES ⑮

Table 15.3 Blood Pressure Levels for Girls by Age and Height Percentile—cont'd

Age (yr)	BP Percentile	Systolic BP (mm Hg)						
		Percentile of Height						
		5th	10th	25th	50th	75th	90th	95th
8	50th	95	95	96	98	99	100	101
	90th	108	109	110	111	113	114	114
	95th	112	112	114	115	116	118	118
	99th	119	120	121	122	123	125	125
9	50th	96	97	98	100	101	102	103
	90th	110	110	112	113	114	116	116
	95th	114	114	115	117	118	119	120
	99th	121	121	123	124	125	127	127
10	50th	98	99	100	102	103	104	105
	90th	112	112	114	115	116	118	118
	95th	116	116	117	119	120	121	122
	99th	123	123	125	126	127	129	129
11	50th	100	101	102	103	105	106	107
	90th	114	114	116	117	118	119	120
	95th	118	118	119	121	122	123	124
	99th	125	125	126	128	129	130	131
12	50th	102	103	104	105	107	108	109
	90th	116	116	117	119	120	121	122
	95th	119	120	121	123	124	125	126
	99th	127	127	128	130	131	132	133
13	50th	104	105	106	107	109	110	110
	90th	117	118	119	121	122	123	124
	95th	121	122	123	124	126	127	128
	99th	128	129	130	132	133	134	135
14	50th	106	106	107	109	110	111	112
	90th	119	120	121	122	124	125	125
	95th	123	123	125	126	127	129	129
	99th	130	131	132	133	135	136	136
15	50th	107	108	109	110	111	113	113
	90th	120	121	122	123	125	126	127
	95th	124	125	126	127	129	130	131
	99th	131	132	133	134	136	137	138

The 90th percentile is 1.28 SD, 95th percentile is 1.645 SD, and the 99th percentile is 2.326 SD over the mean.

Diastolic BP (mm Hg)

Percentile of Height						
5th	**10th**	**25th**	**50th**	**75th**	**90th**	**95th**
57	57	57	58	59	60	60
71	71	71	72	73	74	74
75	75	75	76	77	78	78
82	82	83	83	84	85	86
58	58	58	59	60	61	61
72	72	72	73	74	75	75
76	76	76	77	78	79	79
83	83	84	84	85	86	87
59	59	59	60	61	62	62
73	73	73	74	75	76	76
77	77	77	78	79	80	80
84	84	85	86	86	87	88
60	60	60	61	62	63	63
74	74	74	75	76	77	77
78	78	78	79	80	81	81
85	85	86	87	87	88	89
61	61	61	62	63	64	64
75	75	75	76	77	78	78
79	79	79	80	81	82	82
86	86	87	88	88	89	90
62	62	62	63	64	65	65
76	76	76	77	78	79	79
80	80	80	81	82	83	83
87	87	88	89	89	90	91
63	63	63	64	65	66	66
77	77	77	78	79	80	80
81	81	81	82	83	84	84
88	88	89	90	90	91	92
64	64	64	65	66	67	67
78	78	78	79	80	81	81
82	82	82	83	84	85	85
89	89	90	91	91	92	93

(continued)

Table 15.3 Blood Pressure Levels for Girls by Age and Height Percentile—cont'd

Age (yr)	BP Percentile	Systolic BP (mm Hg) Percentile of Height						
		5th	10th	25th	50th	75th	90th	95th
16	50th	108	108	110	111	112	114	114
	90th	121	122	123	124	126	127	128
	95th	125	126	127	128	130	131	132
	99th	132	133	134	135	137	138	139
17	50th	108	109	110	111	113	114	115
	90th	122	122	123	125	126	127	128
	95th	125	126	127	129	130	131	132
	99th	133	133	134	136	137	138	139

The 90th percentile is 1.28 SD, 95th percentile is 1.645 SD, and the 99th percentile is 2.326 SD over the mean.

Table 15.4 Blood Pressure Levels for Boys by Age and Height Percentile

Age (yr)	BP Percentile	Systolic BP (mm Hg) Percentile of Height						
		5th	10th	25th	50th	75th	90th	95th
1	50th	80	81	83	85	87	88	89
	90th	94	95	97	99	100	102	103
	95th	98	99	101	103	104	106	106
	99th	105	106	108	110	112	113	114
2	50th	84	85	87	88	90	92	92
	90th	97	99	100	102	104	105	106
	95th	101	102	104	106	108	109	110
	99th	109	110	111	113	115	117	117
3	50th	86	87	89	91	93	94	95
	90th	100	101	103	105	107	108	109
	95th	104	105	107	109	110	112	113
	99th	111	112	114	116	118	119	120

From National Heart, Lung, and Blood Institute as a part for the National Institutes of Health and the U.S. Department of Health and Human Services. Available at *http://www.nhlbi.nih.gov/guidelines/hypertension/child_tbl.pdf*. Accessed July 22, 2009.
The 90th percentile is 1.28 SD, 95th percentile is 1.645 SD, and the 99th percentile is 2.326 SD over the mean.

Diastolic BP (mm Hg)

Percentile of Height						
5th	**10th**	**25th**	**50th**	**75th**	**90th**	**95th**
64	64	65	66	66	67	68
78	78	79	80	81	81	82
82	82	83	84	85	85	86
90	90	90	91	92	93	93
64	65	65	66	67	67	68
78	79	79	80	81	81	82
82	83	83	84	85	85	86
90	90	91	91	92	93	93

Diastolic BP (mm Hg)

Percentile of Height						
5th	**10th**	**25th**	**50th**	**75th**	**90th**	**95th**
34	35	36	37	38	39	39
49	50	51	52	53	53	54
54	54	55	56	57	58	58
61	62	63	64	65	66	66
39	40	41	42	43	44	44
54	55	56	57	58	58	59
59	59	60	61	62	63	63
66	67	68	69	70	71	71
44	44	45	46	47	48	48
59	59	60	61	62	63	63
63	63	64	65	66	67	67
71	71	72	73	74	75	75

(continued)

Table 15.4   Blood Pressure Levels for Boys by Age and Height Percentile—cont'd

| Age (yr) | BP Percentile | Systolic BP (mm Hg) | | | | | | |
| | | Percentile of Height | | | | | | |
		5th	10th	25th	50th	75th	90th	95th
4	50th	88	89	91	93	95	96	97
	90th	102	103	105	107	109	110	111
	95th	106	107	109	111	112	114	115
	99th	113	114	116	118	120	121	122
5	50th	90	91	93	95	96	98	98
	90th	104	105	106	108	110	111	112
	95th	108	109	110	112	114	115	116
	99th	115	116	118	120	121	123	123
6	50th	91	92	94	96	98	99	100
	90th	105	106	108	110	111	113	113
	95th	109	110	112	114	115	117	117
	99th	116	117	119	121	123	124	125
7	50th	92	94	95	97	99	100	101
	90th	106	107	109	111	113	114	115
	95th	110	111	113	115	117	118	119
	99th	117	118	120	122	124	125	126
8	50th	94	95	97	99	100	102	102
	90th	107	109	110	112	114	115	116
	95th	111	112	114	116	118	119	120
	99th	119	120	122	123	125	127	127
9	50th	95	96	98	100	102	103	104
	90th	109	110	112	114	115	117	118
	95th	113	114	116	118	119	121	121
	99th	120	121	123	125	127	128	129
10	50th	97	98	100	102	103	105	106
	90th	111	112	114	115	117	119	119
	95th	115	116	117	119	121	122	123
	99th	122	123	125	127	128	130	130

The 90th percentile is 1.28 SD, 95th percentile is 1.645 SD, and the 99th percentile is 2.326 SD over the mean.

Diastolic BP (mm Hg)

Percentile of Height

5th	10th	25th	50th	75th	90th	95th
47	48	49	50	51	51	52
62	63	64	65	66	66	67
66	67	68	69	70	71	71
74	75	76	77	78	78	79
50	51	52	53	54	55	55
65	66	67	68	69	69	70
69	70	71	72	73	74	74
77	78	79	80	81	81	82
53	53	54	55	56	57	57
68	68	69	70	71	72	72
72	72	73	74	75	76	76
80	80	81	82	83	84	84
55	55	56	57	58	59	59
70	70	71	72	73	74	74
74	74	75	76	77	78	78
82	82	83	84	85	86	86
56	57	58	59	60	60	61
71	72	72	73	74	75	76
75	76	77	78	79	79	80
83	84	85	86	87	87	88
57	58	59	60	61	61	62
72	73	74	75	76	76	77
76	77	78	79	80	81	81
84	85	86	87	88	88	89
58	59	60	61	61	62	63
73	73	74	75	76	77	78
77	78	79	80	81	81	82
85	86	86	88	88	89	90

(continued)

Table 15.4 Blood Pressure Levels for Boys by Age and Height Percentile—cont'd

Age (yr)	BP Percentile	Systolic BP (mm Hg)						
		Percentile of Height						
		5th	10th	25th	50th	75th	90th	95th
11	50th	99	100	102	104	105	107	107
	90th	113	114	115	117	119	120	121
	95th	117	118	119	121	123	124	125
	99th	124	125	127	129	130	132	132
12	50th	101	102	104	106	108	109	110
	90th	115	116	118	120	121	123	123
	95th	119	120	122	123	125	127	127
	99th	126	127	129	131	133	134	135
13	50th	104	105	106	108	110	111	112
	90th	117	118	120	122	124	125	126
	95th	121	122	124	126	128	129	130
	99th	128	130	131	133	135	136	137
14	50th	106	107	109	111	113	114	115
	90th	120	121	123	125	126	128	128
	95th	124	125	127	128	130	132	132
	99th	131	132	134	136	138	139	140
15	50th	109	110	112	113	115	117	117
	90th	122	124	125	127	129	130	131
	95th	126	127	129	131	133	134	135
	99th	134	135	136	138	140	142	142
16	50th	111	112	114	116	118	119	120
	90th	125	126	128	130	131	133	134
	95th	129	130	132	134	135	137	137
	99th	136	137	139	141	143	144	145
17	50th	114	115	116	118	120	121	122
	90th	127	128	130	132	134	135	136
	95th	131	132	134	136	138	139	140
	99th	139	140	141	143	145	146	147

The 90th percentile is 1.28 SD, 95th percentile is 1.645 SD, and the 99th percentile is 2.326 SD over the mean.

Diastolic BP (mm Hg)

Percentile of Height

5th	10th	25th	50th	75th	90th	95th
59	59	60	61	62	63	63
74	74	75	76	77	78	78
78	78	79	80	81	82	82
86	86	87	88	89	90	90
59	60	61	62	63	63	64
74	75	75	76	77	78	79
78	79	80	81	82	82	83
86	87	88	89	90	90	91
60	60	61	62	63	64	64
75	75	76	77	78	79	79
79	79	80	81	82	83	83
87	87	88	89	90	91	91
60	61	62	63	64	65	65
75	76	77	78	79	79	80
80	80	81	82	83	84	84
87	88	89	90	91	92	92
61	62	63	64	65	66	66
76	77	78	79	80	80	81
81	81	82	83	84	85	85
88	89	90	91	92	93	93
63	63	64	65	66	67	67
78	78	79	80	81	82	82
82	83	83	84	85	86	87
90	90	91	92	93	94	94
65	66	66	67	68	69	70
80	80	81	82	83	84	84
84	85	86	87	87	88	89
92	93	93	94	95	96	97

16 GROWTH CHARTS

Birth to 36 months: Boys
Length-for-age and Weight-for-age percentiles

NAME _____

RECORD # _____

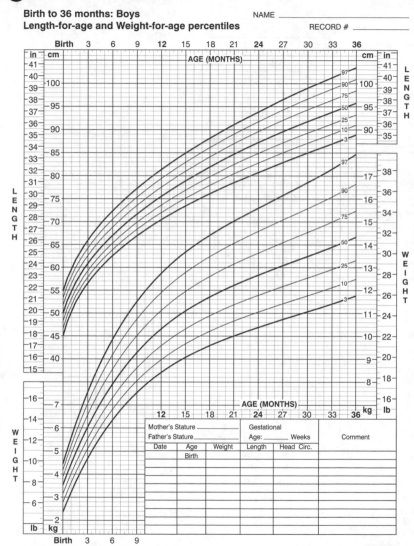

Published May 30, 2000 (modified 4/20/01).
SOURCE: Developed by the National Center for Health Statistics in collaboration with
the National Center for Chronic Disease Prevention and Health Promotion (2000).
http://www.cdc.gov/growthcharts

SAFER·HEALTHIER·PEOPLE™

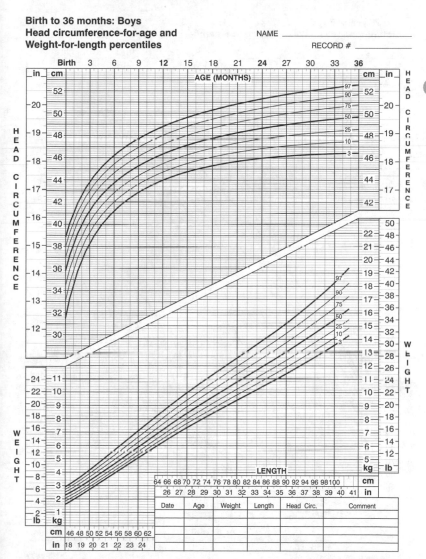

Birth to 36 months: Boys
Head circumference-for-age and
Weight-for-length percentiles

NAME _____

RECORD # _____

Published May 30, 2000 (modified 10/16/00).
SOURCE: Developed by the National Center for Health Statistics in collaboration with
the National Center for Chronic Disease Prevention and Health Promotion (2000).
http://www.cdc.gov/growthcharts

SAFER · HEALTHIER · PEOPLE™

2 to 20 years: Boys
Stature-for-age and Weight-for-age percentiles

NAME _____

RECORD # _____

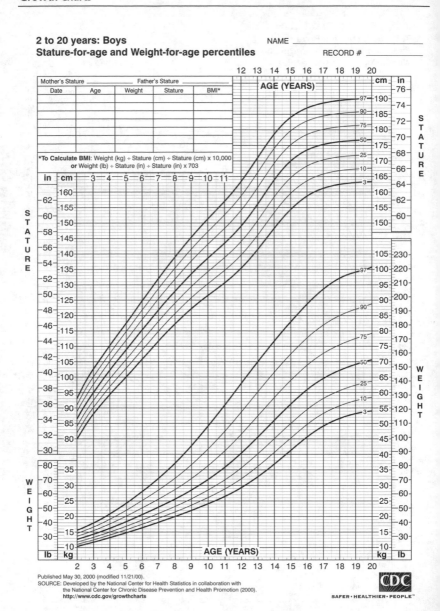

Published May 30, 2000 (modified 11/21/00).
SOURCE: Developed by the National Center for Health Statistics in collaboration with
the National Center for Chronic Disease Prevention and Health Promotion (2000).
http://www.cdc.gov/growthcharts

SAFER · HEALTHIER · PEOPLE™

2 to 20 years: Boys
Body mass index-for-age percentiles

NAME _____

RECORD # _____

Date	Age	Weight	Stature	BMI*	Comments

*To Calculate BMI: Weight (kg) ÷ Stature (cm) ÷ Stature (cm) x 10,000
or Weight (lb) ÷ Stature (in) ÷ Stature (in) x 703

AGE (YEARS)

BMI — kg/m²

Percentile lines: 97, 95, 90, 85, 75, 50, 25, 10, 3

Published May 30, 2000 (modified 10/16/00).
SOURCE: Developed by the National Center for Health Statistics in collaboration with
the National Center for Chronic Disease Prevention and Health Promotion (2000).
http://www.cdc.gov/growthcharts

SAFER · HEALTHIER · PEOPLE™

GROWTH CHARTS 16

Birth to 36 months: Girls
Length-for-age and Weight-for-age percentiles

NAME _____

RECORD # _____

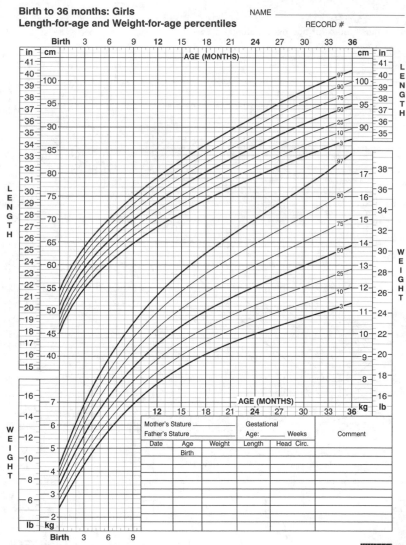

Published May 30, 2000 (modified 4/20/01).
SOURCE: Developed by the National Center for Health Statistics in collaboration with
the National Center for Chronic Disease Prevention and Health Promotion (2000).
http://www.cdc.gov/growthcharts

SAFER · HEALTHIER · PEOPLE™

Birth to 36 months: Girls
Head circumference-for-age and
Weight-for-length percentiles

NAME _____

RECORD # _____

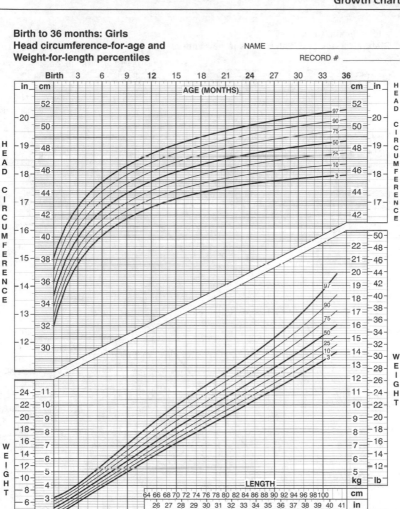

Published May 30, 2000 (modified 10/16/00).
SOURCE: Developed by the National Center for Health Statistics in collaboration with
the National Center for Chronic Disease Prevention and Health Promotion (2000).
http://www.cdc.gov/growthcharts

GROWTH CHARTS **16**

2 to 20 years: Girls
Stature-for-age and Weight-for-age percentiles

NAME _____

RECORD # _____

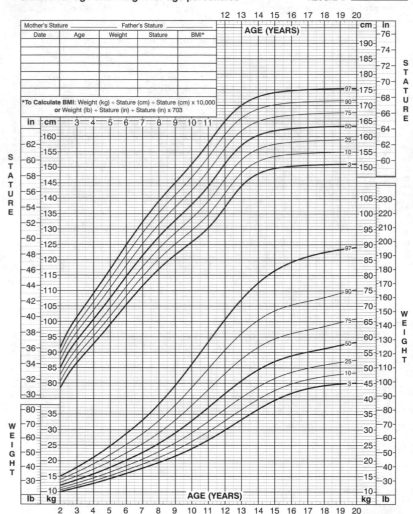

Published May 30, 2000 (modified 11/21/00).
SOURCE: Developed by the National Center for Health Statistics in collaboration with
the National Center for Chronic Disease Prevention and Health Promotion (2000).
http://www.cdc.gov/growthcharts

2 to 20 years: Girls
Body mass index-for-age percentiles

NAME _____

RECORD # _____

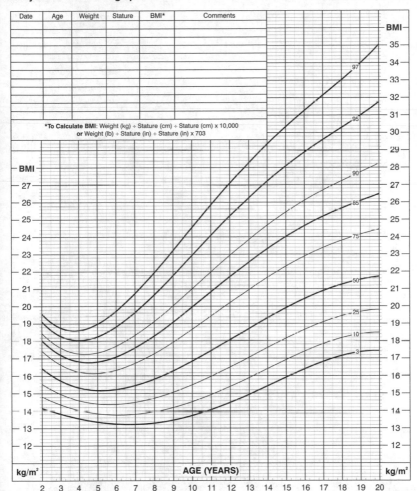

Date	Age	Weight	Stature	BMI*	Comments

*To Calculate BMI: Weight (kg) ÷ Stature (cm) ÷ Stature (cm) x 10,000
or Weight (lb) ÷ Stature (in) ÷ Stature (in) x 703

AGE (YEARS)

Published May 30, 2000 (modified 10/16/00).
SOURCE: Developed by the National Center for Health Statistics in collaboration with
the National Center for Chronic Disease Prevention and Health Promotion (2000).
http://www.cdc.gov/growthcharts

SAFER·HEALTHIER·PEOPLE™

GROWTH CHARTS 16

Growth Charts

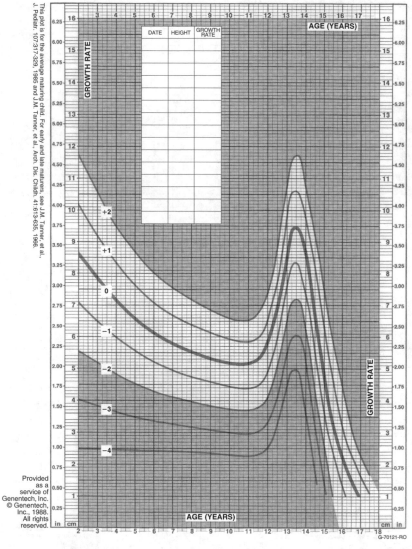

BOYS: 2 TO 18 YEARS
YEARLY GROWTH RATE
MEANS AND STANDARD DEVIATIONS

NAME _____ RECORD # _____
DATE OF BIRTH _____

GROWTH RATE

AGE (YEARS)

DATE	HEIGHT	GROWTH RATE

+2
+1
0
−1
−2
−3
−4

GROWTH RATE

AGE (YEARS)

G-70121-RO

450

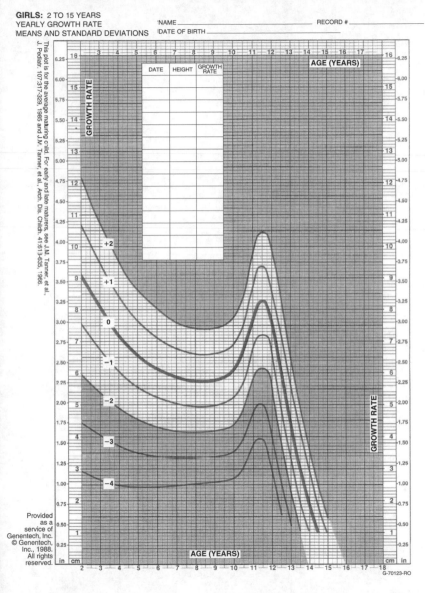

GIRLS: 2 TO 15 YEARS
YEARLY GROWTH RATE
MEANS AND STANDARD DEVIATIONS

NAME _____ RECORD # _____

DATE OF BIRTH _____

This plot is for the average maturing child. For early and late maturers, see J.M. Tanner, et al., J. Pediatr. 107:317-329, 1985 and J.M. Tanner, et al., Arch. Dis. Childh. 41:613-635, 1966.

DATE	HEIGHT	GROWTH RATE

GROWTH RATE

AGE (YEARS)

G-70123-RO

17 GLOSSARY

alpha (α) cells Glucagon-secreting cells of pancreatic islets

ACTH (adrenocorticotropic hormone) Hormone produced by the pituitary gland that in turn stimulates the adrenal glands to produce cortisol and androgens

acanthosis nigricans Diffuse hyperplasia and thickening of the epidermis with gray to black pigmentation, chiefly in body folds, as in the sides of neck, axillae, and groin. It is a sign of insulin resistance

adenocarcinoma Gland-like malignant epithelial tissue neoplasm

adenoma Gland-like benign epithelial tissue neoplasm

adrenal medulla Inner part of adrenal gland. Releases norepinephrine, epinephrine, dopamine, and opiate peptides

adrenarche Changes that usually occur at time of puberty resulting from increased release of adrenocortical hormone ACTH (i.e., pubic hair, axillary hair)

agenesis Failure of an organ or part to develop or grow

aldosterone Hormone that helps to regulate sodium and fluid balance; produced by the adrenal glands

alopecia Absence of hair

amenorrhea Absence or abnormal stoppage of the menses

analog Usually designates a substance chemically related to a naturally occurring regulator. Can be receptor antagonist; agonist that differs from the natural hormone in potency, resistance to degradation, specificity, etc.; or metabolic inhibitor

androgens Testosterone and related steroids that stimulate male reproductive organs and secondary sex characteristics, invoke masculinization in females

anosmia Absence of the sense of smell

arachnodactyly Long fingers

arthralgia Joint pain

beta (β) cells Insulin-secreting cells of the pancreatic islets

BIA (bioelectrical impedance analysis) Measurement of electrical resistance in the body to a tiny imperceptible current

BMI (body mass index) Weight in kilograms divided by height in cm^2

brachycephaly Having a short, wide head

brachydactyly Having short fingers

Brushfield spots Gray or pale yellow spots sometimes present at the periphery of the iris of children with Down syndrome

canthus The angle at either end of the slit between the eyelids (internal and external)

carbohydrate Main source of energy for all body functions; necessary for metabolism of other nutrients; includes sugar, starch, cellulose, and gum; stored in the form of glycogen

CATCH 22 syndrome Cardiac defect, abnormal face, thymic hypoplasia, cleft palate, hypocalcemia

champagne cork Cork-appearing aspect on chest X-ray indicative of vitamin D deficient rickets

Chvostek's sign A technique used to determine hypocalcemia. The facial nerve is tapped with a fingertip (as a hammer), 1-2 cm anterior to the earlobe below the zygomatic process. The local spasm of the facial nerve muscles is graded as (1) twitching of the upper lip (at the corner) only, (2) twitching of the lower extended portion of the lateral wall of the nose as well, (3) contraction of the muscle around the opening or the orbit of the eye as well, and (4) contraction of all the muscles on that side. A sign ≥grade 2 suggests hypocalcemia. The greater the grade, the more serious the condition

clinodactyly Having curvature of the fingers

coloboma A lesion or defect of the eye, usually a fissure or cleft of the iris, ciliary body, or choroid. May involve the eyelid. Congenital, pathological, or surgical

consanguinity The mating of related individuals

corticosteroid Any steroid hormone produced by the adrenal cortex

cortisol Principal glucocorticoid hormone

cryptorchism (cryptorchidism) Retention of testes within the abdominal cavity of humans and other species in which descent to the scrotum normally occurs. Associated azoospermia attributed to high temperature of abdominal cavity

CT (computed tomography) X-ray technique involving cross-sectional method for evaluating tissue structure

cubitus valgus A deformity of the arm in which the forearm deviates laterally; may be congenital or caused by injury or disease. May be present in Turner syndrome

cutis marmorata Transitory purplish discoloration of skin on exposure to the cold

diuresis Increased urine flow

DXA (dual energy X-ray absorptiometry) Radiologic imaging of the soft tissue and bone; estimates total body composition and bone density

dyslipidemias Disturbance in fat metabolism resulting in abnormal lipid levels

dysmenorrhea Painful menstruation

dysmorphology The study of human congenital malformations (birth defects)

dysplasia Abnormal cellular development

electrolytes An element or compound that when melted or dissolved is able to conduct an electrical current. The human body requires adequate levels of certain principal electrolytes and a balance between them for normal metabolism and body function

empty sella syndrome Pituitary hormone deficiency or dysfunction associated with absence of hypophyseal tissue in the sella turcica region

enuresis Incontinence of urine

epiphyses Growing ends of long bones that undergo calcification

estrogens Steroid hormones possessing aromatic A ring, 18 carbons. Produced in largest quantities by the ovaries. Includes estradiols, estrones, and estriol

euthyroid A state describing a normally functioning thyroid gland

exophthalmos Abnormal protrusion of the eye

exostosis A benign bony growth projecting outward from the surface of a bone, characteristically capped by cartilage

fluorescence in situ hybridization (FISH) A molecular cytogenetic technique in which labeled probes are hybridized with chromosomes and then visualized under a fluorescence microscope. Used to identify missing, additional, or rearranged chromosomal material

FSH (follicle-stimulating hormone) Adenohypophyseal glycoprotein. Stimulates growth, maturation of ovarian follicular and testicular Sertoli cells

GABA (gamma aminobutyric acid) An amino acid that acts as a neurotransmitter in the central nervous system

GAD (glutamic acid decarboxylase) Enzyme used as a marker for GABA synthesis

galactorrhea Milk secretion. Associated with hyperprolactinemia that can occur with normal pregnancy and lactation or pituitary tumors/dysfunction

genotype The genetic makeup of an individual

glucocorticoid An adrenocortical steroid hormone that increases the formation of glycogen from fatty acids and proteins, has an antiinflammatory effect, and has many body functions

glycosuria Sugar loss via urine. Usually associated with high blood glucose (>180 mg/dL) such as that in diabetes mellitus, stress, or use of corticosteroids. Renal dysfunction can impair resorption

17

GLOSSARY

goiter Enlargement of the thyroid gland, causing swelling in the front of the neck

gonadotropin Luteinizing hormone (LH) and follicle-stimulating hormone (FSH)

growth potential An individual's potential height, taking parental height, genetic factors, and concurrent illness into consideration

growth rate Incremental height changes over a specific time period

gynecomastia Breast enlargement in males. Usually linked with hormone imbalance, e.g., hyperprolactinemia, high estrogen levels, Klinefelter's syndrome

hemochromatosis A genetic disorder of iron metabolism characterized by excess deposition of iron in the tissues, especially in the liver and pancreas, and by bronze pigmentation of the skin, cirrhosis, diabetes mellitus, and associated bone and joint changes

hemosiderosis A focal or general increase is tissue iron stores without tissue damage

hermaphrodite An individual possessing ovary and testicle, two of each, ovotestes or ovotestis plus ovary or testicle

hirsutism Excessive body and facial hair (usually described in women). Associated with excess ovarian, adrenocortical defects or tumors affecting secretion, metabolism, or responses to androgens

histiocytosis X An abnormal amount of histiocytes in the blood, as in disease of Langerhans cell histiocytes in which these cells characteristically cause granulomas. Many variations of signs/symptoms dependent on location and how well spread they are. Not limited to any one organ system

hormone Highly potent chemical messenger synthesized within the organism that invokes responses after binding to a target cell receptor. Endocrine hormone molecules are secreted directly into the bloodstream, whereas exocrine hormones are secreted into a duct

hyperhidrosis Excessive sweating

hyperkalemia Excessively high levels of blood potassium

hypernatremia Excessively high levels of blood sodium

hyperphagia Excessive food intake

hyperpigmentation Darkening of the skin. Can be caused by heredity, sun exposure, drugs, or adrenal insufficiency

hypertelorism Abnormally long distance between eyes or any two paired organs

hypertrophy Cell enlargement, or the associated growth of tissues and organs

hypogonadism Defective/inadequate secretion of sex steroids from the gonads

hyponatremia A lower than normal concentration of sodium in the blood

hypophyseal portal system The series of vessels that lead from the hypothalamus to the anterior lobe of the pituitary. The releasing and inhibiting hormones are carried to the anterior pituitary via this system

hypophysectomy Removal of the pituitary gland

hypophysis The pituitary gland. Includes adenohypophysis and neurohypophysis

hypoplasia Incomplete or underdevelopment of tissue or organ

hypospadias Defect in which the urethral orifice is located on the undersurface of a poorly developed penis. Usually associated with androgen receptor defect

hypothalamus Portion of the brain that stimulates the pituitary gland to secrete hormones

hypotonia Loss of tonicity of the muscles

idiopathic Usually refers to a disorder for which the cause is not established (e.g., idiopathic short stature)

infundibulum Funnel-like structure connecting the hypothalamus with the hypophysis

inhibin Peptides made by Sertoli and ovarian follicular cells. Low concentrations inhibit FSH release

IGF-1 (insulin-like growth factor 1) Peptide that exerts insulin-like action. Also referred to as somatomedin C. Promotes growth of cartilage and bone as well other cell types

insulinoma Insulin-secreting tumor

islets of Langerhans Endocrine cell clumps within the pancreas. Various types secrete insulin, glucagon, somatostatin, pancreatic polypeptide, and other regulators

karyotype Chromosome characteristics of a cell (or an individual)

ketones/ketone bodies Acetoacetate, β-hydroxybutyrate, and acetone. Formed when fatty acid catabolism leads to acetyl coenzyme A accumulation

lactate Made when pyruvate is not rapidly converted to acetyl-coenzyme A, amino acids, or glucose

lactotrophs Prolactin-secreting adenohypophyseal cells

Leydig cells Interstitial cells of testis that secrete androgens. Stimulated by LH

LH (luteinizing hormone) Glycoprotein secreted by gonadotropes/gonadotrophs. Stimulates steroidogenesis, exerts other effects on ovaries and testes

libido Sexual desire

lymphangiogram Radiograph of the lymphatic vessels

lymphedema An abnormal accumulation of tissue fluid in the interstitial spaces

macroadenoma A glandular tumor greater than 10 mm in diameter

macrocephaly Abnormally large size of the head

macroglossia Hypertrophied condition of the tongue; congenital disorder

menarche Initiation of menstrual cycles

menorrhagia Excessive blood loss during menstruation

methylation In genetics, involves the addition of methyl groups to cytosine bases, forming 5-methylcytosine. Correlates with reduced transcription of genes. Methylation testing includes a technique used in diagnosing chromosomal abnormalities

microcephaly Abnormal smallness of the head; often seen in mental retardation

microdeletion A chromosome deletion too small to be visible under a microscope. DiGeorge syndrome and Prader-Willi syndrome are examples of diseases resulting from a chromosomal microdeletion

microdontia Having abnormally small teeth or a single small tooth

micrognathia Abnormal smallness of the jaws, especially the lower jaw

microphallus Undersized, poorly developed penis, usually attributed to androgen receptor defect or growth hormone deficiency

mineralocorticoid Steroid secreted by the adrenal cortex; its primary purpose is to promote sodium retention, potassium excretion, and a positive water balance. Primary mineralocorticoid is aldosterone

MODY (maturity-onset diabetes of youth) An acronym that describes inherited forms of type 2 diabetes mellitus

mosaic The presence in an individual of cells of two or more different genetic types. Can result from problems arising during fertilization and/or cleavage. XX/XY, XX/XO, XXX/XX, and other sex chromosome patterns are identified in humans

MRI (magnetic resonance imaging) Diagnostic tool that uses a static magnetic field instead of radiation. Provides exquisite anatomic detail of images including reconstruction of images in three views: axial, coronal, and sagittal

myalgia Muscle pain

myopia Nearsightedness; an error in refraction in which light rays are focused in front of the retina, enabling the person to see distinctly for a short distance

myxedema Subcutaneous accumulation of glycosaminoglycans attributed to thyroid hormone deficiency. Can also indicate severe hypothyroidism in adults

neonatal period Of or pertaining to the first 28 days of life

nephrogenic Arising in the kidney. Applied to conditions linked with renal dysfunction (e.g., nephrogenic diabetes insipidus)

nocturesis Incontinence of urine at night

nystagmus An involuntary rapid movement of the eyeball, which may be horizontal, vertical, rotary, or mixed

obesity An increase in body weight beyond the limitation of the skeletal and physical requirement from an excessive accumulation of fat in the body

oligomenorrhea Markedly diminished menstrual flow; relative amenorrhea

oligospermia Deficiency in the number of spermatozoa in the semen

osteomalacia "Softening" of bones in adults attributed to vitamin D deficiency

osteopenia Reduced bone mass

osteoporosis Thinning of the bones with loss of tensile strength. Resorption proceeds more rapidly than bone formation. Causes in endocrine patients may include glucocorticoid therapy for asthma, untreated growth hormone deficiency, prolonged GnRH agonist therapy, ovarian/testicular failure (hypogonadism)

ovotestis Gonad with both ovarian and testicular components

oxytocin Neurohypophyseal peptide. Stimulates mammary gland myoepithelial cells, uterine muscle. Contributes to parturition, protects against postpartum hemorrhage. Affects water balances. May contribute to ejaculation. Brain oxytocin affects maternal behavior

parathyroidectomy Surgical removal of the parathyroid gland

pectus carinatum Pigeon breast

pectus excavatum A congenital condition in which the sternum is abnormally depressed

philtrum The median groove on the external surface of the upper lip

polycystic ovaries Ovaries containing large, fluid-filled cysts. Attributed to conditions (e.g., hormone imbalance) that arrest follicle maturation before it is completed, or that block ovulation

polydipsia Excessive drinking (e.g., in diabetes mellitus or diabetes insipidus)

prolactin Secreted mostly by lactotropes. Affects mammary glands, gonadotropin receptors, corpus luteum survival, steroid metabolism, secretion of many hormones, amphibian "water drive," water and electrolyte balance, behavior, other functions

prolactinoma A benign pituitary neoplasm that secretes prolactin

GLOSSARY 17

pseudotumor cerebri A condition caused by cerebral edema, marked by raised intracranial pressure with headache, nausea, vomiting, and papilledema without neurological signs except occasional sixth-nerve palsy. Also called benign intracranial hypertension

ptosis Drooping of the upper eyelid from paralysis of the third nerve or from sympathetic innervation

rachitic rosary Beading of the ribs, a row of beading at the junction of the ribs with their cartilages

receptors Cell components binding hormones or other regulators with high affinity and specificity in a manner coupled to changes in cell function

retrognathia Location of the mandible behind the frontal plane of the maxilla

sarcoidosis A chronic, progressive, generalized granulomatous reticulosis of unknown etiology, involving almost any organ or tissue. Laboratory findings may include hypercalcemia and hypergammaglobulinemia

seborrhea Excessive secretion of sebum

secretagogue Agent that invokes or augments secretion

Sertoli cells Major nongerminal seminiferous tubule cells. Support spermatogenesis, spermiogenesis; participate in spermiation. Take up, metabolize steroids; synthesize androgen-binding proteins, inhibin; FSH promotes maturation, regulates some functions

serum T4 Total serum thyroxine (T4)

somatotrophs Adenohypophyseal cells. Secrete growth hormone (somatotropin)

steatorrhea Fat in the stool. Most commonly seen in disorders with pancreatic insufficiency

strabismus Deviation of the eye which the patient cannot overcome

syndactyly Fusion of two or more fingers or toes

tachycardia Abnormally rapid heart rate

TBG (thyroxine-binding globulin) A thyroid binding protein which binds the majority of thyroid hormone

teratogenesis The development of abnormal structures in an embryo

testosterone Major androgen. Largest amounts synthesized by testicular interstitial cells, smaller ones by ovaries, adrenal cortex. Secretion stimulated by LH. Acts directly on some targets, requires conversion (e.g., dihydrotestosterone, estradiol) in others

thyroglobulin A glycoprotein found in the thyroid follicles. One of the thyroid autoantigens

thyroglobulin antibody (TG Ab or antithyroglobulin) An autoantibody formed against thyroglobulin

thyroid peroxidase antibody (TPO Ab or anti-TPO) An autoantibody formed against thyroidal peroxidase (a thyroid autoantigen)

thyrotoxicosis The condition resulting from the effect of elevated amounts of thyroid hormones on body tissues

thyrotrophs Adenohypophyseal cells. Secrete thyroid-stimulating hormone (TSH)

thyroxine An iodine-containing hormone secreted by the thyroid gland. Its main function is to increase the rate of cell metabolism. A synthetic form is used to treat hypothyroidism

thyroxine, free (free T4) The metabolically active component of thyroid hormone which is unbound to thyroid proteins

TRH (thyrotropin-releasing hormone) The hormone produced by the hypothalamus to stimulate the pituitary gland to produce and release thyroid-stimulating hormone (TSH)

triiodothyronine (T3) A thyroid hormone derived from peripheral conversion of T4 and thyroid gland secretion

Trousseau's sign Carpal (wrist) spasm. Invoked by occlusion of arterioles supplying the forearm in hypocalcemic subjects. Seen in parathyroid hormone deficiency

truncal obesity Increase in adipose tissue in the trunk of the body and not the extremities

TSH (thyroid-stimulating hormone) The hormone produced by the pituitary gland to stimulate the thyroid gland

Turner syndrome Sex differentiation disorder. Usually associated with XO sex chromosomes, poorly developed female phenotype. Features can include streak gonads, short stature, cubitus valgus; shield-shaped chest; webbed neck; facial deformities, malformed aorta and kidney

uniparental disomy Condition in which two copies of one chromosome are derived from a single parent, and no copies are derived from the other parent (e.g., Prader-Willi syndrome)

vasopressin Antidiuretic hormone secreted by the posterior lobe of the pituitary gland

17

GLOSSARY

violaceous striae Linear pinkish or purplish, scarlike lesions that later become white, occurring on the abdomen, breasts, buttocks, and thighs. They are due to weakening of the elastic tissues, and are associated with pregnancy, excessive obesity, rapid growth during puberty and adolescence, Cushing's syndrome, or topical or prolonged use of corticosteroids

VIP (vasoactive intestinal peptide) Chemically related to gastric inhibitory peptide, glucagon. Neurotransmitter or neuromodulator in intestine and brain. Affects blood pressure, flow; gut motility, secretion; release of prolactin, growth hormone, and insulin; pineal functions. Antagonizes some somatostatin effects

virilization Masculinization. Can designate acquisition of male characteristics by genetic females (growth of facial hair, enlargement of the clitoris, etc.)

vitiligo Lighter patches in normally pigmented skin regions associated with loss of functioning melanocytes. Often attributed to autoimmune processes

Abbreviations and Acronyms

ACE Angiotensin-converting enzyme
ACTH Adrenocorticotropic hormone
ADH Antidiuretic hormone (vasopressin)
AGHD Adult growth hormone deficiency
ALL Acute lympocytic leukemia
ALT (SGPT, GPT) Alanine aminotransferase
AS Angelman syndrome
ASD Atrial septal defect
AST (SGOT, GOT) Aspartate aminotransferase
AVP Arginine vasopressin
BMD Bone mineral density
BMI Body mass index
BP Blood pressure
CAD Coronary artery disease
CAH Congenital adrenal hyperplasia
CATCH 22 Syndrome of **c**ardiac defect, **a**bnormal facies, **t**hymic hypoplasia, **c**left palate, and **h**ypocalcemia (DiGeorge 22q11.2 deletion syndrome)
CBG Cortisol-binding globulin
CD8+ Cytotoxic T cell
CDGP Constitutional delay of growth and puberty
CF Cystic fibrosis
CHD Congenital heart disease
CHF Congestive heart failure
CKD Chronic kidney disease
CMV Cytomegalovirus
CNS Central nervous system
CRF Corticotropin-releasing factor
CRH Corticotropin-releasing hormone
CRP C-reactive protein
CT Computed tomography
DBP Diastolic blood pressure
DCCT Diabetes Control and Complications Trial
DHEA-S Dehydroepiandrosterone sulfate
DI Diabetes insipidus
DKA Diabetic ketoacidosis

GLOSSARY 17

DM Diabetes mellitus
DNA Deoxyribonucleic acid
DOC Deoxycorticosterone
DXA Dual energy X-ray absorptiometry
ESRD End-stage renal disease
FG Fasting glucose
FH Familial hypercholesterolemia
FISH Fluorescence in situ hybridization
FNA Fine-needle aspiration
FPG Fasting plasma glucose
FSH Follicle-stimulating hormone
FSS Familial short stature
GAD Glutamic acid decarboxylase
GH Growth hormone
GHD Growth hormone deficiency
GHRH Growth hormone–releasing hormone
GnRH Gonadotropin-releasing hormone
HC Head circumference
HCG Human chorionic gonadotropin
HCO₃ Bicarbonate
HDL High-density lipoprotein
HEENT Head, eyes, ears, nose, throat
HgbA1c Hemoglobin A1c (human)
HPI/ROS History of present illness/review of systems
hPL High placental analog of prolactin
3β-HSD 3-Beta hydroxysteroid dehydrogenase
ICMA Immunochemiluminometric assay
ICP Intracranial pressure
IgA Immunoglobulin A
IGF-1 Insulin-like growth factor 1
IGFBP-3 Insulin-like growth factor–binding protein 3
IGFD Insulin-like growth factor deficiency
IFG Impaired fasting glucose
IgG Immunoglobulin G
IRMA Immunoradiometric assay
ISS Idiopathic short stature

IUGR Intrauterine growth retardation
17-KS 17-Ketosteroid
LDL-C Low-density lipoprotein cholesterol
LH Luteinizing hormone
LHRH Luteinizing hormone–releasing hormone
MEN Multiple endocrine neoplasia
MODY Maturity onset diabetes of the young
MPHD Multiple pituitary hormone deficiencies
MRI Magnetic resonance imaging
NCEP National Cholesterol Education Program
NGSP National Glycohemaglobin Standardization
NHANES National Health and Nutrition Examination Survey
NHL Non-Hodgkin's lymphoma
NIDDM Non-insulin dependent diabetes mellitus
OCP Oral contraceptive pill
OGTT Oral glucose tolerance test
17-OHCS 17-Hydroxycorticosteroid
OTC Over the counter
PCOS Polycystic ovarian syndrome (Stein-Leventhal syndrome)
PDA Patent ductus arteriosus
PG Plasma glucose
PNET Primitive neurectodermal tumor
POMC Pro-opiomelanocortin
PRL Prolactin
PSS Psychosocial short stature
PTH Parathyroid hormone
PTU Propylthiouracil
PWS Prader-Willi syndrome
rhIGF-1 Recombinant human insulin-like growth factor-1
RSS Russell-Silver syndrome
SBP Systolic blood pressure
SCFE Slipped capital femoral epiphysis
SDS Standard deviation scores
SGA Small for gestational age
SHBG Sex hormone–binding globulin
SHOX Short-stature homeobox–containing gene

17

GLOSSARY

SIADH Syndrome of inappropriate secretion of antidiuretic hormone
SMBG Self-monitoring blood glucose
SOD Septo-optic dysplasia
SSKI Potassium iodide
TBG Thyroxine-binding globulin
TBI Total body irradiation
TG Triglyceride
TORCH Toxoplasmosis, other infections, rubella, cytomegalovirus, herpes simplex virus
TRH Thyrotropin-releasing hormone
TSH Thyroid-stimulating hormone

⑱ REFERENCES AND SUGGESTED READINGS

1 GENERAL ENDOCRINE ASSESSMENT
References

1. Namour N. Adolescent medicine. In Johns Hopkins Hospital, Custer JW, Rau RE, et al, eds. The Harriet Lane Handbook, 18th ed. St Louis: Mosby Elsevier, 2009.
2. Hall JG, Froster-Iskenius UG, Allanson JE. Handbook of Normal Physical Measurements. Oxford, England: Oxford University Press, 1989.
3. Custer JW, Rau RE, eds. The Harriet Lane Handbook, 18th ed. St Louis: Mosby Elsevier, 2009.
4. Murray PA, Davis HA, Hamp M. Pediatric and adolescent gynecology. In Zitelli BJ, Davis HW, eds. Atlas of Pediatric Physical Diagnosis, 3rd ed. St Louis: Elsevier, 1997.
5. Feigelman S. The first year. In Kliegman RM, Behrman RE, Jenson HB, et al, eds. Nelson Textbook of Pediatrics, 18th ed. Philadelphia: Saunders, 2007.
6. Carrillo AA, Lifshitz F. Reference charts used frequently by endocrinologists. In Lifshitz F, ed. Pediatric Endocrinology, 5th ed. New York: Informa Healthcare, 2007.
7. Frazier A, Pruette CS. Cardiology. In Custer JW, Rau RE, eds. The Harriet Lane Handbook, 18th ed. St Louis: Mosby Elsevier, 2009.
8. Dawood FS. Pulmonology. In Custer JW, Rau RE, eds. The Harriet Lane Handbook, 18th ed. St Louis: Mosby Elsevier, 2009.
9. National Heart Lung and Blood Institute. Blood pressure tables for children and adolescents. Available at *www.nhlb.nih.gov/guidelines/hypertension/child_tabl.pdf*.

2 ADRENAL DISORDERS
References

1. Porterfield S, ed. Endocrine Physiology. St Louis: Mosby–Year Book, 1997.
2. New M, Ghizzoni L, Speiser PW. Update on congenital adrenal hyperplasia. In Lifshitz F, ed. Pediatric Endocrinology, 3rd ed. New York: Marcel Dekker, 1996.
3. Pang SY, Lerner AJ, Stoner E, et al. Late-onset adrenal steroid 3 beta-hydroxysteroid dehydrogenase deficiency. I. A cause of hirsutism in pubertal and postpubertal women. J Clin Endocrinol Metab 60:428-439, 1985.
4. New MI, del Balso P, Crawford C, et al. The adrenal cortex. In Kaplan S, ed. Clinical Pediatric Endocrinology. Philadelphia: WB Saunders, 1990.
5. Cerasuolo K. The child with endocrine dysfunction. In Hockenberry MJ, Wilson D, eds. Wong's Nursing Care of Infants and Children, 8th ed. St Louis: Mosby Elsevier, 2007.

Suggested Readings

Custer JW, Rau RE, eds. The Harriett Lane Handbook, 18th ed. Philadelphia: Mosby Elsevier, 2009.
Donohoue PA. Adrenal disorders. In Kappy MS, Allen DB, Geffner ME, eds. Pediatric Practice: Endocrinology. New York: McGraw-Hill, 2010.
Styne DM. Pediatric Endocrinology. Philadelphia: Lippincott Williams & Wilkins, 2004.

Voorhess ML. Urinary catecholamine excretion by healthy children. I. Daily excretion of dopamine, norepinephrine, epinephrine, and 3-methoxy-4-hydroxymandelic acid. Pediatrics 39:252-257, 1967.

Weetman RM, Rider PS, Oei TO, et al. Effect of diet on urinary excretion of VMA, HVA, metanephrine, and total free catecholamine in normal preschool children. J Pediatr 88:46-50, 1976.

3 BONE MINERALIZATION AND METABOLIC DISORDERS

References

1. Moll GW. A Medical Student's Guide to Pediatric Endocrinology [unpublished manual]. Jackson, MS, 1992.
2. David L. Common Vitamin D Deficiency Rickets. Nestle Nutrition Workshop Series, vol 21. New York: Raven Press, 1991.
3. Mace SE. Rickets: reemergence of an old disease with a strategy for prevention. J Clin Outcomes Manag 3:23-31, 1996.
4. Dimitri P, Bishop N. Rickets: new insights into a re-emerging problem. Curr Opin Orthop 18:486-493, 2007.
5. Nield LS, Mahajan P, Joshi A, et al. Rickets: not a disease of the past. Am Fam Physician 74:619-626, 2006.
6. Henderson A. Vitamin D and the breastfed infant. J Obstet Gynecol Neonatal Nurs 34:367-372, 2005.
7. Ward LM, Gaboury I, Ladhani M, et al. Vitamin D-deficiency rickets among children in Canada. CMAJ 177:161-166, 2007.
7a. Wagner CL, Greer FR. Prevention of rickets and vitamin D deficiency in infants, children and adolescents. Pediatrics 112:1142-1152, 2008.
8. Hartman JJ. Vitamin D deficiency rickets in children: prevalence and need for community education. Orthop Nurs 19:63-67; quiz 67-69, 2000.
9. Glorieux FH, Chabot G, Tau C. Familial Hypophosphatemic Rickets: Pathophysiology and Medical Management. Nestle Nutrition Workshop Series, vol 21. New York: Raven Press, 1991.
10. McBride A, Edwards M, Monsell F, et al. Vitamin D-resistant rickets (X-linked hypophosphataemic rickets). Curr Orthop 21:369-399, 2007.
11. Haffner D, Nissel R, Wühl E, et al. Effects of growth hormone treatment on body proportions and final height among small children with X-linked hypophosphatemic rickets. Pediatrics 113:593-596, 2004.
12. Carpenter TO. New perspectives on the biology and treatment of X-linked hypophosphatemic rickets. Pediatr Clin North Am 44:443-466, 1997.
13. Goodyer PR, Kronick JB, Jequier S, et al. Nephrocalcinosis and its relationship to treatment of hereditary rickets. J Pediatr 111:700-704, 1987.

14. Verge CF, Lam A, Simpson JM, et al. Effects of therapy in X-linked hypophosphatemic rickets. N Engl J Med 325:1843-1848, 1991.
15. Glorieux FH. Rickets, the continuing challenge. N Engl J Med 325:1875-1877, 1991.
16. Lips P, van Schoor NM, Bravenboer N. Vitamin D dependent rickets. In Rosen CJ, ed. Primer on the Metabolic Bone Diseases and Disorders of Mineral Metabolism, 7th ed. Philadelphia: JW Wiley, 2008.
17. Perheentupa J. Hypoparathyroidism and mineral homeostasis. In Lifshitz F, ed. Pediatric Endocrinology, 4th ed. New York: Marcel Dekker, 2003.
18. Rivkees SA, Carpenter TO. Hyperparathyroidism in children. In Lifshitz F, ed. Pediatric Endocrinology, 4th ed. New York: Marcel Dekker, 2003.
19. Sheth DP. Hypocalcemic seizures in neonates. Am J Emerg Med 15:638-641, 1997.
20. Koo WWK. Neonatal calcium and phosphorus disorders. In Lifshitz F, ed. Pediatric Endocrinology, 4th ed. New York: Marcel Dekker, 2003.
21. Gertner JM. Calcium control in the newborn. Presented at the Serono Symposia USA and the Lawson Wilkins Pediatric Endocrine Society International Symposium: A Current Review of Pediatric Endocrinology. Washington, DC, April/May 1997.
22. Gertner JM. Metabolic bone disease. In Lifshitz F, ed. Pediatric Endocrinology, 4th ed. New York: Marcel Dekker, 2003.
23. Rauch F, Bishop N. Juvenile osteoporosis. In Rosen CJ, ed. Primer on the Metabolic Bone Diseases and Disorders of Mineral Metabolism, 7th ed. Philadelphia: JW Wiley, 2008.
24. Moshang T. Osteoporosis. In Moshang T, ed. Pediatric Endocrinology: The Requisites in Pediatrics. St Louis: Mosby Elsevier, 2005.
25. Weinstein RS. Glucocorticoid-induced osteoporosis. In Rosen CJ, ed. Primer on the Metabolic Bone Diseases and Disorders of Mineral Metabolism, 7th ed. Philadelphia: JW Wiley, 2008.
26. Ward L, Tricco AC, Phuong P, et al. Bisphosphonate therapy for children and adolescents with secondary osteoporosis. Cochrane Database Syst Rev CD005324, 2007.
27. Hamdy NA. Osteoporosis: other secondary causes. In Rosen CJ, ed. Primer on the Metabolic Bone Diseases and Disorders of Mineral Metabolism, 7th ed. Philadelphia: JW Wiley, 2008.

Suggested Readings

Gafni RI. Measuring bone density in children. Contemp Pediatr 25:64-71, 2008.
Kalkwarf HJ, Zemel BS, Gilsanz V, et al. The bone mineral density in childhood study: bone mineral content and density according to age, sex, and race. J Clin Endocrinol Metab 92:2087-2099, 2007.
Steelman J, Zeitler P. Treatment of symptomatic pediatric osteoporosis with cyclic single-day intravenous pamidronate infusions. J Pediatr 142:417-423, 2003.

4 DISORDERS OF GLUCOSE METABOLISM

References

1. Cryer PE. Glucose homeostasis and hypoglycemia. In Kronenburg HM, Melmed S, Polonsky KS, et al, eds. Williams Textbook of Endocrinology, 11th ed. Philadelphia: Saunders Elsevier, 2008.

2. Langdon DR, Stanley CA, Sperling MA. Hypoglycemia in the infant and child. In Sperling MA, ed. Pediatric Endocrinology. Philadelphia: Saunders Elsevier, 2008.

3. American Diabetes Association Position Statement. Diagnosis and Classification of Diabetes Mellitus. Diabetes Care 33(Suppl 1):S62-S69, 2010.

4. Cooke DW, Plotnick L, Dabelea D, et al. Diabetes mellitus. In Kappy MS, Allen DB, Geffner ME, eds. Pediatric Practice: Endocrinology. New York: McGraw Hill Medical, 2010.

5. American Diabetes Association Consensus Statement. Type 2 Diabetes in Children and Adolescents. Diabetes Care 23:381-389, 2000.

6. Gallo l, Silverstein JH, Winter W. Other specific types of diabetes mellitus and causes of hyperglycemia. In Kappy MS, Allen DB, Geffner ME, eds. Pediatric Practice Endocrinology. New York: McGraw Hill Medical, 2010.

7. American Diabetes Association Position Statement. Standards of Medical Care in Diabetes—2011. Diabetes Care 33(Suppl 1):S11-S61, 2011.

8. Franz MJ. Nutrition. In Funnell MM, Hunt C, Kulkarni K, et al, eds. A Core Curriculum for Diabetes Education, 3rd ed. Chicago: American Association of Diabetes Educators, 1998.

9. Sperling MA, Weinzimer SA, Tamborlane WV. Diabetes mellitus. In Sperling MA, ed. Pediatric Endocrinology. Philadelphia: Saunders Elsevier, 2008.

10. Ballal SA, McIntosh P. Endocrinology. In Custer JW, Rau RE, eds. The Harriet Lane Handbook. St Louis: Mosby Elsevier, 2009.

11. Chase HP, Banion C. Low blood sugar (hypoglycemia or insulin reaction). In Chase HP, ed. Understanding Diabetes: A Handbook for People Who Are Living With Diabetes, 11th ed. Denver: Paros Press, 2006.

12. Trence DL. Hyperglycemia. In Mensing C, McLaughlin S, Halstenson C, eds. The Art and Science of Diabetes Self-Management Education Desk Reference, 2nd ed. Chicago: American Association of Diabetes Educators, 2011.

13. Tomky DM, Kulkarni K. Intensifying insulin therapy: multiple daily injections to pump therapy. In Mensing C, ed. The Art and Science of Diabetes Self-Management Education: A Desk Reference for Healthcare Professionals. Chicago: American Association of Diabetes Educators, 2006.

14. Chase HP, Gaston J, Messer L. Who should use continuous glucose monitoring (CGM)? In Chase HP. Understanding Insulin Pumps and Continuous Glucose Monitors. Denver: Children's Diabetes Foundation, 2007.

15. Bode BW, Tamborlane WV, Davidson PC. Insulin pump therapy in the 21st century. Strategies for successful use in adults, adolescents, and children with diabetes. Postgrad Med 11:69-78, 2002.

16. Kaufman FR, Halvorson M, Carpenter S, et al. Pump therapy for children: weighing the risks and benefits: view 2: insulin pump therapy in young children with diabetes. Diabetes Spectr 14:84-89, 2001.

Suggested Readings

American Diabetes Association Position Statement. Diabetes Care in the School and Day Care Setting. Diabetes Care 33:(Suppl 1)S70-S74, 2010.

Nabors L, Troillett A, Nash T, et al. School nurse perceptions of barriers and supports for children with diabetes. J Sch Health 75:119-124, 2005.

Nathan DM, Balkau B, Bonora E, et al. International Expert Committee report on the role of the A1C assay in the diagnosis of diabetes. Diabetes Care 32:1327-1334, 2009.

National Diabetes Education Program. Helping the Student with Diabetes Succeed: A Guide for School Personnel. Bethesda, MD: National Institutes of Health (NIH publication no. 03-5127), 2003.

Owen S. Pediatric pumps: barriers and breakthroughs. Diabetes Educ 32(Suppl 1):S29-S38, 2006.

5 OBESITY

References

1. Centers for Disease Control and Prevention. Health, United States, 2010: Available at *www.cdc.gov/nchs/data/hus/hus10.pdf.*

2. Epstein LH, Myers M, Raynor H, et al. Treatment of pediatric obesity. Pediatrics 101:554-570, 1998.

3. Barlow SE, Dietz WH. Obesity evaluation and treatment: expert committee recommendations. Pediatrics 102;1-11, 1998.

4. International Obesity Task Force (IOTF) 2008. Available at *www.archive2.official-documents.co.uk/documents/deps/doh/survey02/hcyp/tables/hcypt159.htm.*

5. Institute of Medicine, Preventing Childhood Obesity: Health in Balance. Washington, DC: The Institute, 2005.

6. Barlow SE, Dietz WH. Obesity evaluation and treatment: Expert Committee recommendations. The Maternal and Child Health Bureau, Health Resources and Services Administration and the Department of Health and Human Services. Pediatrics 102:E29, 1998.

7. Krebs NF, Himes JH, Jacobson D, et al. Assessment of child and adolescent overweight and obesity. Pediatrics 120(Suppl 4):S193-S228, 2007.

8. Goran MI. Measurement issues related to studies of childhood obesity: assessment of body composition, body fat distribution, physical activity, and food intake. Pediatrics 101:505-518, 1998.

9. Freedman DS, Mei Z, Srinivasan SR, et al. Cardiovascular risk factors and excess adiposity among overweight children and adolescents: the Bogalusa Heart Study. J Pediatr 150:12-17, 2007.

10. Bristol-Myers Squibb Co. Glucophage (metformin hydrochloride tablets) and Glucophage XR (metformin hydrochloride extended-release tablets). Prescribing information, 2008.

11. Hill JO, Trowbridge FL. Childhood obesity: future directions and research priorities. Pediatrics 101:570-574, 1998.

12. Welch MJ, Harbaugh BL. End the epidemic of childhood obesity...one family at a time. Am Nurse Today 3:26-31, 2008.
13. Freemark M. Pharmacotherapy of childhood obesity: an evidence-based, conceptual approach. Diabetes Care 30:395-402, 2007.
14. Deglin JH, Vallerand AH. Davis Drug Guide for Nurses , 11th ed. Philadelphia: FA Davis, 2008, p 913.
15. Alli. The truth about treatment effects. Available at *www.myalli.com.*

6 HYPERLIPIDEMIA

References

1. Kwiterovich PO. Cut points for lipids and lipoproteins in children and adolescents: should they be reassessed? Clin Chem 54:1113-1115, 2008.
2. Kavey RE, Allada V, Daniels SR, et al. Cardiovascular risk reduction in high-risk pediatric patients: a scientific statement from the American Heart Association Expert Panel on Population and Prevention Science; the Councils on Cardiovascular Disease in the Young, Epidemiology and Prevention, Nutrition, Physical Activity and Metabolism, High Blood Pressure Research, Cardiovascular Nursing, and the Kidney in Heart Disease; and the Interdisciplinary Working Group on Quality of Care and Outcomes Research: endorsed by the American Academy of Pediatrics. Circulation 114:2710-2738, 2006.
3. Wald DS, Bestwick JP, Wald NJ. Child-parent screening for familial hypercholesterolaemia: screening strategy based on a meta-analysis. BMJ 335:599, 2007.
4. Nicholls DP, Cather M, Byrne C, et al. Diagnosis of heterozygous familial hypercholesterolaemia in children. Int J Clin Pract 62:990-994, 2008.
5. Kwiterovich PO Jr. Recognition and management of dyslipidemia in children and adolescents. J Clin Endocrinol Metab 93:4200-4209, 2008.
6. Sigfússon G, Fricker JF, Bernstein D, et al. Long-term survivors of pediatric heart transplantation: a multicenter report of sixty-eight children who have survived longer than five years. J Pediatr 130:862-871, 1977.
7. de Ferranti S, Ludwig DS. Storm over statins—the controversy surrounding pharmacologic treatment of children. N Engl J Med 359:1309-1312, 2008.
8. van der Graaf A, Rodenburg J, Vissers MN, et al. Atherogenic liproprotein particle size and concentrations and the effect of pravastatin in children with familial hypercholesterolemia. J Pediatr 152:873-878, 2008.
9. RxList: The Internet Drug Index, 2009. Available at *www.rxlist.com.*
10. Pfizer, Inc. Lipitor (atorvastatin calcium). Available at *www.lipitor.com.*
11. Hill JO, Trowbridge FL. Childhood obesity: future directions and research priorities. Pediatrics 101(3 Pt 2):570-574, 1998.
12. Deglin JH, Vallerand AH. Davis's Drug Guide for Nurses, 11th ed. Philadelphia: FA Davis Company, 2009.

13. Soriano-Guillén L, Hernández-García B, Pita J, et al. High-sensitivity C-reactive protein is a good marker of cardiovascular risk in obese children and adolescents. Eur J Endocrinol 159:R1-R4, 2008.
14. Thompson GR; HEART-UK LDL Apheresis Working Group. Recommendations for the use of LDL apheresis. Atherosclerosis 198:247-255, 2008.
15. Palcoux JB, Atassi-Dumont M, Lefevre P, et al. Low-density lipoprotein apheresis in children with familial hypercholesterolemia: follow-up to 21 years. Ther Apher Dial 12:195-201, 2008.
16. Martino F, Loffredo L, Carnevale R, et al. Oxidative stress is associated with arterial dysfunction and enhanced intima-media thickness in children with hypercholesterolemia: the potential role of nicotinamide-adenine dinucleotide phosphate oxidase. Pediatrics 122:e648-e655, 2008.

7 PITUITARY DISORDERS

References

1. Porterfield SP, ed. Endocrine Physiology, 2nd ed. St Louis: Elsevier, 2001.
2. Reiter EO, Rosenfeld RG. Normal and aberrant growth. In Wilson JD, Foster DW, Kronenberg HM, eds. Williams Textbook of Endocrinology, 9th ed. Philadelphia: WB Saunders, 1998.
3. Molitch ME, Clemmons DR, Malozowski S, et al. Evaluation and treatment of adult growth hormone deficiency: an Endocrine Society Clinical Practice Guideline. J Clin Endocrinol Metab 91:1621-1634, 2006.
4. Cohen P, Rogol AD, Deal CL, et al. Consensus statement on the diagnosis and treatment of children with idiopathic short stature: a summary of the Growth Hormone Research Society, the Lawson Wilkins Pediatric Endocrine Society, and the European Society for Paediatric Endocrinology Workshop. J Clin Endocrinol Metab 93:4210-4217, 2008.
5. Toumba M, Bacopoulou I, Savva SC, et al. Efficacy of combined treatment with growth hormone and gonadotropin releasing hormone analogue in children with poor prognosis of adult height. Indian Pediatr 44:497-502, 2007.
6. Mauras N, Gonzalez de Pijem L, Hsiang HY, et al. Anastrozole increases predicted adult height of short adolescent males treated with growth hormone: a randomized, placebo-controlled, multicenter trial for one to three years. J Clin Endocrinol Metab 93:823-831, 2008.
7. Bakker B, Frane J, Anhalt H, et al. Height velocity targets from the national cooperative growth study for first year growth hormone responses in short children. J Clin Endocrinol Metab 93:352-357, 2007.
8. Chernausek SD, Backeljauw PF, Frane J, et al. Long-term treatment with recombinant insulin-like growth factor (IGF)-1 in children with severe IGF-1 deficiency due to growth hormone insensitivity. J Clin Endocrinol Metab 92:902-910, 2001.

Suggested Readings

Altschuler SM, Ludwig S, eds. Pediatrics at a Glance. Philadelphia: Current Medicine, 1998.

Backeljauw P, Bang P, Clayton PE, et al. Diagnosis and management of primary insulin-like growth factor-1 deficiency: current perspectives and clinical update. Pediatr Endocrinol Rev 7(Suppl 1):S154-S170, 2010.

Bercu BB. Disorders of GH neurosecretion. In Lifshitz F, ed. Pediatric Endocrinology, 3rd ed. New York: Marcel Dekker, 1996.

Bhangoo A, Anahlt H, Rosenfeld RG. Idiopathic short stature. In Lifshitz F, ed. Pediatric Endocrinology, 5th ed. New York: Informa Healthcare, 2007.

Blizzard RM, Bulatovic A. Syndromes of psychosocial short stature. In Lifshitz F, ed. Pediatric Endocrinology, 3rd ed. New York: Marcel Dekker, 1996.

Blizzard RM, Johanson A. Disorders of growth. In Kappy MS, Blizzard RM, Migeon CJ, eds. Wilkins—The Diagnosis and Treatment of Endocrine Disorders in Childhood and Adolescence, 4th ed. Springfield, IL: Charles C Thomas, 1994.

Bode HH, Crawford JD, Danon M. Disorders of antidiuretic hormone homeostasis. In Lifshitz F, ed. Pediatric Endocrinology, 3rd ed. New York: Marcel Dekker, 1996.

Castro-Magana M, Angulo M. Lectures on growth hormone deficiency, growth hormone excess, hyperprolactinemia. Presented at the Endocrinology Rounds, Mineola, NY, Oct 1999.

Clayton PE, Cianfarani S, Czernichow P, et al. Management of the child born small for gestational age through to adulthood: a consensus statement of the International Societies of Pediatric Endocrinology and the Growth Hormone Research Society. J Clin Endocrinol Metab 92:804-810, 2007.

Fisher DA, Ladenson PW, eds. The Corning Endocrine Manual: A Guide to Selection and Interpretation of Endocrine Tests. San Juan Capistrano, CA: Corning Nichols Institute, 1996.

Grimberg A. Worrisome growth. In Lifshitz F, ed. Pediatric Endocrinology, 5th ed. New York: Informa Healthcare, 2007.

Growth Hormone Research Society. Consensus guidelines for the diagnosis and treatment of growth hormone (GH) deficiency in childhood and adolescence: summary statement of the GH Research Society. J Clin Endocrinol Metab 85:3990-3993, 2000.

Nathan BM, Allen DB. Growth hormone treatment. In Lifshitz F, ed. Pediatric Endocrinology, 5th ed. New York: Informa Healthcare, 2007.

Newman CB, Kleinberg DL. Adult growth hormone deficiency. Endocrinologist 8:78-186, 1998.

Nishi Y. Hereditary growth hormone deficiency and growth hormone insensitivity syndrome. In Lifshitz F, ed. Pediatric Endocrinology, 3rd ed. New York: Marcel Dekker, 1996.

Porterfield SP. Endocrine Physiology. St Louis: Mosby–Year Book, 1997.

Reiter EO, Rosenfeld RG. Normal and aberrant growth. In Kronenberg HM, Melmed S, Polonsky HK, et al, eds. Williams Textbook of Endocrinology, 11th ed. Philadelphia: Saunders Elsevier, 2007.

Root AW, Diamond FB. Overgrowth syndromes: evaluation and management of the child with excessive linear growth. In Lifshitz F, ed. Pediatric Endocrinology, 5th ed. New York: Informa Healthcare, 2007.

Rosenbloom AL, Connor EL. Hypopituitarism and other disorders of the growth hormone and insulin-like growth factor axis. In Lifshitz F, ed. Pediatric Endocrinology, 5th ed. New York: Informa Healthcare, 2007.

Rosenfeld R. A review of IGF-1 deficiency: from molecular mechanisms to clinical experience and appropriate patient selection. Horm Res 65(Suppl 1):S1-S34, 2006.

Shiminski-Maher T. Diabetes insipidus and syndrome of inappropriate secretion of anti-diuretic hormone in children with midline suprasellar brain tumors. J Pediatr Oncol Nurs 8:106-111, 1991.

Siberry GK, Iannone R, eds. The Harriet Lane Handbook. St Louis: Mosby–Year Book, 2000.

Vance ML. New directions in the treatment of hyperprolactinemia. Endocrinologist 7:153-159, 1997.

8 DISORDERS OF SEXUAL DEVELOPMENT

References

1. Brito VN, Latronico AC, Arnhold IJ, et al. Update on the etiology, diagnosis and therapeutic management of sexual precocity. Arq Bras Endocrinol Metabol 52:18-31, 2008.

2. Cools BL, Rooman R, Op De Beeck L, et al. Boys with a simple delayed puberty reach their target height. Horm Res 70:209-214, 2008.

3. MacGillivray MH. Induction of puberty in hypogonadal children. J Pediatr Endocrinol Metab 17(Suppl 4):S1277-S1287, 2004.

4. Laituri CA, Garey CL, Ostlie DJ, et al. Treatment of adolescent gynecomastia. J Pediatr Surg 45:650-654, 2010.

5. Physicians' Desk Reference, 65th ed. Monvale, NJ: Medical Economics, 2011.

6. Package insert for Protropin. Genentech, Inc, San Francisco, 1995.

7. Lee P, Houk C. Puberty and its disorders. In Lifshitz F, ed. Pediatric Endocrinology, 5th ed. New York: Informa Healthcare, 2007.

8. Fulghesu A, Magnini R, Portoghese E, et al. Obesity-related lipid profile and altered insulin incretion in adolescents with polycystic ovary syndrome. J Adolesc Health 46:474-481, 2010.

9. Witchel S. Hirsutism and polycystic ovary syndrome. In Lifshitz F, ed. Pediatric Endocrinology, 5th ed. New York: Informa Healthcare, 2007.

10. Rotterdam ESHRE/ASRM-Sponsored PCOS consensus workshop group. Revised 2003 consensus on diagnostic criteria and long-term health risks related to polycystic ovary syndrome (PCOS). Hum Reprod 19:41-47, 2004.

Suggested Readings

Ergun-Longmire B, Maclaren NK. Insulin resistance syndrome in childhood and beyond. In Lifshitz F, ed. Pediatric Endocrinology, 5th ed. New York: Informa Healthcare, 2007.

Martin KA, Change RJ, Ehrmann DA, et al. Evaluation and treatment of hirsutism in premenopausal women: an endocrine society clinical practice guideline. J Clin Endocrinol Metab 93:1105-1120, 2008.

Needlmen RD. Adolescence. In Behrman RE, Kliegman RM, Jenson HB, eds. Nelson Textbook of Pediatrics, 17th ed. Philadelphia: WB Saunders, 2004.

Root AW. Precocious puberty. Pediatr Rev 21:10-19, 2000.

Styne DM. Disorders of puberty. In Fitzgerald PA, ed. Handbook of Clinical Endocrinology. Norwalk, CT: Appleton & Lange, 1992.

Zeitler PS, Travers S, Kappy MS. Advances in the recognition and treatment of endocrine complications in children with chronic illness. Adv Pediatr 46:101-149, 1999.

9 THYROID DISORDERS

References

1. Van Vliet G, Polak M. Thyroid disorders in infancy. In Lifshitz F, ed. Pediatric Endocrinology, 5th ed. New York: Informa Healthcare, 2007.

2. Fisher DA, Grueters A. Disorders of the thyroid in the newborn and infant. In Sperling MA, ed. Pediatric Endocrinology, 3rd ed. Philadelphia: Saunders Elsevier, 2008.

3. Styne DM. Disorders of the thyroid gland. In Styne DM, ed. Pediatric Endocrinology. Philadelphia: Lippincott Williams & Wilkins, 2003.

4. LaFranchi SH, Austin J. How should we be treating children with congenital hypothyroidism? J Pediatr Endocrinol Metab 20:559-578, 2007.

5. Larson CA. Congenital hypothyroidism. In Radovick S, MacGillivray MH, eds. Contemporary Endocrinology: A Practical Clinical Guide. Totowa, NJ: Humana Press, 2010.

6. Fisher DA, Grueters A. Thyroid disorders in children and adolescents. In Sperling MA, ed. Pediatric Endocrinology, 3rd ed. Philadelphia: Saunders Elsevier, 2008.

7. Brook CG, Brown RS, eds. Handbook of Clinical Pediatric Endocrinology. Malden, MA: Blackwell, 2008.

8. Huang SA. Hypothyroidism. In Lifshitz F, ed. Pediatric Endocrinology, 5th ed. New York: Informa Healthcare, 2007.

9. Huang SA, Reed PR. Autoimmune thyroid disease. In Radovick S, MacGillivray MH, eds. Contemporary Endocrinology: Pediatric Endocrinology: A Practical Clinical Guide, Totowa, NJ: Humana Press, 2010.

10. Dallas JS, Foley TP Jr. Hyperthyroidism. In Lifshitz F, ed. Pediatric Endocrinology, 5th ed. New York: Informa Healthcare, 2007.

11. Rivkees SA, Mattison DR. Propylthiouracil (PTU) hepatotoxicity in children and recommendations for discontinuation of use. Int J Pediatr Endocrinol 2009:132041, 2009.

12. Huang S. Thyromegaly. In Lifshitz F, ed. Pediatric Endocrinology, 5th ed. New York: Informa Healthcare, 2007.

13. LaFranchi S. Thyroid hormone in hypopituitarism, Graves' disease, congenital hypothyroidism, and maternal thyroid disease during pregnancy. Growth Horm IGF Res 16(Suppl A):S20-S24, 2006.
14. Halac I, Zimmerman D. Thyroid tumors in children. In Lifshitz F, ed. Pediatric Endocrinology, 5th ed. New York: Informa Healthcare, 2007.
15. Halac I, Zimmerman D. Thyroid nodules and cancers in children. Endocrinol Metab Clin North Am 34:725-744, 2005.
16. Sklar CA, La Quaglia MP. Thyroid cancer in children and adolescents. In Radovick S, MacGillivray MH, eds. Contemporary Endocrinology: Pediatric Endocrinology: A Practical Clinical Guide. Totowa, NJ: Humana Press, 2010.
17. Hanna CE, LaFranchi SH. Adolescent thyroid disorders. Adolesc Med 13:13-35, 2002.

Suggested Readings

Beck-Peccoz P, Persani L, LaFranchi S. Safety of medications and hormones used in the treatment of pediatric thyroid disorders. Pediatr Endocrinol Rev 2(Suppl 1):124-133, 2004.

Cohen RN. Resistance to thyroid hormone and TSH receptor mutations. In Radovick S, MacGillivray MH, eds. Contemporary Endocrinology: Pediatric Endocrinology: A Practical Clinical Guide. Totowa, NJ: Humana Press, 2010.

DeBoer MD, LaFranchi SH. Pediatric thyroid testing issues. Endocrinol Rev 5(Suppl 1):S570-S577, 2007.

Ballal SA, McIntosh P. Endocrinology. In Custer JW, Rau RE, eds. The Harriet Lane Handbook, 18th ed. St Louis: Mosby Elsevier, 2009.

Rovet J. Congenital hypothyroidism. In Rourke B, ed. Syndrome of Nonverbal Learning Disabilities: Neurodevelopmental Manifestations. New York: Guilford Press, 1995.

Rovet J, Walker W, Bliss B, et al. Long-term sequelae of hearing impairment in congenital hypothyroidism. J Pediatr 128:776-783, 1996.

Selva KA, Harper S, Downs A, et al. Neurodevelopmental outcomes in congenital hypothyroidism: comparison of initial T4 dose and time to reach target T4 and TSH. J Pediatr 147:775-780, 2005.

Selva KA, Mandel SH, Rien L, et al. Initial treatment dose of L-thyroxine in congenital hypothyroidism. J Pediatr 141:775-780, 2005.

Takemoto C, Hodding JH, Kraus DM, eds. Pediatric Dosage Handbook, 13th ed. Hudson, OH: Lexi-Comp Inc, 2011.

10 EFFECTS OF CANCER THERAPY AND CHRONIC ILLNESS

References

1. Sklar C, Boulad F, Small T, et al. Endocrine complications of pediatric stem cell transplantation. Front Biosci 6:G17-G22, 2001.
2. Gleeson HK, Shalet SM. Endocrine complications of neoplastic diseases in children and adolescents. Curr Opin Pediatr 13:346-351, 2001.
3. Nandagopal R, Laverdière C, Mulrooney D, et al. Endocrine late effects of childhood cancer therapy: a report from the Children's Oncology Group. Horm Res 69:65-74, 2008.

4. Rappaport R, Thibaud E. Endocrine problems after cancer therapy. In Lifshitz F, ed. Pediatric Endocrinology, 3rd ed. New York: Marcel Dekker, 1996.
5. Stanhope R, Papodimitriou A, Chessills JM, et al. Precocious and premature puberty following prophylactic cranial irradiation in acute lymphoblastic leukemia. In Green DB, D'Angio GJ, eds. Late Effects of Treatment for Childhood Cancer. New York: Wiley-Liss, 1992.
6. Pieters RS. Side effects of radiation therapy in children and their prevention and management. In Ablin AR, ed. Supportive Care of Children With Cancer. Baltimore: The Johns Hopkins University Press, 1997.
7. Bottomley SJ. Central nervous system. In Hockenberry-Eaton MJ, ed. Essentials of Pediatric Oncology Nursing: A Core Curriculum. Glenview, IL: Association of Pediatric Oncology Nurses, 1998.
8. Hobbie W, Brophy P. Hypothalamic-pituitary axis. In Hockenberry-Eaton MJ, ed. Essentials of Pediatric Oncology Nursing: A Core Curriculum. Glenview, IL: Association of Pediatric Oncology Nurses, 1998.
9. Muller J. Disturbances of pubertal development after cancer treatment. Best Pract Res Clin Endocrinol Metab 16:91-103, 2002.
10. DeSantes K, Quinn JJ. The care of the pediatric patient after hematopoietic stem cell transplantation. In Ablin AR, ed. Supportive Care of Children With Cancer. Baltimore: The Johns Hopkins University Press, 1997.

Suggested Readings

Alvarez JA, Scully RE, Miller TL, et al. Long-term effects of treatments for childhood cancers. Curr Opin Pediatr 19:23-31, 2007.

Bhatia S, Landier W. Evaluating survivors of pediatric cancer. Cancer J 11:340-354, 2005.

Dickerman JD. The late effects of childhood cancer therapy. Pediatrics 119:554-568, 2007.

Eshelman D, Landier W, Sweeney T, et al. Facilitating care for childhood cancer survivors: integrating Children's Oncology Group long-term follow-up guidelines and health links in clinical practice. J Pediatr Oncol Nurs 21:271-280, 2004.

Landier W, ed. Establishing and enhancing services for childhood cancer survivors: long-term follow-up program resource guide. Chidlren's Oncology Group, 2007. Available at: www.childrensoncologygroup.org/disc/le/pdf/LTFUResourceguide.pdf.

Landier W, Wallace WH, Hudson MM. Long-term follow-up of pediatric cancer survivors: education, surveillance, and screening. Pediatr Blood Cancer 46:149-158, 2006.

Laverdière C, Cheung NK, Kushner BH, et al. Long-term complications in survivors of advanced stage neuroblastoma. Pediatr Blood Cancer 45:324-332, 2005.

Nunez SB, Mulrooney DA, Laverdière C, et al. Risk-based health monitoring of childhood cancer survivors: a report from the Children's Oncology Group. Curr Oncol Rep 9:440-452, 2007.

Rodrigo L. Celiac disease. World J Gastroenterol 12:6585-6593, 2006.

Rutter MM, Rose SR. Long-term endocrine sequelae of childhood cancer. Curr Opin Pediatr 19:480-487, 2007.

Stasi AV, Trecca A, Triniti B. Osteoporosis in celiac disease and in endocrine and repro-ductive disorders. World J Gastroenterol 14:498-505, 2008.

Wasilewski-Masker K, Kaste SC, Hudson MM, et al. Bone mineral density deficits in survivors of childhood cancer: long-term follow-up guidelines and review of the literature. Pediatrics 121:e705-e713, 2008.

Watterberg KL, Shaffer ML, Mishefske MJ, et al. Growth and neurodevelopmental outcomes after early low-dose hydrocortisone treatment in extremely low birth weight infants. Pediatrics 120:40-48, 2007.

11 SYNDROMES

References

1. Jones KL, ed. Smith's Recognizable Patterns of Human Malformation, ed. 6. Philadelphia: Saunders Elsevier, 2006.
2. Hall JG, Froster-Iskenius UG, Alanson JE, eds. Handbook of Normal Physical Measurements. Oxford: Oxford University Press, 1989.
3. Dietz HC. Marfan syndrome. In Pagon RA, Bird TD, Dolan CR, et al, eds.GeneReviews. Seattle: University of Washington, 1993. Available at *www.genereviews.org*.
4. Feuillan P, Calis K, Hill S, et al. Letrozole treatment of precocious puberty in girls with the McCune-Albright syndrome: a pilot study. J Clin Endocrinol Metab 92:2100-2106, 2007.
5. Liens D, Delmas PD, Meunier PJ. Long-term effets of intravenous pamidronate in fibrous dysplasia of bone. Lancet 343:953-954, 1994.
6. Romano AA, Dana K, Bakker B, et al. Growth response, near-adult height, and patterns of growth and puberty in patients with Noonan syndrome treated with growth hormone. J Clin Endocrinol Metab 94:2338-2344, 2009.
7. Butler M, Lee P, Whitman B, eds. Management of Prader-Willi Syndrome, 3rd ed. New York: Springer, 2006.
8. Prader-Willi Syndrome Association Advisory Board Consensus Statement 2003 for Recommendations for Evaluation of Breathing Abnormalities Associated With Sleep in Prader-Willi Syndrome. Available at *www.pwsausa.org/syndrome/recevalsleepapnea.htm*.
9. Prader-Willi Syndrome Association (USA). Medical Alert: Stomach Problems Can Signal Serious Illness. Available at *www.pwsausa.org/syndrome/medical_alert_Stomach.htm*.
10. Mogul HR, Lee PD, Whitman BY, et al. Growth hormone treatment of adults with Prader-Willi Syndrome and growth hormone deficiency improves lean body mass, fractional body fat, and serum triiodothyronine without glucose impairment: results from the United States multicenter trial. J Clin Endocrinol Metab 93:1238-1245, 2008.
11. Silver HK, Kiyasu W, George J, et al. Syndrome of congenital hemihypertrophy, shortness of stature, and elevated urinary gonadotropins. Pediatrics 12:368-376, 1953.
12. Russell A. A syndrome of intra-uterine dwarfism recognizable at birth with craniofacial dysostosis, disproportionately short arms, and other anomalies (5 examples). Proc R Soc Med 47:1040-1044, 1954.

13. Braak Salam J. RSS/SGA: A Comprehensive Guide: Understanding Aspects of Children Diagnosed With Russell-Silver Syndrome or Born Small-for-Gestational-Age. Chico, CA: Quadco Printing, 2009. Available at *www.rss-sga-guidebook.com.*
14. Monk D, Wakeling EL, Proud V, et al. Duplication of 7p11.2-p13, including GRB10 in Silver-Russell syndrome. Am J Hum Genet 66:36-46, 2000.
15. Bondy C, Turner Syndrome Study Group. Care of girls and women with Turner syndrome: a guideline of the Turner Syndrome Study Group. J Clin Endocrinol Metab 92:10-25, 2007.
16. Menke LA, Sas TC, de Muinck Keizer-Schrama SM, et al. Efficacy and safety of oxandrolone in growth hormone-treated girls with Turner syndrome. J Clin Endocrinol Metab 95:1151-1160, 2010.

Suggested Readings

Angulo MA, Castro-Magana M, Lamerson M, et al. Final adult height in children with Prader-Willi syndrome with and without human growth hormone treatment. Am J Med Genet 143A:1456-1461, 2007.
Bolar K, Hoffman AR, Maneatis T, et al. Long-term safety of recombinant human growth hormone in Turner syndrome. J Clin Endocrinol Metab 93:344-351, 2008.
Carrel AL, Myers SE, Whitman BY, et al. Benefits of long-term GH therapy in Prader-Willi syndrome: a 4-year study. J Clin Endocrinol Metab 87:1581-1585, 2002.
Davenport ML. Approach to the patient with Turner syndrome. J Clin Endocrinol Metab 95:1487-1495, 2010.
Loeys BL, Dietz HC, Braverman AC, et al. The revised Ghent nosology for the Marfan syndrome. J Med Genet 47:476-485, 2010.
The Magic Foundation for Children's Growth. Available at *www.magicfoundation.org.*
On-line Mendelian Inheritance in Man. Available at *www.ncbi.nlm.nih.gov/Omim.*
Prader-Willi Syndrome Medical Alerts by Medical Specialists in Prader-Willi Syndrome. Sarasota, FL: Prader-Willi Syndrome Association (USA), 2012. Available at *www.pwsausa.org/support/medalert.htm.*
Scales R, Weber C. Turner syndrome: do not miss the diagnosis. J Pediatr Nurs 25:66-68, 2010.

12 STIMULATION TESTING

References

1. Achermann JC, Fluck CE, Miller WL. The adrenal cortex and its disorders. In Sperling M, ed. Pediatric Endocrinology, 3rd ed. Philadephia: Saunders Elsevier, 2008.
2. Carrillo A, Bao Y. Hormonal dynamic tests and genetic tests used in pediatric endocrinology. In Lifshitz F, ed. Pediatric Endocrinology, vol 2, 5th ed. New York: Informa Healthcare, 2007.
3. Osher E, Stern N. Protocols for stimulation and suppression tests commonly used in clinical endocrinology. In Lavin N, ed. Manual of Endocrinology and Metabolism, 4th ed. Boston: Lippincott Williams & Wilkins, 2009.
4. Sperling M, ed. Pediatric Endocrinology, 3rd ed. Philadelphia: Saunders Elsevier, 2008.

5. Osher E, Stern N, Tucker ML. The adrenal cortex and mineralocorticoid hypertension. In Lavin N, ed. Manual of Endocrinology and Metabolism, 4th ed. Boston: Lippincott Williams & Wilkins, 2009.

6. Ranke MB. Diagnostics of Endocrine Function in Children and Adolescents, 3rd ed. Basel, Switzerland: Karger, 2003.

7. Pagana KD, Pagana TJ. Mosby's Diagnostic and Laboratory Test Reference. St Louis: Mosby Elsevier, 2009.

8. Ballal SA, McIntosh P. Endocrinology. In Custer JW, Rau RE, eds. The Harriet Lane Handbook, 18th ed. St Louis: Mosby Elsevier, 2009.

9. Fisher DA, Salameh W. Quest Diagnostics Manual Endocrinology: Test Selection and Interpretation. San Juan Capistrano, CA: Quest Diagnostics Nichols Institute, 2007.

10. Buckway CK, Guevara-Aguirre J, Pratt KL, et al. The IGF-I generation test revisited: a marker of GH sensitivity. J Clin Endocrinol Metab 86:5176-5183, 2001.

11. Miller BS, Hong McAtee I. Endocrine testing. In Sarafoglou K, ed. Pediatric Endocrinology and Inborn Errors of Metabolism. Endocrine Testing. New York: McGraw Hill Medical, 2009.

13 LABORATORY TESTING
Suggested Readings

Eisenbarth GS, Verge CF. Immunoendocrinopathy syndromes. In Wilson JD, Foster DW, Kronenberg HM, et al, eds. Williams Textbook of Endocrinology, 9th ed. Philadelphia: WB Saunders, 1998.

Endocrine Series. Endocrinology Expected Values and SI Unit Conversion Tables. Calabasas Hills, CA: Endocrine Sciences, 2011.

Jones KL, ed. Smith's Recognizable Patterns of Human Malformation, ed. 6. Philadelphia: Saunders Elsevier, 2006.

14 PEDIATRIC ENDOCRINE MEDICATIONS
Suggested Readings

Lee P, Houk C. Puberty and Its Disorders. In Lifshitz F, ed. Pediatric Endocrinology, 5th ed. New York: Informa Healthcare, 2007.

Nurse Practitioners' Prescribing Reference. New York: Prescribing Reference, 2012.

Package insert for Androderm patch. Watson Pharma Inc, 2012.

Package insert for AndroGel 1%. Unimed Pharmaceuticals, Marietta, GA.

Physicians' Desk Reference, 65th ed. Montvale, NJ: Medical Economics Co, 2011.

Sissan E, Cornell S. Pharmacology for glucose management. In Mensing C, ed. The Art and Sciences of Diabetes Self-Management Education Desk Reference, 2nd ed. Chicago, IL: American Association of Diabetes Educators, 2011.

Thornton PS, Finegold DN, Stanley CA, et al. Hypoglycemia in the infant and child. In Sperling MA, ed. Pediatric Endocrinology. Philadelphia: WB Saunders, 2002.

Walsh P, ed. Physicians' Desk Reference, 55th ed. Montvale, NJ: Medical Economics Co, 2001.

15 CONVERSIONS/FORMULAS/TABLES

References

1. Rosner B, Prineas R, Loggie J, et al. Percentiles for body mass index in U.S. children 5 to 17 years of age. J Pediatr 132:211-222, 1998.
2. Siberry GK, Iannone R, eds. The Harriet Lane Handbook, 15th ed. Philadelphia: Elsevier, 1999.
3. Hall JG, Froster-Iskenius UG, Allanson JE. Handbook of Normal Physical Measurements. Oxford, England: Oxford University Press, 1989.
4. National Heart Lung and Blood Institute. Blood pressure tables for children and adolescents. Available at *www.nhlbi.nih.gov/guidelines/hypertension/child_tbl.pdf*.

16 GROWTH CHARTS

Charts on pp 442-449 were developed by the National Center for Health Statistics in collaboration with the National Center for Chronic Disease Prevention and Health Promotion (2000). Available at *www.cdc.gov/growthcharts*.

INDEX

A

INDEX